Praise for *The Baby Boomer Diet*

"A few years ago I attended a weeklong workshop with Donna Gates. It was an eye-opening experience, as she shared simple but powerful principles for attaining and maintaining a superhealthy body. One of the most important things in the workshop was that Donna fed us breakfast and lunch. We were able to taste and experience how delicious the fermented foods were. Everyone enjoyed her way of cooking and was delighted to take her recipes and probiotic nutrition home with them. I have been a follower ever since, and at 84 am enjoying vibrant health. Thank you, Donna Gates."

— **Louise L. Hay,** *New York Times* best-selling author of *You Can Heal Your Life* and co-author of *You Can Create an Exceptional Life*

"I love this book! Our national health has become an emergency, and Donna Gates provides the solution. As Boomers, we've pioneered it all, and now we're leading the way in new approaches to aging. Scientifically and clinically based, this book provides a user-friendly, comprehensive handbook for our care and feeding into healthy longevity. Read it and stay young."

— **Hyla Cass, M.D.,** author of *8 Weeks to Vibrant Health*

---

*"Donna Gates packs every page of **The Baby Boomer Diet** with health principles and nutrition advice that help rejuvenate your life and allow you to actually grow younger based on the latest breakthrough natural-health technologies. This inspiring book empowers your healing, improves your life experience, and gives you tools to live over 100—all while having 'the best day ever' every single day!"*

— **David Wolfe,** creator of The LongevityNOW Program; author of *Superfoods: The Food and Medicine of the Future, Eating for Beauty,* and *Amazing Grace*

The
Baby Boomer Diet

Also by Donna Gates

THE BODY ECOLOGY DIET: Recovering Your Health and Rebuilding Your Immunity (with Linda Schatz)

━∿━

Hay House Titles of Related Interest

YOU CAN HEAL YOUR LIFE, the movie, starring Louise L. Hay & Friends (available as a 1-DVD program and an expanded 2-DVD set) Watch the trailer at: **www.LouiseHayMovie.com**

THE SHIFT, the movie, starring Dr. Wayne W. Dyer (available as a 1-DVD program and an expanded 2-DVD set) Watch the trailer at: **www.DyerMovie.com**

━∿━

THE AGE OF MIRACLES: Embracing the New Midlife, by Marianne Williamson

THE BEAUTY BLUEPRINT: 8 Steps to Building the Life and Look of Your Dreams, by Michelle Phillips

CONSTANT CRAVING: What Your Food Cravings Mean and How to Overcome Them, by Doreen Virtue

FACE IT: What Women Really Feel as Their Looks Change, by Vivian Diller, Ph.D., and Jill Muir-Sukenick, Ph.D.

THETAHEALING® DISEASES AND DISORDERS, by Vianna Stibal

THE VITAMIN D REVOLUTION: How the Power of This Amazing Vitamin Can Change Your Life, by Soram Khalsa, M.D.

YOU CAN CREATE AN EXCEPTIONAL LIFE, by Louise Hay and Cheryl Richardson

━∿━

All of the above are available at your local bookstore, or may be ordered by visiting:

Hay House USA: **www.hayhouse.com®**
Hay House Australia: **www.hayhouse.com.au**
Hay House UK: **www.hayhouse.co.uk**
Hay House South Africa: **www.hayhouse.co.za**
Hay House India: **www.hayhouse.co.in**

The
Baby Boomer Diet

Body Ecology's Guide to Growing Younger

Donna Gates
with
Lyndi Schrecengost

HAY HOUSE, INC.
Carlsbad, California • New York City
London • Sydney • Johannesburg
Vancouver • Hong Kong • New Delhi

Published and distributed in the United States by: Hay House, Inc.: www
.hayhouse.com • *Published and distributed in Australia by:* Hay House
Australia Pty. Ltd.: www.hayhouse.com.au • *Published and distributed in the
United Kingdom by:* Hay House UK, Ltd.: www.hayhouse.co.uk • *Published and
distributed in the Republic of South Africa by:* Hay House SA (Pty), Ltd.: www
.hayhouse.co.za • *Distributed in Canada by:* Raincoast: www.raincoast.com •
Published in India by: Hay House Publishers India: www.hayhouse.co.in

Cover design and typesetting: John T. Davidson: jrocket77@mac.com
Interior design: Kenneth Storey
Indexer: Stephanie Marr

Library of Congress Control Number: 2011923242

Hardcover ISBN: 978-1-4019-3545-0
Digital ISBN: 978-1-4019-3546-7

14 13 12 11   4 3 2 1
1st edition, October 2011

Printed in the United States of America

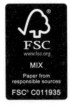

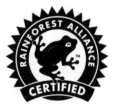

*T*his book is dedicated to my delightful, charming, and very wise granddaughter, Mia, and to the billions of children who will be born generations from now. You inspire me to do the work I do and motivate me to want to live a long, healthy life and be here to see the amazing world you will create upon this earth.

My prayer is that this book will spark our generation into action and create for you an opportunity to inherit strong physical bodies and brilliant minds that are in harmony with your already-radiant souls.

Contents

—⚬—

PART I: A New Way of Life for Our Generation

PART II: The End of the Road for All "Diets"

PART III: 7 Universal Principles—Guideposts to Anti-Aging

Foreword

I have known Donna Gates for nearly a decade. During this time we have worked together with many families who have children with serious conditions, including autism and autism spectrum disorders. I have watched her tirelessly and selflessly work for these kids and their families, teaching them about the foods and methods of her Body Ecology program.

My background is in gastrointestinal surgery and health, and Donna and I have often consulted together to find the best ways to communicate the principles and advantages of Body Ecology to multiple audiences, particularly to health practitioners who are seeking to understand the medical underpinnings of the program and share it with their patients.

Donna and I have lectured and conducted several seminars together on the principles of Body Ecology for the lay public, physicians, and other health-care professionals, as well as for students planning a career as Body Ecology consultants. At some point, we became aware that this program would be a solid foundation for most anyone dealing with any type of illness, and that it would be particularly beneficial for people who are beginning to experience some of the effects and possibly the health concerns associated with aging . . . the Baby Boomers.

Body Ecology includes whole, organic foods, either raw or cooked gently so as to maximize the nutrient content. In addition, there is a strong emphasis on fermented foods, while eliminating simple sugars. Such a program will balance and heal the gut lining, optimize gut flora, and minimize intestinal candida, thereby promoting good intestinal health. Today, science has shown that many conditions such as arthritis, allergies, autoimmunity, and neuroinflammatory ailments, as well as several forms of cancer, have significant connections to an unhealthy intestinal tract. Throughout this book, you will see how the Body Ecology program confronts many of the diseases and concerns of aging, from cosmetic issues such as wrinkles to more serious health problems, such as Alzheimer's.

I was pleased to be asked to serve as the medical consultant on this project, and was eager to share my perspective on the benefits and applications of the Body Ecology program as seen through the eyes of someone intimately involved in health and wellness, and who has witnessed the power of this program firsthand.

— **Leonard Smith, M.D.,**
medical advisor to Donna Gates & Body Ecology

Preface

We live on an amazing planet. What new, undiscovered worlds wait to entice us? A tranquil lake in the Canadian Rockies? A painting on a wall of the Louvre? A smile of recognition on our new grandchild's face? Will we have the chance to enjoy these "mountaintop experiences," or will time run out for us?

What if we knew in advance what our final years would look like? Can we imagine a day when we are too frail to drive our cars? Can we imagine a time when we can no longer recognize a place we've been to a thousand times before, or can no longer hear our granddaughter's sweet voice? Can we imagine not doing all the things we've worked our whole lives to be able to do? The great irony of aging is that we may finally have everything we need materially, but no longer be able to enjoy it and share it with those we love most.

We Baby Boomers have redefined every phase of life we've passed through. I believe we will redefine aging as well. We will choose how we will live our later years; we will choose how modern medicine will treat us; we will even choose how we will die. The loss of dignity that so often characterizes later life is something we Baby Boomers will confront, challenge, and transform.

Today, despite the current statistics and the common belief that tells us we are living longer, healthier lives, it is clear that we are not. Degenerative conditions such as heart disease, cancer, diabetes, obesity, osteoporosis, and stroke are causes of serious concern. Aging is also a degenerative disease. Fading vitality, wrinkles, sagging skin, obesity, gray hair or no hair, and diminished sex drive are just a few of the symptoms of an unhealthy body. The signs of aging began decades ago, but they went unnoticed. Aging happens quietly and cunningly, and it speeds up with time, startling us with its abrupt and dramatic changes that weren't there yesterday but are here today.

As for heart disease, cancer, diabetes, obesity, osteoporosis, and stroke, the statistics favor the odds that many of us will suffer from at least one of these conditions. I believe that unlike our parents, who accepted these as unavoidable, we

Baby Boomers in our hearts are passionately committed to not going there. As a result of this intense desire, we are drawing new forms of health-care technology, from both traditional and complementary medicine, into our realm. We are also being allowed to rediscover precious ancient knowledge to empower us to achieve what we so strongly desire.

The information in this book is truly groundbreaking, an advance in how to resolve the problems of aging and disease. No other system of wellness is as balanced or as complete. As health educators, my team of Body Ecologists and I have been on the front lines of some of the most challenging issues facing people today, from autism to obesity to immunological disorders. Because we work every day with real people with real problems, we are intimately aware of emerging health trends and concerns.

The Body Ecology Way of Life is not my creation. Around our offices we always say that you can see "the hand of God" in this work. This knowledge is here because it's time. It's time for us to understand the missing pieces that create *genuine* health, not the illusory idea of health we currently have. We age because of ignorance, because of choice, because we live in a world that supports early aging and degenerative conditions. Body Ecology has been given the mission to change ignorance to understanding when it comes to the way we eat and care for our bodies. We exist to be a catalyst for creating a paradigm shift toward the true science of health and healing in this world—a paradigm shift that will benefit our children, grandchildren, and great-grandchildren for generations to come.

— **Donna Gates**

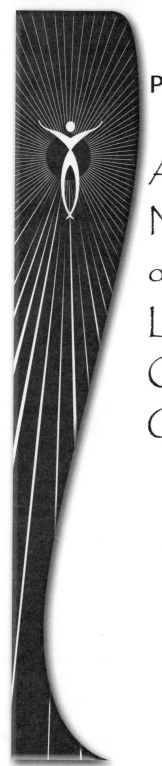

PART I

A New Way of Life for Our Generation

Chapter 1

Baby Boomers: Forever Young

Born in prosperity, harbingers of change,
Baby Boomers have made a significant impact on
the world. But what will be our final legacy?

It's been nearly 40 years since the Baby Boomers arrived at Max Yasgur's 600-acre alfalfa field to attend *Woodstock,* an outdoor festival that was as much a counterculture "happening" as it was a celebration of music. Area residents didn't know what to make of these "hippies" in bohemian dress who abandoned their cars and walked for miles to stand before the concert stage. Woodstock's political provocation, defiance of convention, and back-to-nature innocence would make it one of the defining moments of an entire generation. Now, 78 million strong and approaching retirement, we Baby Boomers are showing few signs of slowing down.

The Baby Boomer generation is usually defined as those individuals born between 1946 and 1964, and today we comprise more than one-quarter of the entire U.S. population. The "first wave," or Boomers who were born in the decade between 1946 and 1957, arrived soon after millions of servicemen returned home from war. Between 1945 and 1946, the number of U.S. marriages doubled to more than 2.2 million; and 92 percent of the women who could have children, did. A flourishing economy encouraged couples to have large families, and in 1946, 3.4 million babies were born in the U.S., 20 percent more than the previous year. For the next decade, the annual total would hover above the four million mark, and the surge in births would continue until 1964. In that final Boomer year, the first wave hit college, the Beatles arrived in New York for their first U.S. tour, and Congress passed the Gulf of Tonkin Resolution, authorizing an escalation of the war in Vietnam. The youth movement had begun, and we Baby Boomers were coming of age.[1]

Why This Book? Why Now?

Although Boomers rode into the world on a wave of optimism and promise, we also inherited some of the worst ills and environmental crimes of the century. In his book *The Hundred-Year Lie: How Food and Medicine Are Destroying Your Health,* journalist Randall Fitzgerald notes how many of his fellow Baby Boomers are afflicted with diseases that used to be reserved for "old age," from multiple sclerosis to cancer to Parkinson's and Crohn's disease. He describes the extent to which Baby Boomers have been duped by the myth of "better living through chemistry."

A famous commercial that aired during the 1970s promoted a relatively new product called "margarine," which looked and tasted very much like real butter. Mother Nature, played by a memorably indignant Dena Dietrich, is not pleased that she, too, has been fooled by this deceptive substitute. Amid a fury of thunder and lightning, the commercial concludes: "It's not *nice* to fool Mother Nature." Today, in so many ways, the irony of this visionary statement is coming to terrible fruition.

The petrochemical era that was born along with the Baby Boomers initiated an onslaught of toxins that are exacting a

Although Boomers rode into the world on a wave of optimism and promise, we also inherited some of the worst ills and environmental crimes of the century.

heavy price on this and subsequent generations. The incidence of neural disorders has tripled in Western countries; and researchers have begun to link it to exposure to crop pesticides, synthetic chemicals, processed foods, and industrial chemicals.[2] As Fitzgerald notes, between 1952 and 1987, the production and use of synthetic pesticides in the U.S. increased 13 times faster than before the war. From genetically modified foods to sex hormones, from industrial contaminants that pollute our air and water, to overuse of antibiotics and inoculations, seemingly inescapable toxins have besieged the bodies of Baby Boomers for decades.

Baby Boomers are the first generation to experience the devastating assaults of the chemical era.

The Mission

Baby Boomers were born during a period of unprecedented prosperity not witnessed since the Gilded Age. A growing number of our parents were truly living the American dream; they purchased nice homes, sent many of us to college, financed trips to Europe, and provided us with an ever-increasing array of luxury items largely beyond the reach of earlier generations. Critics of Baby Boomers point out that this emphasis on materialism and immediate gratification created a generation of overindulged "Peter Pans" who are slow to accept the realities of the adult world. Baby Boomers, they complain, feel a sense of *entitlement* rather than a sense of *responsibility*. But others defend Baby Boomers as idealistic free spirits who broke boundaries, catalyzed social change, and helped make the world more tolerant and open.

Regardless of how the experts might argue these points, most agree that Boomers' adaptability, focus on fulfillment, and never-ending quest to look and feel young are changing the way age is defined, and fundamentally altering the face of health care in America.

Although I was never a flower child and chose to bypass the drug scene of the '60s, I have always identified with many of the generational values we Baby Boomers share. I understood how important it was to break free from what our parents had taught us and to find the courage to follow our own unique path, even if that journey was a lonely one at times. What I identify with most about Baby Boomers is our openness to change and our empowering pursuit of self-fulfillment. We are very much a generation that believes: *If you don't like something, change it.* And we have. This is why I believe we have the creativity and the obligation to transform the way we take care of ourselves and the planet.

Who Are We Kidding?

Sixty-one percent of Boomers surveyed by AARP in 2004 said they felt younger than their age. Yet two in ten of these cited physical health as the one area of their lives they would most like to change, while three in ten said that their physical health was worse than they expected it to be at this point in their lives. Only a little more than half thought they were likely to achieve their goal of improved physical health.[3] *The Washington Post* reported that a number of recent large surveys are showing some surprising feedback from Boomers who appear to be less healthy than their forebears were at the same age. In spite of their gym memberships, Boomers are less physically active than their parents and grandparents, due in part to long commuting times and jobs that keep them in front of a computer screen all day. Although there are fewer smokers in our generation, more of us are likely to report chronic pain, drinking and psychiatric problems, high blood pressure and cholesterol, and debilitating levels of stress.[4]

One wonders if we Baby Boomers feel young in spirit, in spite of what our bodies may be telling us. Or do we just have higher expectations for ourselves? The reality is, despite our optimism, our greater prospects, and the millions of dollars we will spend on our health, we Boomers will confront new and often premature health threats simply because of the world we've been living in and the choices we've made.

Our bodies were not designed to absorb synthetic chemicals, even in small doses, throughout an entire lifetime. Environmental toxins alter our DNA. They damage our immune systems. They increase our predisposition to illness and disease. And they are passed on, through the umbilical cord and blood of the mother, to our children and grandchildren. In fact, from the moment sperm and egg cells come together, toxins are already present. Children born today are coming into the world with serious infections, weakened immune systems, and increased susceptibilities to certain diseases.

Baby Boomers grapple with new psychological stresses as well. Since the 1970s, globalization and other economic developments have seriously eroded the kind of job security that was the norm in the decades following World War II. Today, Baby Boomers are particularly vulnerable to these economic shifts, and are often among the first to be laid off and the last to be rehired by employers who perceive them as more expensive and less flexible than younger workers. Once again, our generation is faced with redefining itself; and, for some, this will literally mean starting over. Rising life expectancy, aging parents, and faulty pension plans mean that many of us will need to work much longer than our parents did, whether we want to or not. This makes our continued good health not wishful thinking but a practical necessity.

Regardless of how the experts argue over them, most agree that Boomers' adaptability, focus on fulfillment, and never-ending quest to look and feel young are changing the way age is defined . . .

As we Boomers struggle to stay young, many of us have turned to quick-fix solutions—cosmetic procedures, anti-aging hormones, and extreme diets to stave off the aging process. But these methods are akin to repainting a dilapidated car. At first glance, these cosmetic changes may improve the appearance, but they don't account for more important and deep-seated issues. These can only be addressed through an understanding of our inner ecosystem; and how diet, food purity and selection, and lifestyle choices can lessen the effects of aging, giving us not just *longer* lives, but *better* ones.

We Baby Boomers are celebrated for our independence, for ignoring and even defying convention, and for our unswerving idealism. We are a generation of trendsetters. Staying healthy and vital is not just a pipe dream for us; *it is our calling.* We have long been the forerunners of social, political, and environmental change. Now it is vital that we also bring about a revolution in health and develop truly revolutionary roles for maturity. It is time that we harnessed our resources—our sheer numbers, our money, our wisdom, and our will—to heal our bodies and our planet.

Our greatest mission lies ahead.

Chapter 2

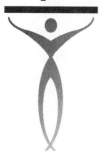

Our Thoughts and Intentions: Anything Is Possible

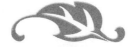

Baby Boomers will live longer than any previous generation. Will we live <u>better</u>?

My grandfather used to say that man would never walk on the moon. I remember him sitting in his favorite green chair in the living room, grumbling about all the tax dollars we were wasting on what he thought was an arrogant and futile attempt to achieve the impossible. Before long, millions of Boomers were crowding around their television sets to watch Neil Armstrong take his first tentative step onto that beautiful orb we had only observed from afar. We experienced the impossible that day, and it was one of the first signs that we Baby Boomers were in for an exciting journey.

Since then, our generation has experienced an avalanche of change. We've seen the emergence of thousands of new technologies, from microwave ovens and VCRs to cell phones and the Internet. We've witnessed the first successful heart transplants, and lasers that correct eye defects. In the early '70s, physicians began using MRI and CAT scan technology to detect brain abnormalities. We now have prosthetics that enable formerly wheelchair-bound athletes to break world records, and scientists are currently developing handheld sensing devices that will "sniff out" lung and breast cancers in the same amazingly accurate way dogs are now trained to do. And doctors are now able to repair holes in the diaphragms of fetuses, a genetic defect, while they are still in the womb.

In 1953, Watson and Crick discovered the double-stranded DNA in our chromosomes and were later awarded the Nobel Prize in medicine. This meant that we had literally discovered the "recipe book" for how to create a living form. And with the advent of computers, teams of scientists all around the world began competing with each other to actually read these recipes, with an eye to manipulating and fixing genetic problems.

Of equal importance, the new developments on the frontiers of stem-cell research will allow us to heal many damaged areas of the body. Because it is imminent, Boomers can also expect to see doctors doing gene-transfer procedures on fetuses in utero and curing babies of genetic conditions using stem cells.

We are a generation that rises to new health challenges with commitment and invention. Epidemics such as autism and AIDS have given us an important opportunity to study and understand the immune system. They have provided new insights into cellular intelligence and the important role our inner ecosystem plays in the prevention of disease. Autism, in particular, allows us to look at the connection between the gut and the brain . . . and we now know that pesticides; chemicals; and heavy metals such as mercury, lead, and aluminum are dangerous neurotoxins that weaken our children before they are even born.

Out of much pain and uncertainty have come enlightenment and discovery, and there are more world-changing breakthroughs ahead. I believe that a whole new level of science will emerge because of our desire to know and harness the positive forces of nature to create health and longevity. Baby Boomers can help bring about a revolution in how we heal ourselves and in how we address, and even defy, aging.

Science Supports Our Intention to Stay Young and Healthy

Consider this: had you been born in the late 1800s, your life expectancy would have been about 45. That doesn't seem like much time to live a full life. As many of us Baby Boomers are just now hitting our mid-40s, it might seem inconceivable that had we lived a little more than a century ago, life might almost be over.

We've come so far! It is a brilliant time to be alive, because there is so much more that we know today about how to stay young and healthy. Baby Boomers are the first generation to truly reap the benefits of medical breakthroughs—and also holistic and nutritional advances—that make agelessness not just conceivable, but a *reality*. We will live longer than any previous generation, and we have the *potential* to live better—with the opportunity to reinvent what it means to be in our "golden years."

Here are just a few of the medical advances that may change our world, the way we view disease, and how we age.

Resistance to Disease

In 2003, a team of scientists at Wake Forest University discovered a mouse that was immune to injected cancer. From this one miracle mouse they bred and produced many generations of healthy, cancer-free mice who lived normal life spans. The Wake Forest mouse had an unusual immune system—the ability to flood its system with massive amounts of white blood cells that destroyed the cancer.

Scientists were led to wonder why this genetic mutation is not seen in other mammals or even in other mice. It may be that as mammals evolved over time, they did not live long enough to develop cancer. Instead, they were succumbing to other diseases or circumstances that took evolutionary precedence. For example, a mouse might be eaten by a fox long before the mouse had a chance to develop cancer.

Soon we will not only be able to regenerate tissues and cells with healthy food, supplements, herbs, and alternative therapies; but advances in stem-cell research are also unfolding that offer even more exciting possibilities for reversing the aging process.

11

Scientists must now figure out how this genetic mutation works at the molecular level, but the "mouse model" offers exciting possibilities for future therapies. Research suggests that the body's natural ability to protect itself against cancer—*host resistance*—declines with age, which explains why many cancers surface in later years when the body's immune system is not as strong. Fortunately, according to researchers, it will probably be easier to develop rejuvenating cell-therapy treatments for the immune system than for other systems of the body.[1] Four major U.S. research institutions are now working together in an effort to accelerate this discovery into potential cancer therapy for humans.

Body Ecology offers you an exciting way to build immunity right here and right now with food and lifestyle changes.

Regeneration & Renewal

Even though many of us are unaware of this, our bodies were created with a marvelous capacity for self-regulation and self-repair. Soon we will not only be able to regenerate tissues and cells through healthy food, supplements, herbs, and alternative therapies; but advances in stem-cell research, offering even more exciting possibilities for reversing the aging process, are also unfolding.

Adult stem cells come from our bone marrow and fat stores; as well as from amniotic fluid, menstrual blood, and umbilical cords. These adult cells are different from the politically charged human *embryonic stem cells* that in some cases have been implicated in cancer.

Adult stem cells are *unspecialized* and retain the ability throughout life to give rise to cells that will become *specialized*. They can also take the place of any type of cell that is lost or dies. Stem cells contribute to the body's ability to renew and repair its tissues. Unlike mature cells, which are permanently committed to their fate, stem cells can both renew themselves and create new cells at the same time. They are also remarkably "plastic," meaning that those from one tissue can generate functional cell types of another tissue. Stem-cell therapies show great promise to repair nervous-system conditions such as Parkinson's, brain and spinal-cord damage from trauma or stroke, epilepsy, autism, Alzheimer's, Lou Gehrig's disease, and more.[2]

A team at Newcastle University in England has grown mini-livers from umbilical-cord stem cells. Two scientists, Dr. Nico Forraz and Professor Colin McGucklin, collaborated with scientists at NASA to make the miniature livers, which can be used for drug testing and erase the need to test on animals and humans. In ten years, they believe they will be able to build a full-sized liver, and within as little as five years, pieces of this "stem-cell-produced" tissue could be used to repair organs damaged by disease, injury, alcohol abuse, and paracetamol overdose. The scientists project that in 15 years we could have entire transplants with livers grown in a lab.[3]

On a more cosmetic level, stem-cell research can also make some of those formerly unavoidable signs of aging a thing of the past. For example, until very recently we had to accept that problems with our teeth would only worsen as we aged. When we aren't undergoing major repairs to our teeth, we face the possibility of losing them or replacing them with artificial versions. In the Western world, an estimated 85 percent of adults have had some form of dental treatment. After age 50, most of us will have lost an average of 12 teeth. In theory, a natural tooth made from a person's own tissue and grown in its intended location would make the best possible replacement.

Armed with knowledge, medical evolution, and the power of our own minds and wills, our generation can literally transform how we live the last innings of our lives, as well as the legacy we leave future generations.

But these "bioteeth" have, until recently, been more conjecture than reality. This is changing, however.

Researchers are now using advances in stem-cell biology and tissue reengineering to fashion new teeth out of old ones. Their approach is based on the fact that living tissues are made of cells that constantly signal to one another and move around in a kind of community (in Chapter 7, I'll discuss how this applies to bacteria as well). Each cell knows its place and role in the larger group that forms and maintains a functional tissue. So, it stands to reason that if you could find the right mix of dissociated cells and reaggregate (regroup) them, they should instinctively re-form the tissue or organ to which they belong. We are now closer than ever to replacing a lost tooth with a new one made from our own stem cells.[4] The potential for these medical innovations gives us hope that we may indeed live longer. But will we live *better*?

How do we Boomers become "a model for living"—a generation that feels, looks, and behaves with vitality? The answer lies in our diet, our lifestyle choices, and very important . . . our *intentions*. Wouldn't it be a worthwhile mission to leave this world in better shape than it was when we first entered it? To have the energy to do this, we must reclaim the vitality of our youth.

Embracing the Mind's Potential

While science continues to redefine the future, we are becoming more and more aware that in our own individual lives and bodies there is unlimited potential as well. The groundbreaking work of many scientists is revealing that we are masters of our genetic code. Biologist Bruce Lipton's pioneering research in the area of cell science indicates that the environment—and, more specifically, our perception and interpretation of the environment—directly controls the activity of our genes, giving credibility to the phenomenon of "mind over matter."

In his book *The Biology of Belief: Unleashing the Power of Consciousness, Matter & Miracles,* Lipton speaks of how the energy of our thoughts can actually activate or inhibit a cell's functioning. His studies of the cell membrane revealed that this outer layer of the cell functions rather like a computer chip—the equivalent of a brain.[5] Far from the hardwired machine we've always assumed it was, the brain is a continually changing organ with the power to rejuvenate itself.

Lipton asserts that we humans have billions of regenerative cells in our bodies that are designed to repair or replace damaged tissues and organs. The activity and fate of these cells, says Lipton, "are profoundly influenced by our thoughts and perceptions about the environment. Hence our beliefs about aging can either interfere with or enhance stem-cell function, causing our physiological regeneration or decline."[6]

Armed with knowledge, medical advances, and the power of our own minds and wills, our generation can transform how we live the last innings of our lives, as well as the legacy we leave future generations.

Health and Vitality . . .
a Birthright and an Intention

Myriad philosophers and thinkers have noted how we humans tend to attract what we think. If we think negatively, we attract negativity back. This "law of attraction," or what psychologists call the self-fulfilling prophecy, can have a tremendous impact on how we live and enjoy our lives. We have 60,000 thoughts a day, and every one of them has a frequency. But instead of the "good vibrations" that Beach Boy Brian Wilson sang about, too often our thoughts are pessimistic and come from a place of deficiency and discouragement: *I'll never own my dream house, I'll never meet my soul mate, I'll never have a career that fulfills me,* or *I'll never feel as good as I did when I was 25.* And yet, affirmative thought is a hundred times more powerful than these "bad vibes."

When we focus on lack, that's what we attract. Many of us ask ourselves why we keep ending up in the same unsatisfying relationships, playing out the same self-destructive patterns, enduring the same never-ending cycle of calamity and recovery. We wonder if we will ever have what our hearts desire. Most of us experience this type of life because we are not visualizing what we want in a limitless universe; we are visualizing what we *don't* want in a universe of negative returns. This is the message that the universe hears, and it honors our intentions accordingly.[7]

But there is another, better way; and it can literally transform our reality.

My friend Louise Hay is a wonderful example of how thinking "different" can change the future. I first met Louise when she attended a Body Ecologist workshop. I was quickly inspired by her balanced way of taking care of her own growth and needs while helping the world and seeking the truth. Her openness and availability to new ideas keeps her perennially young and engaging. She follows the Body Ecology Way of Life, and it is wonderful to see how her body and demeanor are in harmony with her youthful spirit.

Louise has faced some hard challenges in her life, beginning with a traumatic and impoverished childhood. Still in her teens when she ran away from home, she ended up in New York City, where she became a model and married a prosperous businessman. Although it appeared that her life had turned around, it was not until the marriage ended 14 years later that her healing really began.

Baby Boomers will be encouraged to know that Louise's personal mission and life's work began when she was 52, an age when most of us start to slow down. In the '70s, she attended meetings at the Church of Religious Science and began training in the ministerial program. She became a popular speaker at the church and soon began counseling clients. This work quickly blossomed into a full-time career. After several years, Louise compiled a reference guide detailing the mental causes of physical ailments, and she developed positive thought patterns for reversing illness and creating health. This compilation was the basis for her 1976 book, *Heal Your Body,* a bestseller that has been translated into 42 different languages and sold in 132 countries.

Louise was able to put her philosophies into practice when she was diagnosed with cancer years ago. She considered alternatives to surgery and drugs; and developed an intensive program of affirmations, visualization, nutritional cleansing, and psychotherapy. Within six months, she was completely healed.

Considered one of the founders of the self-help movement, Louise has helped millions of people create their hearts' desires. In 1985, she began her famous support group, "The Hayride," with six men diagnosed with AIDS. By 1988, the group had grown to a weekly gathering of 800 people and had moved to an auditorium in Santa Monica. Louise now heads Hay House, one of the fastest-growing publishing houses in the world. Her passionate intention to help the world heal emotionally, spiritually, and physically began as a small venture in the living room of her home. Today, it has turned into a prosperous corporation that has sold millions of books (including this one) and audio programs since its inception.

Louise is a great inspiration to me, and a powerful model for those of us in our generation who may think getting older means limitations rather than opportunities.

Like Louise, I found that my own healing and happiness evolved out of a very personal health crisis and recovery. I was born with a sensitive constitution. It seemed as a child I was always coming down with lung infections and suffering stomachaches, and many of the foods I ate didn't agree with me. When I was 15, my skin began to break out, and a well-meaning but misguided dermatologist prescribed antibiotics. Fifteen years later, frequent use of antibiotics had weakened my body to the point where I had almost no functional immune system, and my stomach burned whenever I ate anything. By the time I was 30, I could tolerate only about five foods.

This launched me on a personal quest; and I began to explore every kind of diet available, including vegetarian, raw, macro, natural hygiene, and high protein. I also spent a fortune on supplements and found real value in neuromuscular massage, acupuncture, colonics, and craniosacral therapy. Everything helped, but I still felt weak, and my digestion never improved.

At the age of 38, confused and uncertain as to where to turn next, I found that fate intervened. I met Dr. William Crook, who had just written *The Yeast Connection*. After reading his book, I realized that I had a classic case of an extremely common systemic infection called *candidiasis*. The infection and its toxins had seriously compromised my digestive, immune, and endocrine systems.

After much study and trial and error, I eventually created an entire system of health and healing centered around repairing and restoring my inner ecosystem—killing off the bad yeast and the accompanying viruses and then recolonizing my intestines with friendly microflora, thus restoring proper digestion.

More than anything else, I am a teacher, so naturally I began to share what I was learning with others. I knew my discoveries needed to reach more people, and in 1994, the first edition of *The Body Ecology Diet* was self-published. Slowly the book made its way around the world to the people who needed it. I also founded a nutrition company called Body Ecology, Inc.

Two decades later, the system of health and healing I was guided to create, step by step, is now providing answers to many other health challenges, not just candidiasis. Unbelievably, this book, currently in its 11th edition and now published by Hay House, has helped tens of thousands of people return to optimal health. To this day I can see so clearly a happier, healthier world. And I have embarked on an even larger mission to change the way the world eats. Like Louise Hay, I will never stop believing it will happen.

Our thoughts and emotions are always reassembling and reorganizing, but they follow our instructions! We can transform our reality if we change our beliefs. In fact, the body acts like a puppet to our thoughts, and it has a tremendous capacity for self-healing *if* we focus on health, not disease.

Our Thoughts Produce Results

Have you been resigned to or obsessing over the changes in your body? If this continues to be your focus, you will certainly find more and more signs of aging with each passing year. Instead, I encourage you to begin—right this moment—to direct your thoughts to how it looks and feels to be young. Focus on what you want to *become,* not on what you currently *are.* Your body will begin to respond with new health and vitality.

Now, imagine if 78 million of us collectively start to concentrate our thoughts on how it looks and feels to be young. Our cells will respond immediately, and the universe will begin to give us what we want. Why would it do this? Because the universe wants this, too! If millions of us remain young and healthy, we can be of much greater service to the world. We can begin the work we have come here to do.

This is our generation's last, but truly most important, mission. With our great numbers—our collective wisdom, resources, and insight—we can begin right now to correct the mistakes of the past. It's time . . . and timing is everything.

It is my greatest hope that this book will become the first in a series of "inspired thoughts" that will guide you to take your own "moon walk" to a younger, healthier, and even happier you.

Chapter 3

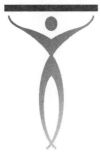

Why We Age: Finding the Fountain of Youth Within

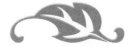

Armed with new knowledge about what accelerates aging and disease, Baby Boomers will transform the way we view, experience, and treat getting older.

Cultures around the world—from Spain and the 16th-century explorer Ponce de León, who believed he'd found the waters of agelessness in Florida; to Shangri-la, where longevity was embodied in a mythical, mystical paradise where anything was possible—have sought the fountain of youth. Have you, too, ever wished that you possessed the secret of eternal youth? I certainly have. Wouldn't it be wonderful if it were as simple as a magical elixir or potion . . . or perhaps the perfect antiwrinkle cream?

Theories of Aging

There are many theories on aging, and while it is beyond the scope of this book to provide them in much detail, a brief overview of the more popular ones is quite interesting. Each offers valuable insights into the role that food, nutrition, and lifestyle play in longevity. Understanding *why* we age will give us the knowledge we need to *prevent* aging and, just as important, to *reverse* the already existing signs of aging.

— The **genetic** or **DNA theory of aging** argues that we were born with a blueprint encoded within the DNA we received from our parents that predetermined our physical and mental weaknesses and strengths, and now regulates the rate at which we age. By far the most well known of all the theories, it is also sometimes referred to as the *planned-obsolescence theory* . . . a rather depressing idea, isn't it? It paints a pessimistic picture: We are predestined to follow in the footsteps of our ancestors and, therefore, have very little choice over how we age. If our parents and grandparents entered their decline early, so will we. And what if they lived to a ripe old age but were quite ill and feeble? This might be our fate as well.

The good news is that this theory is not as fatalistic as it sounds. DNA can be positively or negatively affected by diet, toxins, lifestyle, environment, and even our thoughts (see the previous chapter). In other words, our choices—past, present, and future—can accelerate DNA damage or slow it down. The reins are in our hands.

— The **free-radical theory of aging** was developed in the 1950s by Dr. Denham Harman, who also developed the mitochondrial theory of aging (explained later). This theory maintains that aging is due to the accumulation of free radicals—very small molecules containing the oxygen atom. Their effect is called "oxidative damage."

Free radicals are a natural by-product of life when you breathe, eat and burn glucose for energy, detoxify dangerous chemicals, are injured, or do strenuous exercise. They are around everywhere in the form of radiation, chemicals, and heavy metals. If you have a poor diet, drink too much alcohol, smoke tobacco, are under chronic stress, are exposed to radiation, and/or push yourself too hard when you exercise, you are accelerating your body's production of free radicals. As most of us are under stress and exposed to radiation and x-rays against our will, free radicals appear to be unavoidable.

Healthy cells can overcome minor attacks from free radicals. But when those attacks become more intense, our cells begin to die, speeding up the aging of the body and brain, perhaps even causing premature cell death, known as *necrosis*. Normally, when a cell is in the process of dying, it sends signals to the immune system that a "cleanup crew" will be needed. The cleanup crew consists of white blood cells called *phagocytes* that arrive immediately to eat up the dead cell. Necrosis occurs when this chemical signal is never sent, causing a buildup in dead tissue and cell debris. Cells dying by necrosis also release harmful enzymes into the surrounding tissue, causing a chain reaction that leads to the death of more cells and eventually to gangrene.[1]

In addition to damaging cells and the way they communicate, free radicals create metabolic waste products that interfere with DNA, RNA, and protein synthesis. Free radicals also cause inflammation, lower our energy levels, and generally disturb vital chemical processes throughout the body. In short, they accelerate aging, and the most obvious sign of their handiwork is wrinkles.

The large market for antioxidants (which help the cell defend itself against free radicals) seems to suggest that people are more aware today of what free-radical damage can do. And, fortunately, there are many antioxidant-rich foods, probiotic liquids, and even special waters available that you can consume every day to help combat the damage of free radicals.

The Body Ecology Diet, with its delicious foods and liquids, is the quintessential antioxidant diet.

— The **inflammation theory of aging** has received a lot of press of late. Integrative physician Mark Hyman defines inflammation as "the activation of the immune system due to the presence of some kind of intruder," such as an infection (viral, fungal, or bacterial) or allergen (mold, for instance, or ragweed) or toxin (heavy metals, pesticides, and xenoestrogens). This inflammation can be obvious, such as eczema or psoriasis, or it can be more subtle, working deep inside us at the cellular level (for example, inflammation of the arteries, leading to heart disease).[2] Inflammation breaks down the body—every ache, pain, and disease is connected to chronic inflammation.

When we don't eat properly, when we fail to hydrate or get enough sleep, when we allow ourselves to become overweight, when we are overcome by stress or besieged by environmental toxins, and when we avoid sunlight and become deficient in vitamin D, we increase inflammation in the body.

While inflammation makes us more susceptible to aging, aging in turn makes us more susceptible to inflammation. To break free from this vicious cycle, we must trigger a "youthening" in our cells. *Diet is one way we can either fuel or cool the fires of inflammation*, reducing tissue breakdown.

Baby Boomers are the first generation to become aware of inflammation, and are forced to cope with its serious consequences. Unfortunately, the damage has been done, and we must now "cool" what Chinese medicine calls "heat" in the body. A lifetime of bad fats, especially trans-fatty acids found in margarine and fried and processed fast foods, has left its mark. We turned from grass-fed to corn- and soy-fed animals, losing essential fatty acids that cool the fires of inflammation. Refined carbohydrates and acid-forming foods that strip minerals from the body head the list of enemies that contributes to age-related diseases such as osteoporosis, Alzheimer's, and arthritis.

Although I tend to view inflammation as a symptom rather than a cause of aging, I definitely agree that it quickens this process. While a poor diet is certainly a major cause of inflammation, a nutrient-rich one can become your most important tool to reverse it.

— The **hormonal-decline theory of aging** (also called the *neuroendrocrine theory of aging*) involves diminishing levels of critical hormones. Our hormones are secreted by little organs—the hypothalamus, thyroid, adrenals, ovaries, testes, pineal gland, and pituitary glands. As we age, we become more toxic and malnourished, and these glands lose their ability to secrete their respective hormones (estrogen, progesterone, testosterone, DHEA, thyroid, and HGH [human growth hormone]). In addition to this dramatic decline in production, our trillions of cells lose their sensitivity and will no longer "accept the hormones," even if the body is still making them or is taking them exodenously (from an outside source).

As this decline occurs, cortisol and insulin become elevated in our blood. These two hormones work together as a team; as cortisol levels climb and remain high, so do blood sugar and insulin. Our bodies neither want nor need the excess sugar that insulin escorts into our cells.[3]

Our cells can only take in so much at one time, and then they "shut their doors" and refuse to let the sugar in. The excess sugar remains, permeating our bloodstream, causing weight gain, elevated blood pressure, and unremitting acidity of key body fluids. An acidic environment is the perfect home to infections, cancer, and many other health hazards . . . including early aging.

Cortisol is produced when our bodies are under stress, and in today's world, who *isn't* under chronic and intense pressure? As the years go by, this stress usually increases. Dealing with the illness or death of our parents, financial struggles, and our own failing health is more than enough for most of us. Add to that toxins in our environment or in our relationships, along with fears and concerns about our future, and you can see why elevated cortisol levels often remain high in our middle and later years and contribute to early aging.

This combination of elevated cortisol and our cells' resistance to insulin is most likely the underlying cause of what is called "metabolic syndrome," a growing condition in America, which includes increased risk for heart disease, stroke, and diabetes. Early warning signs are high blood pressure, elevated insulin levels, excess body fat around the waist, and abnormal cholesterol levels.

The foods and herbs that are a part of the Body Ecology Way can actually help repair hormone imbalances. Body Ecology's 7 Principles and seven food groups are the ideal solution for dealing with hormonal decline and elevated cortisol and insulin. Foods that are both calming and fortifying will help you through stressful times and will nourish your endocrine organs. These same foods, combined with cleansing practices such as colon therapy, will help remove lifelong accumulation of toxins that are poisoning your endocrine glands.

Yoga, massage, and spa vacations that calm the mind and center us are already becoming some of the most sought-after therapies for our entire generation.

— The **mitochondrial-decline theory of aging** suggests that augmenting and protecting our mitochondria is an essential part of preventing and slowing aging. The mitochondria are organelles (tiny organs) found in every cell of every organ in the body. They are powerful energy generators, using oxygen and sugar (glucose) to create the fuel that every cell needs.

The primary job of the mitochondria is to create adenosine triphosphate (ATP), an important chemical that is essential for repair and regeneration inside our bodies. Unique to the mitochondria is that they have their own DNA. But this is actually a problem in terms of aging. While other kinds of DNA have histone proteins and repair enzymes to protect them, mitochondrial DNA does not, which means the mitochondria are subject to greater free-radical damage. Because they lack the defenses we have in other parts of the body, the mitochondria become larger, more tired, less efficient, and fewer in number as we age.[4]

In addition, very little ATP can be stored in the body. Our reserves are quite small. Thus, the mitochondria have to be very efficient and healthy in order to produce the continuous supply of ATP that we need.[5] The decline in ATP production and loss of mitochondrial efficiency

Body Ecology's 7 Principles and seven food groups are the ideal solution for dealing with hormonal decline and elevated cortisol and insulin levels.

can lead to diseases such as cancer, where it has been shown that the mitochondria in the cells of people who have cancer are not utilizing oxygen the way they should.[6]

The quality and quantity of mitochondria are determined by many factors: heredity, stress, nutrition, and environment. Stress, in particular, puts greater demands on our cells, requiring a greater number of mitochondria to generate more ATP, necessary for the production of more hormones, proteins, and energy balance.

But mitochondria play an even greater role in longevity than we once knew.

A recent study conducted at Harvard Medical School and published in *The Journal of Molecular Evolution* has revealed that our mitochondria are of paramount importance in prolonging life span. These scientists discovered that mitochondria are not static and unchanging; they have actually evolved over time in a way that has "allowed humans to lead longer, healthier lives without the scourge of neurodegenerative disease."[7] As mitochondria are now being viewed as central to the evolution of human longevity, it is important to explore proven methods for supporting and enhancing these organelles.

Daily nutritious foods, sunshine, and water—actively balanced with rest, deep sleep, plus positive thoughts—are the most important determiners of good mitochondrial quality and function.

— Related to the mitochondrial-decline theory is the **glycation theory of aging.** In fact, glycation can reduce the functionality and efficiency of mitochondrial proteins, which in turn promotes cell death. Glycation takes place when the body's proteins or DNA molecules bond chemically with sugar molecules. Eventually these sugars modify again to form rogue molecules called *advanced glycation end-products* (AGEs). In essence, this works in very much the same way as the "caramelization" of sugar. AGEs are "resistant to the body's routine efforts to remove damaged proteins. Ultimately, they will cross-link with adjacent proteins, rendering tissue increasingly stiff and inflexible."[8]

AGEs in tissues increase free-radical production to many, many more times the rate produced by unglycated proteins, which has been associated with accelerated aging. There are obvious physical manifestations of glycation products— wrinkles and sagging skin, to name two.

But it's not just the outside that bears the brunt of the damage. Inside our bodies, glycation can reduce protein flexibility and functionality; and plays a role in a wide range of problems, including cataracts, arthritis, and atherosclerosis.[9,10] AGEs also trigger inflammatory reactions throughout the body, including the brain, where they have been shown to cause certain cells to pump out free radicals that are toxic to neurons. Many scientists believe that AGEs play a significant role in cognitive-decline diseases such as Alzheimer's.[11]

Other theories of aging focus on the structure and behavior of the body's cells:

— The **membrane theory of aging** suggests that as we grow older, the cell membrane becomes less lipidic (watery). This inhibits cell functioning and can lead to accumulation of toxins.

— The **Hayflick limit theory of aging** suggests that the human cell is limited in the number of times it can divide. Dr. Leonard Hayflick theorized that a cell divides approximately 50 times, after which it simply stops dividing and dies. Hayflick's research showed the need to slow down the rate of cell division through diet and lifestyle. In particular, he found that calorie restriction (discussed in Chapter 5) might play a role in the rate at which a cell divides, as underfed cells do so much more slowly than overfed ones.[12]

Let's Simplify

Body Ecology posits two principal causes of aging: (1) an accumulation of toxins in our cells, and (2) nutritional deficiencies in our cells. Both of these factors weaken our cells, resulting in a loss of our core energy and vitality and leading to degenerative disease, including that of aging.

It is interesting—but not surprising—that in every theory of aging, lifestyle and diet have a clear and dramatic impact, both negative and positive, on the aging process. This is also true of the **Chinese medicine theory of aging,** which offers its own unique insights into aging and how to do it more gracefully.

The Chinese Medicine Theory of Aging— Quality of Life Through Increased Energy

In the West, we live in a youth-obsessed culture. We admire the beauty and vitality of younger people, and we don't want to admit that we may have lost our own.

People in the Far East have a very different attitude toward aging. They focus on the quality and vitality of life at any age . . . how to live long, happy, and full of youthful *energy.* They believe that the essence of aging is not in how we *look,* but in how we *live.*

Body Ecology embraces this viewpoint. Remember, what you focus on is what you get. You don't want to focus on aging; you want to put all your thoughts and intentions into creating youthfulness. It's time to leave behind negative (or even resigned) beliefs about aging and instead focus on increasing your vitality and energy.

Ancient Chinese medicine understood that we age when our energy wanes and eventually becomes depleted, causing us to become vulnerable to what Western doctors call "disease." You know it well: cancer, heart disease, osteoporosis, Alzheimer's . . . even aging is now seen by some as a "disease."

Body Ecology avoids the term *disease,* preferring the more positive Eastern concept of *imbalances,* as this model is more empowering. If something is out of balance, the obvious solution is to put it back *into* balance.

Why is there an imbalance? Do you have an infection? Is your digestion weak and your body lacking in vital nutrients? Are there toxins in your system that are interfering with your life force? If yes, then you have it within your own power to address and correct these imbalances.

Let's take a closer look at energy—the vital life force. Where does it come from? How do we get more, and how do we keep our energy balanced?

Jing Energy: A Gift from Our Ancestors

In Chinese medicine our primal life-force energy comes from the inherited prenatal life before we entered this world *(jing)* and from the energy we acquire as we nourish our bodies day by day *(chi).*

Were you born with a strong constitution? Was your fundamental intrinsic energy once quite strong? Jing energy (or essence energy) is the prenatal, primordial energy given to us from our parents, grandparents, and ancestors. If our mothers ate well and had a happy, easy pregnancy with very little stress; and if our ancestors were strong, hardy people, then we would have inherited a strong constitution.

More than anything else, constitutional energy determines longevity and controls the aging process and our resistance to disease. Strong jing generates a long life that is free of degenerative disease. Weak jing shows itself as a failure to thrive (in children) and premature aging (in adults). It determines our ability to rejuvenate. Our sexual vitality and how "sexy" we look and feel is directly related to our prenatal energy.

If our parents did not understand how important it was to eat well, to cleanse their bodies of toxins, and to reduce stress in their lives—both prior to conception and while our physical bodies were being formed—then we were, in truth, victims of the ignorant times into which we were born.

Although our jing energy is fixed and inherited, it can be conserved by our actions throughout the day. Because it is *stored* energy, it provides the reserves we need to adapt to all the various toxins and stresses we encounter in modern life. Jing energy can be steadily depleted as the years go by. For some of us, it was depleted quickly because of our diet and lifestyle choices. If we had been taught to protect it and to even build up these inherited reserves, we would now be seeing a generation of Baby Boomers looking and feeling amazingly youthful.

Think of jing energy like a bank account. Imagine that each of us had a rich uncle, Freddie. Your "Uncle Freddie" gifted you with $5 million on the day you were born. (You inherited a really strong constitution.) *My* Uncle Freddie may have only had $2 million

> *Think of jing energy as a bit like a bank account. You must make daily good investments into the account so that you have something to draw upon in times of added stress and demand.*

to give to me. (My parents were not as healthy as yours.) Let's pretend that from the moment we were born, you and I began to spend our money. You spent yours faster than I did mine because you had more than I did, but even so, by the time we were both in our 50s, we were broke. (Our constitutional energy was depleted, and we could actually feel that it was.)

But my friend Sara, who, like me, only received $2 million, was taught to never draw money from her account unless she also put much of it right back in. (Sara led a busy life, too, but she never ate sugar, and loved fermented foods and vegetables. She also exercised moderately and managed her stress through yoga and meditation.) Not surprisingly, when she reached 50, she still had most of her inherited money. (And she looked and felt 20 years younger than we did.)

Jing is exactly like this. If each day we spend what we've inherited and never replace it, we will reach our older years looking and feeling pretty spent.

If you know that the day ahead calls for a lot of energy, you will want to fuel your body with those foods, herbs, and supplements that give you that needed *extra* energy (see the explanation of "chi" to follow) to get you through that day. You must make *daily* investments into the inherited account so that you have something to draw upon in times of added stress and demand.

We drain our accounts when we smoke, drink alcohol and coffee, or eat a diet of refined foods that contain a lot of sugar and poor-quality fats. Add stress, poor sleeping habits, overwork, too little exercise, and a poor understanding of how to conserve our sexual vitality, and we have a perfect description of today's Baby Boomer. Even chronic and acute illnesses deplete jing. Diminished sexual desire, weight gain, memory loss, graying hair, sagging skin, and poor muscle tone should be seen as evidence of how we've "misplaced" (not lost) this essence of rejuvenation. Sadly, we have taught this way of life to our children, who are now teaching it to our grandchildren.

Chi Energy: A Gift from Ourselves

Chi (sometimes spelled "qi") energy is *acquired* energy. It is our daily life force—it powers us to move and to thrive. It suffuses every living thing; resides within every cell, organ, and tissue; and affects every stage of our growth, from conception to death. When we are healthy, the body is a fountain of constantly circulating chi—a lovely dance of yin and yang that nurtures a sense of balance, harmony, and wellness.

Chi energy is the key to maintenance of health and the prevention of disease. After birth, chi comes from the good things we take into our bodies, along with their proper digestion and transformation. It is the energy we obtain day after day as we feed ourselves nourishing foods. These nutrient-rich fruits, vegetables, herbs and roots, proteins, fats, and seeds have a life force of their own and give us the daily energy we need.

Some foods have no nutritional power unless they are altered in some way to make them easier to digest. In fact, preparing foods in a way that increases their life force so that they, in turn, increase *ours* is an "art." As humans, we have the ability to change the nature of foods by cooking them, fermenting them, and sprouting them to enhance their inherent life force. Many have to be prepared to make them more digestible so that we can "get the most out of them."

As infants—and even as older children—we had very little ability to obtain our acquired chi on a daily basis. Even if our mothers offered us healthier foods, did we really want them? After all, most of us Baby Boomer kids were never taught to care for our bodies. Frozen dinners on aluminum trays, mushy white bread you could roll into a ball, and fake butter were really "cool." They were easy to prepare and tasted great. We were happy with these sweet-tasting, lifeless foods. As adults, we find that these items have become embedded in our cellular memory, and they are now our comfort foods in times of stress.

Chi is energy we create through our daily choices. But there's another kind that must be in place first in order for us to act at all. To live a long and happy life, we must first envision the life we desire and then use our energy and intent to create it. This third kind of energy in Chinese medicine is called *shen,* or spiritual energy.

Shen Energy: A Gift from Our Creator

Chinese masters say that *shen* is an all-embracing love that expresses itself in our hearts. It presides over the emotions and communicates itself outwardly as an all-encompassing compassion, acceptance, and tolerance toward others. Shen energy is our guiding spirit, a wonderful manifestation of our higher nature as humans. When our "shen is off," we are dispirited, brought low by life's stresses, toxins, and traumas. But when we are "full of shen," we dare to live to the fullest! When our intrinsic prenatal energy is restored and meets with the energy in our hearts, our shen energy can open outward so that we act from a place of forgiveness and unconditional love. Amazing changes can be accomplished almost immediately.

Strong shen is essential for well-being; it gives us our willpower. Without it, restoring our prenatal jing and creating daily chi are difficult to achieve. In turn, the interaction of jing and chi leads to vital shen. When shen, jing, and chi are in perfect balance, our minds are strong, our emotions are balanced, and our bodies are vital and healthy.

Jing, Chi, and *Shen*—the Three Treasures

Constitutional energy (jing), daily acquired energy (chi), and spiritual energy (shen) are together called the three heavenly treasures. They are gifts for us to cherish as we live upon this earth in our physical bodies.

Besides the three heavenly treasures, we have been given earthly treasures as well. All over the earth, humankind has been provided with countless wonderful foods, herbs, air, water, and an amazing variety of life experiences with which to nourish ourselves. The 7 Principles and the seven food groups you will discover in this book will provide you with the foundation you need to sort through the limitless possibilities.

Where Do We Go from Here?

Many of us look in the mirror and see that we have not done a very good job of nourishing ourselves. Much of our core intrinsic energy has dissipated, and we don't know how to replenish it. We aren't even aware of how to acquire energy day by day. But we're Baby Boomers . . . and we're determined to stay young.

Each and every Baby Boomer must now ask: "What can I do to restore my depleted *inherited energy?*"

Answer: For each remaining day of your life, you must begin to create—step by step—enough energy to carry you through the day, *plus extra* to replenish the prenatal energy that has been exhausted from a lifetime of neglect and a lack of knowledge.

Whether it is out of fear of becoming old and suffering the pain of aging, or out of vanity because we do not like what we see in the mirror, many of us are ready to take this action.

Each of the chapters in this book will provide you with the valuable tools you need to reverse the signs of aging and rejuvenate your jing and chi.

In the next chapter, we'll look at the "diet phenomenon" in America, what's good about these different dietary approaches and what's not, and how the Body Ecology program offers the critical missing piece.

From the Physician's Desk

"It isn't what you eat that ages you. It's what happens to what you eat that ages you."

*A*ging is due to chronic low-grade systemic inflammation that the body is not managing efficiently. The Body Ecology system is an ideal anti-aging strategy because it manages inflammation through appropriate diet. But it's not just about food. The Body Ecology system is about eating the right kinds of food the right way. Ultimately we want to heal the gut lining so that the life-giving attributes of food have the opportunity to get through and do their best work.

The Body Ecology approach involves many components, including food combining; minimal sugar in the form of organic fruits; and an 80 to 90 percent plant-based diet of organic vegetables, legumes, seeds and nuts, some whole grains, and free-range organic animal products. When these foods enter the small intestine, they help create the ideal environment for optimal intestinal and immune function. Body Ecology foods have the digestive enzymes that are so important for breaking down foods in the proximal small intestine before reaching the colon. This "optimal absorption scenario" is only possible when beneficial bacteria stay in the intestinal tract on a continuous, round-the-clock basis. A vegetable-based diet is more supportive of beneficial bacteria, in terms of how long they stay in the intestinal tract and how well they work. The bacteria interact with the gut lining so that it can optimize food intake without overactivation of the immune system, while feeding the body.

One other important aspect of all of this is managing your psycho-emotional stress. If you are not able to manage the fight-or-flight response, you won't be able to digest properly, and your immune system won't work right. Stress can cause neutral bacteria to transform into "turncoats" (possible pathogenic bacteria).

So, along with the right foods eaten the right way, it's important to find methods for detoxifying and decompressing the stress in our lives. Drinking lots of water, ridding the body of toxic metal poisons using infrared saunas, habitual exercise that sweats the toxins out, regular sleep, and work that fulfills you and makes you happy are simple but tried-and-true methods of managing stress and giving your inner ecosystem the greatest chance of thriving.

— *Leonard Smith, M.D.*

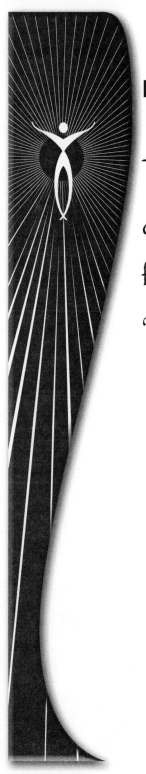

PART II

The End of the Road for All "Diets"

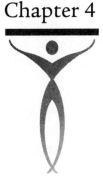

Chapter 4

Diet Madness: Half Truths and Partial Solutions Behind Today's Popular Diets

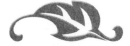

Why do so many diets fail?
Is it possible to lose weight, look younger, and feel healthier without starving ourselves?

About 50 million Americans go on a diet each year, and an estimated $30 billion is spent annually on weight loss. Even more troubling is that after all that money has been spent on diet books, pills, drinks, and plans, large numbers of people—sometimes more than half—drop out within months of beginning their diets. In the minds of many today, *diet* has become an ugly word. You probably cringe a bit when you hear it, and now you hold in your hands another diet book! However, this is not a diet for losing weight. It's not merely about reversing the aging process, either . . . it is much, much more. It's an exciting new way of living . . . a system of health and healing that 78 million Baby Boomers have been yearning to find.

Diets fail because they are about deprivation and denial, rather than life-affirming changes in behavior and great-tasting foods that nourish and sustain the body. Because their focus is typically on *losing pounds* fast rather than on permanent changes in eating behaviors and lifestyle, many of us will often experience short-term success and long-term failure.

Another reason why many diets fail is that they often restrict calories to a dangerous point—a point at which the metabolism actually begins to slow down, ultimately hindering rather than helping weight-loss efforts. In Chapter 5 you will learn about "calorie restriction," and its benefits in stopping and reversing several significant signs of aging. But if not done properly, it can be dangerous.

Perhaps the most important reason many diets fail is that they advocate an all-or-nothing approach. They do not incorporate the *Principle of Uniqueness* (discussed in Chapter 8), particularly important for Baby Boomers who revel in their individuality. The first of Body Ecology's 7 Principles, *Uniqueness* recognizes the distinctiveness of each person and adapts customized protocols to specific health conditions and needs.

You're Not Failing the Diet . . . the Diet Is Failing *You*

Between South Beach and Atkins, the Zone and Weight Watchers, Ayurvedic and macrobiotic, raw diets and e-diets, it's easy to get frustrated and confused with the overabundance of choice. Is it possible to find a diet that meets all of our nutritional needs? We live in an information age, where there are infinite opportunities to educate ourselves about health. Baby Boomers, in particular, have a passion for information and the latest news. But one of the disadvantages of this is that many of us don't have the time or the knowledge to beat a

Diets fail because they are about deprivation and denial, rather than life-affirming changes in behavior and great-tasting foods that nourish and sustain the body.

path through all these competing and conflicting ideas to find the simple truth. What we need are some basic guidelines that fit for us no matter who we are or how our needs change.

Some of the more popular diets today have many valuable things to offer. But as you will discover in Chapter 6, they offer only a partial picture of what your body really needs. They lack a missing piece of information that is essential for inhibiting the aging process for anyone at any age. Let's look at four of these trendsetting diets, with their benefits and drawbacks. . . .

The High-Protein Diet

This dietary approach, which encompasses eating plans such as Atkins and Protein Power, has a large and enthusiastic following. On the upside, these diets have shown some effectiveness in rapid weight loss, because they allow virtually no carbohydrates and sugars, particularly during the initial stages. Given that in some generations as many as 85 percent have a yeast infection called *candidiasis,* a diet that eliminates or greatly restricts sugary foods will start people on the path to wellness.

But that isn't enough to get them all the way home free.

There is a downside to too much animal protein. Most people do not have enough stomach acid to digest all these proteins, and undigested animal protein produces a lot of poisonous waste in the body. Some of these diets condone a high (and imbalanced) consumption of saturated fats. I believe this eating plan is a particularly harsh one for women, whose monthly cycles require more calming and soothing foods.

In addition, people on these diets often suffer from constipation and colon problems. Because they lack a significant source of fiber, it has been suggested that long-term practitioners may have a greater chance of contracting colon cancer. Fiber is extremely important for improving peristaltic movement so that our colons can eliminate waste the way they should.

I've also observed that while on high-protein diets, people often have pallid skin and bad breath, and are angry and irritable from the overconsumption of meat protein, which is contracting. (See Chapter 11: The Principle of Balance.) Many also eventually develop sleep disorders at night, and they appear to be lethargic and listless during the day.

The Macrobiotic Diet

A Japanese educator named George Ohsawa developed the macrobiotic diet and philosophy with his wife, Lima. They taught that simple, natural food eaten in a balanced way was the key to optimal health. I had the privilege of studying with Lima Ohsawa when she was in her 80s. She lived to be just over 100. Looking back, I now realize that she was my first true mentor in anti-aging. I was in my 30s when I met her, yet she was much more resilient and healthy than I. I will never forget following behind her one afternoon to interview her for an article for the *Macrobiotic Journal*. Three long flights up had me gasping for air, but she didn't seem to be the least bit fazed by our rapid climb—a journey she made often to her office.

Of the many things I learned during my five-month macrobiotic tutorial, two stand out:

1. Lima told me that if she had to live her life all over again, she would "take the macrobiotic principles, travel all over the world, and apply them to the foods found in all cultures everywhere." This was her way of telling me that it was the *principles* that were important, not the foods we were eating on macrobiotic diets in the U.S. and Japan. This tiny bit of information has served me well for many years. I began to understand that the universal principles were just that— universal. They could apply to anyone living anywhere, and to all foods.

2. The second thing that Lima taught me had to do with food choice and portion size. Those who knew her well told me that Lima "ate like a bird." Yet what I observed was that she consumed small portions of very healthy foods, especially vegetables. As you will learn in Chapter 5, Lima was properly practicing calorie restriction.

Predominantly vegetarian, the standard macrobiotic diet is a low-fat, high-fiber diet of whole grains; vegetables; and small amounts of fish, legumes, soups, and pickles. The ancient Chinese principle of balance, called *yin and yang,* is the basis for this diet, but this is a complex principle requiring many years of study to fully master. So, although yin and yang are honored in the diet, very few practice it properly.

Many people who do try macrobiotics have found it to be too rigid and restrictive. A heavy reliance on complex carbs from grains . . . mostly brown rice . . . creates high levels of acidity in the body. Brown rice is high in sugar, which is not good for the millions of people who suffer from candida and many other conditions such as cancer. This also promotes early aging. The lack of protein and healthy fats can result in poor energy and will be challenging for people of particular blood types. People with certain digestive conditions, such as colitis, would not be able to tolerate many of the grains on the diet, which are not soaked and prepared properly. Healthy medicinal herbs and antifungal spices are frowned upon; and, quite frankly, the food can be extremely tasteless.

People often complain of digestion problems and extreme fatigue while on the macrobiotic diet. I've observed that those who follow this approach religiously often seem intolerant and inflexible, and are short of temper. The diet contains a lot of salty foods, causing one to become too contracted or "uptight."

Nevertheless, I am extremely grateful for my eight years of training in macrobiotics, both in the U.S. and in Japan. If you are familiar with macrobiotics, you will find it very easy to follow the Body Ecology Way.

The Raw-Foods Diet

Of course, our earliest prehistoric ancestors were "raw food–ists" by default, because they didn't have fire to cook their meals. As a modern-day phenomenon, the raw-foods diet, originally created by Ann Wigmore, became very popular during the '90s. It is currently enjoying a revival, particularly on the West Coast (especially in Hollywood). (Because it is a cooling diet, it can be ideal during the summer months or if you live in a warmer climate such as California, Florida, Arizona, or Hawaii.)

Practitioners consume only uncooked, unprocessed (and often only organic) vegetables, seeds, nuts, and fruit. These nutrient-rich foods are thought to be easier to digest because they maintain the enzymes that are lost during cooking. Because it is primarily vegetarian, another benefit of the raw-foods diet is that it has less of a negative impact on our environment.

But for many, the raw-foods diet is daunting and ultimately not satisfying over the long term, as they miss the taste of cooked food. Over time more serious health problems associated with this approach can begin to surface. Yes, the fruits and vegetables do contain enzymes, but humans cannot break down cellulose, the indigestible fiber in vegetables, and therefore cannot fully extract the nutrients in them. Furthermore, vegetables from the cruciferous family (broccoli, cauliflower, kale, cabbage, and collards) suppress the thyroid when eaten raw. Spinach, beet greens, chard, rhubarb, and almonds are high in oxalates, and when eaten raw, bind calcium, making it unavailable to us.

In addition, there are many vegetables that become *more* nutritious after cooking. For example, when carrots are cooked, their cell structure is softened, which makes their inherent carotene, minerals, and vitamin C more accessible to us. Studies are now showing that cooking some vegetables, such as corn, can actually boost their antioxidant benefits. When people have been on this raw-foods diet for a while, they often become deficient in minerals and even proteins, and are thin and undernourished.

Many nutritionists argue that you risk missing out on important nutrients when you eat *only* uncooked produce. Like most of us, many people on this diet lead busy lives and find themselves grabbing a piece of fruit instead of taking the time to properly prepare a wide variety of foods in their blender, dehydrator, or sprouter. Fruits are high in phosphorus, and over time this will lead to teeth loss because calcium levels must be two and a half times phosphorus levels. Another thing I've noticed about people on a raw-foods diet is that they often appear spacey, unfocused, and a bit out of touch with reality. This is because their diet contains too much sugar, which is expansive. Fruits, raw-food bars, raw-food desserts, and the like contain a great deal of sugar.

Body Ecology also praises the benefits of a raw-foods diet *if* it is practiced properly. People with an active viral infection or cancer will benefit from this diet, but there is a way to do it correctly. Many who incorporate Body Ecology's raw and fermented foods report that they feel more energized, have clearer skin, are able to successfully maintain their weight, and are less susceptible to colds and other viruses.

Body Ecology does "raw" differently. Most important, it includes cultured foods to encourage digestion and to help heal the mucosal lining of the digestive tract. In addition, only very sour fruits are consumed, preferably combined with probiotic foods so that the microflora eat the small amounts of sugar present. Body Ecology also honors food-combining principles, and we utilize a full range of healthy fats.

The Vegetarian Diet

The Baby Boomer Diet is adaptable to fit ever-changing needs. It can certainly be vegetarian if that is best for you. A vegetarian diet can be an excellent diet if it is done properly . . . *Body Ecology*-style. As you read more about each of the 7 Principles and the superfood groups, you will find many tools that vegetarians must know in order to do "veggie" right.

Adapting to the ebb and flow of our lives requires that we be attuned, that we train ourselves to listen and act upon what our bodies are telling us in the here and now.

Vegetarians often choose protein "alternatives," such as beans, nuts, and cheese; and do not understand that these are quite difficult to digest. They often also compensate for the lack of meat protein by consuming a lot of bread carbs and other sugary foods, which is not a balanced way to eat and can lead to weight gain. Many vegetarians are also anemic, often with dangerous iron deficiencies, because they fail to choose high-energy foods such as eggs, leafy-green vegetables, and high-protein grain-like seeds to fortify themselves.

"Digestion is everything," as we say in Body Ecology, and typically as we grow older and our bodies becomes more acidic, our stomachs produce less and less acid. We can no longer digest the animal foods, even if we prefer them, and they will start to make us feel sluggish and tired.

Perhaps over time you will find yourself gradually moving into an easier-to-digest, largely plant-based diet; and Body Ecology can show you how to do this wisely.

Square Pegs in Round Holes

I recognize how these diets have helped many people in many ways, but I also feel that they offer only partial solutions. Body Ecology assimilates the "best of the best" to create a more exciting and fluid dietary approach that works for *all people,* precisely because it isn't a cookie-cutter program.

Many of the foods in the Body Ecology Way of Life are consistent with what people are now calling the Mediterranean diet and the Okinawan diet, with their emphasis on healthy oils, seafood, and a rich variety of vegetables. But greatly enhancing these diets is the inclusion of some powerful superfoods, such as fermented vegetables, probiotic liquids, ocean plants, grain-like seeds, and stevia (an all-natural sweetener). Body Ecology also incorporates unique eating and lifestyle strategies that don't simply drop pounds, but *fundamentally alter the way we feel, look, and age.*

The Body Ecology dietary approach is also quite flexible and can be adapted to those suffering from many health conditions, such as:

- Leaky gut syndrome
- Adrenal fatigue
- Viral infections
- Candida
- Low energy
- Food allergies
- Autism

In addition to addressing these conditions, the Body Ecology Way is the most effective diet for anti-aging and protection against disease. As you begin to delve into the 7 Principles, you'll discover how the Baby Boomer Diet addresses many of the challenges and outward signs of aging.

Learning to Listen to Your Body

Our bodily needs shift all the time. Both men and women go through biological and emotional cycles that require different foods and behaviors at different times. People who live in urban areas have different needs from those who live in rural areas. Climate and seasonal changes affect our choice of foods and supplements and how they are prepared and utilized. We have differences based on our unique blood type and based on our individual levels of toxicity. And, as discussed in the previous chapter, we all have different *jing* energy, or the constitutional energy we inherited from our forebears. All of these factors affect how we tailor our diet and how we make it work from one day to the next.

From year to year and decade to decade, our bodies ask for different things. A type of exercise that may have served us well when we were 25 may be less effective or healthy for us when we're 55. Doctors are now referring to a phenomenon called "boomeritis"—the growing incidence of Baby Boomers who end up in emergency wards from overindulgence in high-risk activities that take a toll on bodies that are expected to behave as they did when they were 18. Aging gracefully doesn't mean giving up what we love, but rather *adapting creatively* to what our bodies are asking of us today.

Baby Boomers who are in their 40s will have different health needs from those in their 60s. Many Boomers in their 40s are focused on family and are still living a very high-energy, on-the-go lifestyle. Older Boomers, while wanting to enjoy greater stamina and vitality, are also more concerned about warding off particular health issues, such as osteoporosis or eye disease.[1] Adapting to the ebb and flow of our lives requires that we be attuned, that we train ourselves to listen and act upon what our bodies are telling us in the here and now. Instead of always trying to conquer nature, our physical selves are asking us to restore our connection with nature and acclimate ourselves intuitively to its rhythms.

Finally, each of us will place a different priority on health. Wonderfully for us Baby Boomers, as we approach retirement or choose more flexible second careers, we will have more time to learn about our bodies, to explore how we feel, and to discover what foods and behaviors will be the most fruitful for us at different points along our journey.

As you progress through this book, you will encounter some foods that will be new to you, as well as innovative and interesting ways of preparing them so that they deliver the most value to your body and soul. Yes, weight loss will come easily as you eat these delicious foods. But the most important reason for mastering this new way of eating is to stay young and healthy for as long as possible.

In the next chapter, we will take a look at calorie restriction, the only intervention proven to extend life span, slow or reverse aging, and reduce the risk for degenerative diseases. But you'll learn how to do it the right way—the Body Ecology Way.

The First Americans—a Dietary Model

*M*ore than half of the food eaten all over the world today is derived from plants originally domesticated by the American Indian, and Native American cookery involves the oldest foods and cooking traditions in North America. Prior to the arrival of Europeans in the 1500s, indigenous peoples primarily ate food that was gathered or hunted, and it was largely eaten while still fresh. As a result, they enjoyed unusual longevity, healthy bone structure, and relative freedom from disease.

Correspondingly, the European introduction of sugar, alcohol, and dairy products to these cultures had a devastating effect on Indian health. These items brought about a significant rise in diabetes, heart disease, lactose intolerance, and dental deterioration. Today, some tribes are trying to find ways to reverse this dietary damage. The Karuk Indians of northwest California, for instance, are waging a public fight for salmon-fishing rights, citing the low incidence of heart disease, obesity, and diabetes among their people prior to World War II—the result of a diet rich in omega-3 fatty acids derived from wild salmon. Many other tribes are returning to more traditional foods and methods of preparation.[i]

Although there were regional differences among America's indigenous peoples, their nutritional choices were almost without exception healthy. Common to all were the foods they did *not* consume, in part because many had not yet been created. Native peoples had no refined sugar in their diet and did not eat lots of refined grains and processed carbohydrates. Trans fats, those killer oils so prevalent in American fast food today, were virtually nonexistent in the Indian diet. Although some tribes fermented their own antioxidant-rich wine, alcohol was relatively rare, and tobacco (naturally grown) was generally used only for ceremonial purposes.

For many tribes, specific foods were highly symbolic and spiritual in nature. Northwestern coastal tribes held the salmon as sacred and important for fertility, while Southwestern tribes venerated corn (as did the Maya in Central America).

Because they lacked modern agricultural methods, Native Americans ate whole, raw, organic foods (no additives, fortifiers, preservatives, or antibiotics), as well as animals that fed on grass rather than corn or other grains. Whatever food was eaten took a great deal of effort to obtain and prepare. Game had to be hunted, killed, cleaned, smoked, and dried. Corn and vegetables were grown, harvested, and made more digestible. Roots, herbs, berries, seeds, and nuts were gathered.

When Americans weren't eating raw, they were slow-cooking their food over very low heat. Foods were not fried, refrigerated, or processed. Fire-pit cooking was the preferred cooking method. A pit was dug and lined with rock. When the fire had burned down to coals, foods were placed in the pit to roast or steam. Since storage was difficult, sun-dried meats were ground between stones and mixed with hot melted fat (suet) and berries into a substance called pemmican. All Indian tribes were very familiar with natural methods of preserving foods, such as fermenting vegetables, and they smoked and dried their game to preserve it for the winter.

The American Indian diet of pure, natural, simply prepared foods, high in essential fatty acids and antioxidants, was the ultimate in preventive medicine.

---

[1]Blaine Harden, "Tribe Fights Dams to Get Diet Back: Karuks Trying to Regain Salmon Fisheries and Their Health, *The Washington Post*, January 30, 2005: A03.

Chapter 5

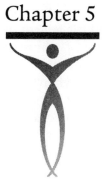

Calorie Restriction: The Right Way

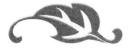

Baby Boomers have lost their spiritual connection to the food they eat. How do we find a balance between eating healthy and eating happy?

Food is truly one of the great and enduring pleasures of life. Many of our earliest childhood memories are tied to the evocative smells, colors, and tastes of our favorite foods; and there are few things more satisfying than a thoughtfully prepared meal shared with the people we love.

Ironically, before food was readily available, it actually had greater intrinsic value. Many backbreaking hours were spent planting, harvesting, storing, and preparing it. Because it came from the sweat of our own labor, food was very precious to us and connected us in an intimate way with the earth. Mealtimes were bonding occasions when the extended family got together, often offering a prayer of thanks for the bountiful food they had been given and asking that it nourish and strengthen them.

Even in the early 20th century, food was still treated in this respectful way. The mass production of food and the advent of the refrigerator in the 1920s and '30s were milestones in human evolution (not unlike the discovery of fire or the invention of the telephone). Refrigeration transformed how, when, and what we ate. Before that time, food was preserved by cooling it with snow and ice or by fermenting, pickling, dehydrating, salting, smoking, or canning.

Food often had the power to bind communities or countries together in times of need. During World War II, people planted "Victory Gardens" in their backyards and on rooftops. These vegetable, fruit, and herb gardens helped reduce the pressure on the food supply brought on by the war effort. After the war was over, many people continued this practice, growing what we might now call "organic" produce. The harvesting of crops in the fall and the preserving of produce for the winter months were often a community effort. It was the season when neighbors and families often gathered together for canning or pickling and preserving foods in large mason jars for the winter. As a Baby Boomer, you might remember your own mother or grandmother devoting an entire day of the week just to baking loaves of bread and pies or putting up casseroles.

Today, food can play many different roles in our lives. We eat what we want, when we want it. Food makes us feel good and satisfies our cravings. It appeases and soothes us in times of stress. Unfortunately, many of the things we eat to satisfy these urgent hungers and emotional voids are *low-vibrational foods* that are stripped of their nutrients and depleted of their life force.

Accordingly, food is no longer appreciated as a source of sustenance. More attention and money are invested in the marketing, packaging, and distribution of food than in its nutritional value. Foods are mass-produced and prepared with an emphasis on how they *taste*, not on how they *nourish*. It would be unthinkable to our ancestors that today's foods—so easily found in the supermarket—contain hundreds of harmful ingredients and chemicals, and give us so little energy to live.

The busy, fun-loving lifestyle of the typical Boomer led to an entirely new industry in America: fast food. It seemed like a great idea at the time—to be able to eat exactly what we wanted, cheaply, and on the go. But we are paying a heavy price for this self-indulgence—our children and grandchildren even more so. Do we ever stop to think about the message we convey to them when we take them to fast-food restaurants? We are telling them that food is merely a means of quick gratification, rather than a way to fortify and sustain us in the days and years ahead. We have taken food for granted, and this thankless attitude is now reflected back to us in the mirror in our appearance and in our behavior. We are not happy, healthy people.

At Body Ecology, we, like our ancestors, view food as energy and fuel for the body. We know that whole, pure foods vibrate with a positive, spiritual life force. These *high-vibrational foods* are the ones that create the greatest *chi*—that optimal youthful energy we so desire. And they can actually restore our constitutional prenatal *jing*. The healthier we are, the more we will vibrate the kind of energy that makes us—and those around us—feel good.

In Part IV, you will be introduced to the foods that can prevent and reverse aging. These foods provide you with the *quality* of nutrients you need to stay young, but what about *quantity*? Does how much you eat matter? If you eat too much or too little, will that affect how well you age?

How We Eat

Most Americans eat far too much—about 12 percent more calories per day than they did in the mid-1980s. With many fast-food restaurants promoting "supersize" options, and most sit-down restaurants offering excessively large portions, it can be challenging to eat moderately today. And even when restaurants do adopt a "smaller-servings strategy," as Ruby Tuesday tried to do a few years back by trimming portion sizes and printing nutritional information on the menu, consumers balk at the change. This is because

> *At Body Ecology, we, like our ancestors, view food as energy and fuel for the body. We know that whole, pure foods vibrate with a positive, spiritual life force.*

we've become accustomed to a "Bigger is better" mentality that associates food value with size. The more you get—we think—the more you get.[1]

Most of us are mindful that we should be limiting the calories we consume each day to a certain quantity, and most weight-loss diets involve some kind of calorie restriction. But many people become quickly frustrated or even obsessed with having to curb what they eat all the time. They become shackled to their bathroom scales in a never-ending cycle of one step forward, two steps back. But research has clearly shown that there is a connection between longevity and limiting the number of calories you consume in a day. In fact, of all the *research* to date on aging and diet, the most promising option for extending longevity is calorie restriction.

Let's take a look at some of its pros and cons:

The Connection Between Calorie Restriction and Life Extension

The effectiveness of calorie restriction as a weight-loss option was discovered more than 70 years ago. It means a restricted diet that involves the reduction of food consumption by a significant amount—in fact, by as much as 30 to 40 percent compared with what is considered normal for that species.

In a Washington University (St. Louis) study over a three-year period, participants who reduced their calories by 66 percent scored vastly better on all major risk factors for heart disease, including total cholesterol, triglycerides, and blood pressure. All three factors tend to increase with age. Other findings were lower markers for inflammation, which causes disease and aging, and lower body fat. This could mean a reduced risk of type 2 diabetes, with associated obesity.[2]

Some researchers actually believe that calorie restriction is a "biological stressor," something that elicits a defensive reaction in our cells that boosts our chances of survival. As a mild stressor, calorie restriction triggers the longevity genes into action. Once these genes are "switched on," there is an orchestrated shift in our metabolism, including "improved DNA stability, increased repair of DNA damage, improved immune function, prolonged cell survival, and enhanced energy production."[3] These "longevity genes" have been around for as

Intermittent Fasting as an Alternative to Calorie Restriction

*I*ntermittent fasting has been proposed as an alternative to calorie restriction, and some people find it easier to implement than continual calorie restriction. The way intermittent fasting typically works is that you fast every other day. You can eat as much as you'd like on the days you eat, but eat nothing on your fasting days. Studies, mostly on mice, show that intermittent fasting had results similar to calorie restriction, including slowing the progression of Huntington's, Parkinson's, and Alzheimer's disease; and increasing insulin sensitivity and resistance to stress.[i]

The Center for Conservative Therapy (CTC) in California specializes in all-water fasting programs that range from 5 to 40 days. These fasting programs have been found effective in the treatment of hypertension. They have also proven useful in cases of cardiovascular disease, diabetes, and other problems such as arthritis, because they clean the arteries and increase circulation to the joints. But even with these positive results, the CTC recommends fasts of shorter duration and encourages participants to gradually reintroduce food back into their diets after fasting, as this reinforces good nutritional habits. Fasting is not recommended for people with low body mass, those in the end stage of cancer, pregnant women (as it shuts down their milk supply), or people with AIDS.[ii]

---

[i]Jule Klotter, "Fasting & Neurodegenerative Disease," *Townsend Letter for Doctors and Patients,* November 2003: 1.

[ii]Alan Goldhamer, D.C., "Benefits of Fasting," *Well Being Journal,* September/October 2005, **http://www.healthpromoting.com/ Articles/articles/benefit.htm** (accessed October 19, 2009).

long as we have, and have helped us during times of drought or famine or other kinds of environmental stress.

Recently, the discovery of a family of enzymes called *sirtuins* (sir-two-ins) has provided us with another piece of this complex puzzle. Sirtuins appear to play a major role in the life-extending effects of calorie restriction. Found in organisms ranging from baker's yeast to roundworms to humans, they function as cellular "guardian angels" that come to our aid when called upon. They protect cells and enhance their survival. Medical research is under way to develop medications that modulate the activity of sirtuin enzymes; and these would be used to treat certain conditions such as Alzheimer's, diabetes, and heart disease.[4]

Most of the benefits of calorie restriction are likely related to its influence on blood sugar and insulin. Eating *fewer* calories each day *lowers* blood sugar and insulin. Excess insulin depletes your body of essential anti-aging hormones and suppresses your immune system. Normalizing blood sugar and insulin is crucial if you expect to reach your maximum life span. Both, when elevated, lead to acidity and mineral loss, not only causing premature aging, but also making us more prone to diseases such as diabetes, yeast infections, viruses, and cancer.

Eating fewer calories also lowers oxidative stress. We don't "rust" as fast (see the free-radical theory in Chapter 3).

If done properly, calorie restriction not only allows us to live longer but also better. Most neurodegenerative diseases, like Alzheimer's and Parkinson's, are forestalled, and restriction can actually modify our cellular defenses. There is, indeed, an abundance of recent evidence that supports the efficacy of calorie restriction . . . so is it recommended on the Baby Boomer Diet?

The Drawbacks to Calorie Restriction

There is some evidence that we humans are predisposed to calorie restriction, and even periods of fasting, because our early ancestors were forced to go without food for extended periods of time. This was because they may have had plenty of food available at one time of year and a scarcity at others. But this was hardly an ideal state of affairs. Does it serve our needs in this day and age? To starve one day and binge the next is today's dictionary definition of an eating disorder! At Body Ecology we believe that, unlike our early ancestors, modern people have unique stressors that make our bodies ill equipped for lengthy periods of restriction.

Although it is true that calorie restriction positively affects biomarkers of longevity, it is unlikely that most people would be willing or able to adopt a severe calorie-restriction diet. That's why many health professionals are eager to find a "therapeutic intervention" that will produce the same health and longevity effects of calorie restriction without compromising reasonable food intake. Let's look at some of the drawbacks to severe calorie restriction, and how Body Ecology has discovered that optimal therapeutic intervention researchers have been searching for.

1. Calorie Restriction Comes from a Place of Lack and Deprivation

Restricting, fasting, and weight-loss dieting all stem from a place of shortage and self-denial. Chapter 2 talked about how many of us perceive our lives in terms of what we don't have instead of in terms of what we do. Anything that comes from a place of lack has an energy-lowering impact on mind, body, and spirit, making us overcompensate in self-destructive ways.

Long before the Washington University study mentioned in the previous section, a study conducted in the 1950s took 36 healthy, psychologically normal men and restricted their caloric intake by 50 percent for six months. (Keep in mind that this is a smaller cut in calories than the two-thirds reduction used in the calorie-restriction studies on rodents.)

The University of Minnesota study followed the men for three months of normal eating and six months of eating a calorie-restricted diet. Participants lost approximately 25 percent of their former weight. They were then followed for another three months while they resumed their normal caloric intake.

During the six months of "semi-starvation," as it was called, the men became preoccupied with food—thinking, talking, and dreaming about it; and playing with what was on their plate. They even smuggled food out of their rooms so they could take their time eating on their own after group meals.

Coffee and tea consumption increased dramatically, and many of the men admitted to episodes of binge eating, followed by extreme guilt.

Once their normal diets were resumed, it took time for the men to get back to where they had been before the study. Some of them reported a continuous preoccupation with food, including binging and other behaviors associated with eating disorders.[5]

Here we are back to the emotional side of eating again. We can see how when this activity comes from a place of deprivation or unfulfilled cravings, it can have a detrimental effect on how we look at food, and even alter our behavior and mood. As early as 1995, a Johns Hopkins study reported that food restriction was the number one cause of depression and was an unsafe way to lose weight.[6]

2. Calorie Restriction Emphasizes Quantity Rather Than Quality

Many of us define ourselves by our chronological age. We become obsessed with numbers, and we may lie about how old we are. Calories are numbers as well, and we may begin to define our health and our eating habits based on what these figures are saying to us. If you are a calorie counter, do you feel as if your day was good or bad depending on how many calories you consumed? That's no way to live!

A calorie (the amount of heat it takes to raise the temperature of water) is the measure of energy that scientists created as a guideline for determining how much to eat. But counting calories (energy) doesn't tell you how much fuel actually reaches your cells to produce cellular energy.

In fact, you could be eating a *greater amount* of food and still be thin, as long as the foods you're eating are nutritious and well digested. By the same token, you could lower your calorie intake, but if you aren't eating nourishing foods, you could be malnourished.

An excellent example of this is the people of Okinawa, an archipelago southwest of the main island of Japan. Okinawans appear to be the largest and healthiest population of centenarians on Earth. They suffer significantly fewer heart attacks and have an 80 percent lower incidence of breast and prostate cancer. Their rate of diabetes is also lower, and they have far fewer cases of ovarian and colon cancer.

What is their secret? A calorically low, nutrient-dense diet. Okinawans eat fewer calories, but they also eat more food! They consume many vegetables, some of the least calorically dense foods you can eat. Fruits, whole grains, and lean proteins are also calorically low. By contrast, Okinawans avoid caloric-dense foods, such as fatty proteins, oils, and sugars.[7]

The quality of what you eat, the way it is prepared and combined with other foods, and the critical manner in which you digest and assimilate it determine the *quantity* of nutrients that nourish your cells. *A calorie is not a true measure of nourishment!*

3. Calorie Restriction Doesn't Allow for Unique Modern-Day Stresses

By now, most of us Baby Boomers are not healthy enough for extreme calorie reduction or fasting. Poor digestion, infections, toxins, and a high-stress lifestyle have made us too weak to bounce back from periods of food deprivation. Although Body Ecology promotes the idea that eating smaller portions is best (see Chapter 13: The 80/20 Principle), most people are so nutritionally depleted at the cellular level that they would need to *rebuild their bodies first* if they tried to practice true calorie restriction.

For example, the adrenals and thyroid, very small organs responsible for producing the energy in your body, have to be fed and nourished well. Fasting and calorie restriction can have a weakening effect on them. As you get older, you're already experiencing loss of muscle, lean body weight, and bone density, which fasting and calorie restriction can further compromise.

In addition, studies show that people who repeatedly engage in crash diets or yo-yo dieting also radically alter their metabolism, which hinders rather than helps weight loss. This is because over time their bodies become very efficient at conserving calories and storing them as fat. Frequent fluctuations in weight also increase the risk of hypertension and endometrial cancer, and can lead to a preponderance of body fat in the upper body.[8]

4. Calorie Restriction Is Joyless, Aggravating, and Doomed to Fail!

Many people have come to the conclusion that calorie-restriction diets don't work, simply because they are too difficult to maintain over the long term. Dieting also has psychological consequences; and people will often become weak, irritable, and even depressed from chronic food deprivation. In their attempt to restrict calories, some will end up feeling emotionally and socially starved as well, which can create an entirely different category of health issues.

In her excellent book *The Mood Cure*, Julia Ross warns: "The short-term nutrient losses sustained in a diet can easily add up to long-term mood deficits. Dieting, fasting, restricting—all have indelible effects on your brain. There is no such thing as a 'successful' low-calorie diet: dieting starves and literally shrinks your brain." Besides throwing off your blood sugar, restricting food intake also inhibits serotonin and thyroid hormones, causing depression.[9]

Wouldn't it be a lot easier if we could reverse the aging process simply by eating the right foods in the right way?

The Body Ecology Way—
Creating the Energy of Abundance

At Body Ecology we view the theory of calorie counting as unnecessary, unsound, and passé. Clearly the whole idea of measuring our daily intake of food is flawed. Let's say you want to limit your calories to 1,000 per day, so you consume one hamburger, one doughnut, and one slice of turkey. Is that enough? You're reaching your maximum calorie intake, but you haven't come close to covering all the nutritional bases.

Instead of calorie counting, it's far more important for you to evaluate the potential a food has to support your daily physical and mental needs. You must choose foods with the greatest vitality and potential for creating and sustaining life. And now, with your new goal to rejuvenate and reclaim the vitality of your youth, a new way of assigning value to your food choices has never been more critical.

It is better to focus instead on eating smaller amounts of very high-quality foods that are nourishing and that leave you satisfied and fulfilled. This is especially important so that your adrenals and thyroid are fed well, because they must provide you with a constant supply of energy to fuel you throughout the day. Remember, one of the goals of the Baby Boomer Diet is to *restore your constitutional energy.*

Calorie-Count No More

When done correctly—the Body Ecology Way—decreasing your calories is not starvation, but simply a lowering of food intake, while at the same time optimizing nutrition. Like the Okinawan diet, Body Ecology offers you a *calorically low yet nutrient-dense* eating plan—with food choices that are more familiar and readily available to us here in the West.

What's the Secret?

Body Ecology foods are so satisfying, rich, and nourishing that you simply won't want or need as much. While you may eat less, the foods you do eat, such as fermented vegetables, are highly nourishing to every cell in your body. This means that they are properly digested; assimilated; and distributed to cells that remain healthy, active, clean, and pure. In fact, the friendly bacteria in these foods even communicate with each other to ensure they are creating the specific nutrients that your body needs.

As you focus on building your inner ecology, you may find that you reconnect with nature—a key goal of the Body Ecology system of health and healing. You may discover that you become aware of a rhythm to your physical self, just as there is a rhythm in nature. Getting to know your body's signals allows you to tap into your own optimal energy—and align it with the energy that exists in nature. Over time, you will find that you are, in essence, following the principles of calorie restriction because you will need less food to meet your nutritional needs. Instead of feeling deprived, you will be pleasantly surprised to feel *satisfied*—even enjoying a light feeling you may have been missing from your life.

As you follow the Body Ecology Way, you may find that you no longer struggle to determine whether your hunger is emotional or physical, because the foods nourish you on *all levels*. The more you learn to separate emotional from physical hunger—and the more you learn how to nourish your mind, body, and spirit—the less you'll fall back on your former cravings. You'll discover that what you want to eat gradually changes. In fact, your taste buds will begin to change. You'll find that you can actually taste and savor foods properly when they are not masked by sugar, bad oils, and lackluster ingredients.

We can move from counting calories and counting years on the planet to feeling grounded in our health and well-being.

As you will discover in the next chapter, what is most revolutionary about the Body Ecology approach is the way it lays down a "unified theory" of health that no other diet attempts to do. It does so because it embraces the true secret to health and longevity that lies hidden deep within us—a miraculous internal ecosystem that mimics the world around us.

From the Physician's Desk

"To be maximally healthy, happy, and functional, you need to find a balance. You need to honor your own individuality."

*T*he problem I see with many strict calorie-restriction programs is that they are used solely to lose weight. This is an unhealthy approach, because many people who practice calorie restriction aren't exercising. They're not using their hearts, lungs, and muscles actively, so they become targets for tissue breakdown.

Yes, you can certainly lose fat with calorie restriction, but you can also lose strength, aerobic capacity, muscle, endurance, and other important indicators of health. And many people who practice calorie restriction also don't eat properly. So they may be eating less, but what they *are* eating is not optimally nutritious. It's all a question of balance.

It's very true that the biomarkers of aging decrease with calorie restriction. This is because when you stop eating, *sirtuins* (enzymes connected with genes that affect cellular metabolism) will begin to down-regulate (that is, decrease the activity of) the genes that promote inflammation. Calorie restriction lowers from 153 to 144 the number of genes that have been activated by eating too much of the wrong food.

However, if you combine intelligent exercise with moderate restriction of calories, along with optimal nutrition, you will probably come out with biomarkers that are better than those you might get if practicing calorie restriction alone. To be maximally healthy, happy, and functional, you need to find a balance. You need to honor your own individuality.

If your latest medical exam shows elevated LDL (bad cholesterol), triglycerides, blood sugar, and insulin, along with decreased levels of HDL (good cholesterol), this is an indication that your genes are in storage mode, because your body is perceiving itself as being stressed. Your ratios are off, and the game has become one of "storing for the fight for survival that is coming."

Exercise builds skeletal muscle, and this is integral to health, especially as we age. Skeletal muscle is very metabolically active. When we have good muscle mass, the sugar we eat goes directly into the muscles to be used for fuel, instead of turning into fat. In addition, when we exercise, enzymes that break down fat for fuel are released from our muscles into the blood. Lean muscle mass also helps protect us from inflammation and keeps our energy levels high. We were meant to have strong muscles as humans, and to be able to use them . . . *simply a healthier way to live.*

The traditional body mass index that many people use as their guide can be misleading. A person could be obese because he has too much fat *relative* to his muscle. But because he is tall and slim, he might not know it and think he's safe. That's why bioelectrical impedance analysis (BIA) is a much more accurate measurement of body composition and health.

BIA simply involves placing a pad and a wire on your forearm and ankle for a few seconds to measure tissue resistance, which is then picked up as an electrical signal (you can now also get a basic BIA device in bathroom scales). From this the BIA extrapolates interesting information related to lean body mass (which includes bones, organs, and muscles; and is ideally a higher number), as well as fat mass (which should be a lower number). It also measures total body water, along with intra- and extracellular water. Whether you're training for a marathon or just starting on the Body Ecology program, measuring the lean mass/fat ratio and the ratios of hydration allows you to see how diet and lifestyle changes are affecting your body composition, which is far more important than monitoring weight loss.

Why is this so important to Baby Boomers? Because as we age, we confront a condition called *sarcopenia*—the degenerative loss of skeletal muscle mass. From the Greek, meaning "poverty of flesh," sarcopenia is most common among the elderly, but it can be true of anyone with too much body fat and not enough lean muscle mass. Such a person is effectively "malnourished." As we age, most of our hormone levels decrease. We have lower growth hormone, testosterone, DHEAS, and melatonin. Poor sleep, malnutrition, and immune imbalances create a chronic low-grade systemic inflammation that causes chronic increase in cortisol. Increased cortisol further weakens immunity, lowers thyroid function, and breaks down skeletal muscle to raise blood sugar, which increases insulin and promotes further fat storage, which then completes the vicious cycle by promoting more inflammation! Sadly, if we don't maintain enough skeletal muscle, sugar is very easily converted into fat.

A study from the UCLA School of Medicine showed that 28 out of 30 premenopausal women who were at an increased risk of breast cancer had "sarcopenic obesity," or the "too much fat, not enough muscle" syndrome. It is interesting that these women had a normal body mass index, which means they did not appear overweight based on their height-to-weight ratio. So how one looks or what one weighs may not be as important as body composition. Remember, fat leads to inflammation, which in turn leads to all kinds of problems, including cancer.[i]

In the elderly it has been shown that sarcopenia can be reversed by supplementing the diet with the nine essential amino acids: *isoleucine, leucine, valine, lysine, methionine, phenylalanine, threonine, trytophan,* and *histidine.* Dr. Robert Wolf and his team at the University of Texas–Galveston found that adding essential amino acids to the diet was needed to rebuild protein and muscle and help restore normal function.[ii]

In the past, there were two topics of conversation we were told to avoid in polite conversation—religion and politics. Now we can add a third—*diet*—because it generates so much heated controversy today, and there are so many options. People who are focused and passionate can derive benefits from many different diet programs . . . *for a period of time.* But the question is: "How long will it last?"

What is most important is to start with a solid foundation, not a quick-fix weight-loss program. Body Ecology is a good foundational starting point for most people. I have often told patients that they are an "experiment of one." Be honest with yourself, and let your long-term results be your guide.

— *Leonard Smith, M.D.*

---

[i]D. Heber, S. Ingles, J. M. Ashley, M. H. Maxwell, R. F. Lyons, and R. M. Elashoff, "Clinical detection of sarcopenic obesity by bioelectrical impedance analysis," *American Journal of Clinical Nutrition* 64 (1996): 472S–477S.

[ii]E. Volpi, H. Kobayashi, M. Sheffield-Moore, B. Mittendorfer, and R. R. Wolfe, "Essential amino acids are primarily responsible for the amino acid stimulation of muscle protein anabolism in healthy elderly adults," *American Journal of Clinical Nutrition* 78 (2003): 250–258.

Chapter 6

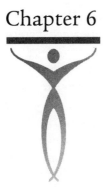

The Missing Piece: A Healthy Inner Ecosystem

Within each of us is a miraculous inner ecosystem. Most of us are ignorant of its existence at all, yet it is essential to our health, immunity, and longevity.

A Return to the Garden

We've explored the vast reaches of space; the dark depths of the ocean; the intricate workings of the brain; and even the beautiful, once-invisible, world of the womb. There is, however, a microscopic universe within our own bodies that has, until now, been largely uncharted and unknown. It is the last, perhaps *greatest, frontier.* At Body Ecology, we call this unexplored secret world the "Missing Piece"—the single most important building block for health, immunity, and, certainly, longevity.

This Missing Piece is our inner ecosystem . . . the intestinal garden that must be established deep inside us as we leave the womb. Visible only with a microscope, it is our delicate inner world, and it requires perfect balance and harmony for us to flourish.

As the term *inner ecosystem* is largely unknown, I've created a definition that describes the ideal, healthy inner ecosystem we should all strive to attain:

A healthy inner ecosystem is a dynamic "garden" of beneficial and neutral bacteria and yeast called microflora. They live and associate with their environment (your intestines), creating a vibrant interrelating community. These energetic microflora are surrounded by your enteric nervous system or "gut brain" (sometimes called your second brain); and are related to the transfer of energy and materials into your nervous system, your brain, and the rest of your body.

The inner ecosystem is so vital to your well-being that as you continue to read this book, you might soon be asking yourself, "Have I overlooked the importance of my own inner garden?"

The word *garden* originates from an old German term, *gart,* meaning "enclosure." A garden can be as simple as a pot of herbs in your kitchen, or it could be as vast as the rain forest in South America, rumored to be an ancient garden from another era. For many, the garden is a sacred space—a place of spiritual connections.

An ancient Chinese proverb says: "If you want to be *happy* all your life, plant a garden." But I'd like to add: "If you want to be *healthy* all your life and *live a longer one,* cultivate and fertilize your sacred inner garden."

Body Ecology believes that the garden inside us should also be lovingly tended and respected as sacred. With careful husbandry, it will protect us from dangerous diseases and the physical effects of aging.

Nature's Secrets Revealed

Humans, fish, birds, and even insects—in fact, all living animals—have an *inner ecosystem in their intestines.*

Unlike plants, which are rooted firmly in soil, animals are in constant movement. We do not stay in one place and, therefore, must carry our "soil" inside our own bodies. A tree acquires its nutrients from the soil in which it was planted, but we humans carry ours around with us *in our gut.* If that precious soil is depleted and stressed, we may develop the human equivalent of root rot, fungal infections, spotty leaves, and so forth. Or we may just fail to thrive and prematurely die.

When you were in the womb, if your mother ate a nutritious diet rich in fermented foods, and if she had strong constitutional *jing* energy, you would have been well nourished during your growth and development. Beneficial microflora would have naturally colonized *in your mother's digestive tract* and *in her birth canal* so that when you entered the world, your own pristine intestines would be *immunized* with the "good little bugs." You would now be able to safely eat and digest your next food: mother's milk.

The natural sugars found in your mother's breast milk would soon stimulate the growth of these indispensable microflora, and in just a few months, this thriving inner world of beneficial beings would be working together to protect and support you so that you could live safely in the outer world once you were born. These microflora would help your body digest nutrients; neutralize toxins; metabolize vitamins; balance hormones; and keep pathogens such as fungi, yeast, and parasites in check.

Sadly, since this was an unheard-of phenomenon (and mostly still is), many of us were deprived of this sound foundation. In fact, by the time Baby Boomers came along, breast-feeding had fallen out of favor. Few people understood the life-giving properties of mother's milk. Breast-feeding was considered inconvenient—even embarrassing—and many fathers were uncomfortable with it.

Paradise Lost

Some of us Baby Boomers may have been fortunate enough to have very enlightened parents who understood the importance of creating a toxin-free, nutrient-rich environment within the womb. But most of us were not that lucky. The wonderful prenatal energy that should be the rightful inheritance of every child was denied us—and now our children and grandchildren.

Before birth, we should have been inoculated with healthy bacteria in the birth canal so that when we emerged from the womb, we would have quickly developed a strong, hardy immune system that would allow us to live in a world that contained pathogenic microbes. We would have also digested our foods properly and have healthy intestines, blood, and cells. We would not crave refined, sugary foods and would be satisfied with the natural sweetness in fruits and vegetables.

Body Ecology views the inner and outer ecosystems as parallel. We all know what happens to the atmosphere, to our water supply, and to our food when environmental pollutants are not kept in check. Our planet becomes inflamed, fatigued, and congested. In the same way, without beneficial microflora present in our inner world we are literally walking about with polluted bodies that *cannot* detoxify, in spite of our best efforts.

Let's return to our soil metaphor . . . fertile soil is *living* soil, containing billions of microorganisms. Baby Boomers may have no memory of a time when all farmers practiced ecological farming—planting different crops every year and rotating them so that the balance in the soil was preserved. Instead of using chemical fertilizers, these "eco-farmers" enriched their fields with manure, putting organic matter back into the soil to reenter the ecological cycle.

Today, farming is controlled mostly by the petrochemical industry, which has had a disastrous effect on the quality of our food and our health. Fritjof Capra, author of the famous book *The Turning Point*, refers to synthetic fertilization as "agricultural chemotherapy," which depletes the humus content in the soil and affects a crop's ability to take up and absorb nutrients.[1] Depleted, overused, and compromised with fertilizers and pesticides, this dry, "dead" soil is more susceptible to wind and water erosion and produces food that has a fraction of the nutritional value it is supposed to have. You cannot expect healthy food to come from wasted ground. In the same way, you cannot expect to enjoy radiant health when your own internal "biological terrain" is weak, stressed, and defenseless.

These parallels between our outer and inner ecosystems are fascinating. When a patch of soil becomes degraded and empty, it has lost the microorganisms that give it life. Earthworms, fungi, bacteria, ants, millipedes, and termites are veritable "ecosystem engineers" that drive soil fertility and support plant health and reproduction. They ward off insect pests and protect plants against invasive kinds of bacterial species. Even the most contaminated forms of soils—those polluted with dangerous materials such as heavy metals, oil, and gases—can be "disarmed" by the introduction of beneficial microorganisms. Some kinds of bacteria can actually break down organic pollutants and turn them into carbon dioxide and water.[2]

Similarly, by replenishing our own inner gardens—the complex and dynamic ecosystems inside our guts—we create an environment that sustains us, driving our health and protecting against disease and the typical assaults of aging.

Paradise Regained—
Finding Our Youthful Secret Garden

I have often wondered why the secret—the "Missing Piece"—has remained hidden from us for so long. I've come to believe that we have finally advanced far enough in our spiritual awareness that we are now asking the right questions of our Creator . . . and receiving the answers. We have recognized the great achievements of modern medicine, but we've also seen its limitations. More and more of us are realizing that all of the state-of-the-art medical advances and technologies in the world will avail us nothing if we've lost our connection with the earth that sustains us. The Missing Piece asks us to reestablish this vital connection, intended for us at conception, but now seemingly lost.

When you build your Body Ecology, you are creating a living, thriving inner ecosystem that supports your health—doing all the work of creating energy and longevity on the inside of your body. Wouldn't it be ironic if the legendary "Fountain of Youth" was not a source of water at all, but rather a "secret inner garden" that holds the answers to life, longevity, and youthfulness? While water is certainly essential for life and longevity, perhaps igniting our digestive *fire* is just as important.

In a previous chapter, you learned how *shen, jing,* and *chi* are critical to health, and how the latter in particular is related to what we take into our bodies. Chi is dependent upon what Taoists call "digestive fire," the ability of the stomach and spleen to "ripen" food, transform it, and turn it into energy. Many foods in the standard American diet, with its emphasis on processed sugars and flours, "dampen" and slow down this digestive fire.

As you will soon discover, the Body Ecology approach encourages balanced but diverse methods of food preparation—

from lightly steaming and low-heat stir-frying to raw techniques and fermenting. These, and the powerhouse foods themselves, will ignite your digestive fire, not only delivering more nutrients, but also making them more "bioavailable" (accessed and used more effectively). And, unlike any other way of eating you may have tried before now, the Body Ecology Way of Life honors and helps create your amazing inner garden, bringing life, vitality, and youthfulness back into the power center of your body—your intestines.

Louis Pasteur's Legacy

More than 100 years ago, Louis Pasteur, a French micro-biologist, proposed a new theory of disease called the "germ theory." It continues to exert a powerful influence on medicine to this day. Peering through his microscope at a sample of spoiled wine, Pasteur observed a colony of active "little unseen bodies" (germs), and determined that if the growth of these germs, or what he called *microorganisms*, were the cause of the spoiled wine, they could just as well be the cause of contagious disease. In Pasteur's mind, these microorganisms were "bad," and it was necessary to prevent them from entering the body.

Pasteur's ideas about germs were partly true. We know that bad, or unfriendly, bacteria and viruses feed and multiply, causing the body to become susceptible to infection, fatigue, and degenerative disease. Pasteur's work led to the development of antiseptic surgical methods that ultimately saved countless lives—in fact, one in three women died in childbirth until doctors began washing their hands before delivering babies.

Pasteur's efforts and discoveries were truly revolutionary, but they were also myopic. He noticed that the little bugs inside the wine were easily destroyed when the wine was heated. From that point on, medicine took on a troubling bias—that disease was caused by outside, invading forces that made victims of us all. It was this largely fear-based germ theory that also led to pasteurization; mass immunization; and, eventually, the discovery of antibiotics.[3]

Working against nature rather than with it has led to the present state of affairs in medicine today. In fact, Pasteur stated in his acceptance speech to the French Academy of Sciences that the experimenter is one who tries continually to conquer nature.[4] Pasteur had a very limited understanding

Here are just a few of the many reasons why beneficial microflora must be present in the gut for us to be healthy:

- **Beneficial microflora ensure that we are well nourished,** and help eliminate nutritional deficiencies that cause our bodies to fail and age quickly.

- **Beneficial microflora assist in the breakdown of foods.** By acting as enzymes, these bacteria support the digestive process.

- **Beneficial microflora produce vitamins.** Vitamins such as B and K are produced deep down inside of us, where they can enter immediately into the body.

- **Beneficial microflora help extract and retain minerals from our foods.**

- **Beneficial microflora prevent toxins from causing damage to the intestinal lining.** This damage leads to disorders such as irritable bowel syndrome, Crohn's disease, and colitis.

- **Beneficial microflora protect us against colon cancer.** Ingestion of viable probiotics and prebiotics—food that nourishes beneficial bacteria (see Chapter 15)—is associated with anticarcinogenic effects, one mechanism of which is the detoxification of genotoxins (agents that damage DNA) in the gut.

- **Beneficial microflora are essential for immunity.** The mechanisms by which probiotic bacteria affect the immune system are not yet fully known, but many microflora are correlated with an increase in the innate or acquired immune response. In fact, 70 to 80 percent of our immune system is located in the gut, where microflora are critical for protection against disease.

of one of the most important universal laws of nature—the *Principle of Balance*. Indeed, we live in a world of opposites. As was mentioned earlier, there is a positive and negative side to everything, including bacteria. Pasteur left out a vital part of the truth.

A hundred years later we are suffering from this one-sided view of nature. Sadly, we have created an entire system of healing called "modern medicine," which is not a system of healing at all. It is a disease-management system based on fear and focused on killing "bad bugs," viruses, and cancer cells with drugs, surgery, and radiation. Modern medicine, with its emphasis on killing and cutting, has taken many lives it might have saved. Iatrogenic disease (a health threat caused by doctors and medicines) is up there within the top ten causes of death in the U.S. According to a study of 37 million patient records by HealthGrades, a health-care quality-assessment company, an average of 195,000 people in the U.S. died due to potentially preventable, in-hospital medical errors in each of the years 2000, 2001, and 2002.[5]

If you focus on the positive, creating a world inside your body of cooperative, constructive, and supporting beneficial microflora, then health, happiness, and longevity will follow.

To a great degree, Pasteur's discoveries led to as many problems as they solved. If only he had noted that the superb wines of France contained beneficial bacteria and yeast, as did sourdough breads, cheeses, and sour-milk products (kefir and yogurt)—and if only he had promoted the benefits of an environment where the good bugs not only ruled but also destroyed the bad bugs—we might be living in a very different world today.

Another Side to the Story

Pasteur's colleagues at the time argued that the *environment* of the blood surrounding the cells was the cause of disease—not the bugs. They believed that something in the environment of the wine allowed the bad bugs to flourish. They were adamant that something happening within the body and blood was allowing pathogenic bacteria, viruses, fungi, and cancer cells to grow. As you will soon learn when you read about the *Principle of Acid and Alkaline* in Chapter 12, Pasteur's colleagues were correct.

A century later, we are beginning to see the negative consequences of Pasteur's "all or nothing" approach to bacteria. Pasteur believed that a healthy body had no bacteria in it.[6] In our society we've been taught to be afraid of bacteria. Bacteria mean "germs." It is a nasty word to many of us, evoking the source of disease and sickness. In truth, however, we live in a world where good and bad exist together, and this is certainly the case in the amazing world of microflora.

In his zeal to eliminate pathogenic bacteria from the world, Pasteur made an unfortunate mistake. His method of pasteurization, developed to prevent milk from spoiling, also prevents it from fermenting into "clabbered" milk (milk that sours and thickens naturally). Because it ferments naturally, clabbered milk contains a much higher number of healthy microflora and is far better for you than just raw milk. Pasteurization, by contrast, robs milk of some of its most life-giving nutrients and destroys naturally occurring friendly flora that cause it to safely ferment.

Why did this mistake occur? Why were people not allowed to know the complete truth? Perhaps it was simply a matter of timing. Perhaps we could not appreciate truth until we had made a devastating blunder first. We humans do tend to learn best from our own mistakes. By experimenting with killing, cutting, and radiating our way to health, we are now ready for another, wiser path to wellness.

In a nutshell: *If you focus on the positive, creating a world inside your body of cooperative, constructive, and supporting beneficial microflora, then health, happiness, and longevity will follow.*

A Closer Look at Microflora—
Warriors on the Intestinal Battlefield

It is certainly true that disease begins in our intestines, but health begins there, too. It is true that bad little bugs can infect and harm us, but good little bugs can protect us and keep us strong and healthy. Pasteur's work, although critically important, came from a place of fear and alarm. It served its purpose in its time. But we are in a different time now, and we must adapt what we know to create a new system of health and healing.

Medical science's 100-year error has provided us with a counterpoint—a unique perspective on what we want and what we do not want. Now our thoughts and intentions can reach out for a better way. Body Ecology offers that "Missing Piece" that Pasteur and the rest of the world weren't allowed to see—a radical (but long-overdue) way of looking at beneficial microflora, the foods that contain them, and the role they play in our digestive tracts and in keeping us young and healthy.

The next chapter will explore how new technologies are giving us exciting insights into the prenatal universe . . . the wisdom of the womb is unfolding before our very eyes! I find it particularly appropriate that as we learn more and more about the magical world of the womb, the mystery of the inner ecosystem is also coming to light. It, too, is a secret hidden *deep inside each of us* where we cannot see it. It is a secret that means the difference between surviving and *thriving*. It is the key to unlocking a longer, healthier, and happier life.

From the Physician's Desk

"All diseases lead to the gastrointestinal tract."

*J*ulius Caesar famously said, "All roads lead to Rome." When it comes to disease, one might say, "All diseases lead to the gastrointestinal tract." This would appear to be the case, as so many medical conditions we see today are largely due to the fact that poor-quality food—which is not digested properly—is sending the wrong information to the intestinal lining, which results in inflammation and increased intestinal permeability. Thus the "leaky gut" allows for more absorption of unwanted food substances, microbial toxins, and bacteria themselves . . . all of which cause the immune system to become imbalanced.

When this happens, your immune cells may produce antibodies affecting different body parts such as the joints and pancreas, which contribute to arthritis and type 1 autoimmune diabetes—and many other conditions as well. The medical term for this is *antigen mimicry,* where antibodies that are being made against food and toxins "cross-react," and then attack normal human tissues. This is just one of many mechanisms whereby damage to the gut lining, with increased permeability, may lead to systemic diseases.

That's why it is important to include probiotics and cultured foods in our diets on a regular basis. As we Baby Boomers get older, we have less and less beneficial bacteria to work with. We begin to have problems such as irritable bowel syndrome (IBS), which is often the result of low-grade bacterial infections that we never quite got over. A study published in the *American Journal of Gastroenterology* discovered an association between abnormal lactulose breath test (LBT) findings and IBS. Researchers estimated the bacteria levels in IBS patients by having them breathe into a bag to measure the gases produced by the bacteria. The study showed that IBS patients had an overgrowth of bacteria in the colon and small intestine. Treated with a nonabsorbable antibiotic, *neomycin,* a high percentage of them quickly got better.[i] Another study showed that by simply removing sugar and animal fat—foods of choice for bad bacteria—from their diets, a high percentage

75

of patients with inflammatory bowel disease (Crohn's or ulcerative colitis) became considerably less symptomatic.[ii]

What's more, a recent study published in the *British Medical Journal* showed that consumption of a readily available probiotic fermented drink containing *Lactobacillus casei, Lactobacillus bulgaricus,* and *Streptococcus thermophilus* twice daily during a course of antibiotics and for one week afterward, reduced the incidence of diarrhea. In addition, the incidence of *C. difficile* (a deadly virulent bacteria) diarrhea was also reduced. The study concluded that use of this type of probiotic had the potential to decrease morbidity and should be used routinely in patients over 50 who were being treated with antibiotics.[iii]

The potential health applications of the Body Ecology program are endless. Some physicians are already using Body Ecology trainers to educate and counsel their patients on diet and food choices. This program can address many of the atopic diseases of childhood, such as allergies, asthma, autism, autoimmune diabetes, and dermatitis. In adults, Body Ecology will be helpful in a wide range of medical conditions, including obesity, metabolic syndrome, diabetes, cardiovascular disease, autoimmune disorders, cancer, neurodegenerative disorders, and more.

Here is one of many ways the Body Ecology program works: The diet includes foods that contain high levels of both soluble and insoluble fiber, as well as fermented foods and drinks. These fermented products are rich in beneficial bacteria (also known as probiotics). When the fiber and bacteria reach the colon, the bacteria spread out and cover the insoluble fiber and eat the soluble fiber, producing short-chain fatty acids (SCFA) in the process. The most notable SCFA is butyrate or butyric acid, which is taken up by the colonic cells and is their major source of nutrition. When well fed by the butyrate, the colon is able to do a good job in water and electrolyte absorption, plus barrier protection from toxins and microbes in the stool, all of which are crucial for good health. In addition, the butyrate feeds information to the cell that helps control inflammation, polyps, and cancer. The World Health Organization has recommended between 20 and 40 grams of fiber daily to maintain optimal health. Sadly, most Americans are lucky if they get in 20 grams of fiber.

More and more, science bears out the overlooked importance of the inner ecosystem. More recently, research is showing a link between obesity and bacteria, known as "infectobesity." This is a new term for the theory that some people who are obese may actually have combinations of bacteria and viruses that cause an immune imbalance, which can lead to greater weight gain and fat storage.

Recent studies have shown that in rats or humans, being placed on a high-fat, high-sugar diet causes increased release and absorption of a bacterial cell-wall toxin known as lipopolysaccaride (LPS). The LPS is absorbed through the intestinal lining, goes into the vascular system, and creates arterial stiffness and endothelial dysfunction (which promotes atherosclerosis). In addition, ongoing inflammation and insulin resistance contribute to further fat storage, which leads to more inflammation. In the rats on this diet, it was discovered that they began to develop fatty livers, with elevated triglycerides and increased markers of inflammation, including TNF-alpha, IL-1, and IL-6, as well as increased risk of type 2 diabetes.

Donna often speaks of beneficial bacteria as "warriors," which dominate the intestinal lining and promote a healthy balance in the gut immune system . . . *and they really do.* These beneficial bacteria communicate directly with the intestinal-lining lymphocytes (white blood cells) and indirectly with the immune cells in the intestinal wall. Through this communication, a balance is established that keeps the immune system flexible in knowing when and when not to attack or react to bacteria or partially digested food. When this balance is not achieved, there can be many problems, ranging from food allergies and IBS to serious recurrent infections—not only of the gut, but of other parts of the body, including the lungs and throat.

What we are seeing today with many children who have chronic colds, viral pneumonias, earaches, swollen tonsils, asthma, multiple food allergies, and autoimmune diabetes is that their immune systems do not have the proper balance and are over- or underreacting. It requires a healthy diet, like Body Ecology, to develop and maintain a flexible and balanced immune system.

I believe we will continue to see new clinical syndromes that will further support the need for Body Ecology and healthy, balanced microflora (Donna's "Missing Piece"), and this will begin to transform health care as we know it.

The Latest Breakthrough in Intestinal Health

Soon we may be integrating beneficial parasites, as well as beneficial bacteria, into our diets. Maybe we will call them proparasitics rather than probiotics. Studies are showing that certain kinds of parasites help alleviate conditions of the intestinal tract. A study conducted by Joel Weinstock, professor of medicine and immunology at Tufts University, showed that the larvae from the porcine whipworm assist in reprogramming the gut lining to down-regulate immune responses. Patients with Crohn's disease and ulcerative colitis who used this parasite have gone into remission.

Dr. Weinstock wrote: "In less developed countries, 100% of children have worms in their gastrointestinal tract. Helminths' [parasitic worms] effects on the immune system are longlasting, with changes detectable a decade after the worms have been removed. You can argue that it's our [industrialized] immune systems that are deviant."[iv]

It has been shown in children from Brazil that they had healthy levels of both the T_h1 and T_h2 cytokines (immune-cell signaling molecules), but most interesting was the discovery that they also had high-normal levels of T_h3 cytokines (known for their regulatory balancing effect). These children were all found to have low-grade parasitic infections, but did not have the usual childhood allergies, asthma, or diabetes. When they were treated for their parasites and were cleared of the parasitic infection, allergies began to develop for the first time!

This is a powerful example of ecological balance in the gut having widespread effects in the body. On the other hand, uncontrolled parasitic infections in anyone can create serious medical problems. So like all things, it is a question of balance. It appears that Dr. Weinstock and his associates have found that balance using the *Trichuris suis* (pig whipworm), as it does not stay and develop harmful long-term problems in humans. This type of "controlled" parasitic infection has also been shown to be beneficial with autism (see **autismtso.com**) and systemic autoimmune illnesses, like sarcoidosis.

This is a very new field of study that I believe provides more insight into the nature of our complex, healthy inner ecosystem.

— Leonard Smith, M.D.

[i]M. Pimentel, E. J. Chow, and H. C. Lin, "Normalization of Lactulose Breath Testing Correlates With Symptom Improvement in Irritable Bowel Syndrome: A Double-Blind, Randomized, Placebo-Controlled Study," *American Journal of Gastroenterology*, 98 (2003): 412–419.

[ii]S. Reif, I. Klein, F. Lubin, M. Farbstein, A. Hallak, and T. Gilat, "Pre-illness dietary factors in inflammatory bowel disease," *Gut*, 40 (1997): 754–760.

[iii]M. Hickson, A. L. D'Souza, N. Muthu, T. R. Rogers, S. Want, C. Rajkumar, and C. J. Bulpitt, "Use of probiotic Lactobacillus preparation to prevent diarrhoea associated with antibiotics: randomized double blind placebo controlled trial," *British Medical Journal*, 335 (June 29, 2007): 80.

[iv]K. Harby, "Pig Whipworm Ova Found Active in Crohn's Disease and Ulcerative Colitis," *Medscape Medical News*, May 19, 2004, **http:// www.medscape.com/viewarticle/478342** (accessed 11/19/09).

Chapter 7

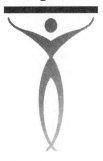

That Gut Feeling: Learning the Lessons of the Womb

What has happened to most of us—and our fatigued and lifeless inner ecosystems—is quite literally a gut-wrenching experience. Without a healthy body ecology, we simply cannot thrive.

For as long as we humans have existed, the inner workings of the womb and the miracle of birth have been shrouded in mystery, superstition, and old wives' tales. The universe inside the womb—like the moon, sun, and stars above us—was obscure and unfathomable. Today, 4-D ultrasound technology allows us a rare glimpse into this remarkable enclosed garden and what takes place there.

We now know that the womb is not a self-contained holding cell where the fetus simply "hangs out" until birth. Instead, it is a highly intricate, fragile, and dynamic environment where every minute of every day, some new piece of the developmental puzzle falls into place. By the time a baby is born, it has tasted, smelled, flexed its muscles, and heard and recognized its mother's voice. Pictures from the womb reveal fetuses smiling, yawning, tugging at their umbilical cords, sticking out their tongues, responding to music, reacting physiologically to their mothers' stress, and using the walls of the uterus as a trampoline to practice their "stepping reflex."

These miraculous glimpses also show us firsthand how the biological and emotional interplay between mother and unborn child is critical, not just to the baby's survival, but to its future vitality and longevity. From as early as day 15 after conception, we observe this vital connection at work, as the tiny embryo begins to develop nerve cells and the mother's blood volume increases to compensate for the new life inside. At two months, the placenta becomes the baby's life-support system; and the fetus obtains everything it needs from its mother's bloodstream—water, oxygen, and food. By 18 weeks, its digestive system becomes active, and we see it actually tasting and sipping the amniotic fluid in which it floats.[1]

As these pictures inside the womb clearly demonstrate, what happens during the gestation period plays a dramatically important role in later health. But we also know that the birthing process itself becomes a significant stage in the infant's future vitality and longevity.

What Should Have Happened

During childbirth—and often several days before—the mother's cervix will open slowly. It will dilate approximately ten centimeters—large enough for the still immaturely developed infant to enter the world. When this happens, microflora from the mother's birth canal inoculate the amniotic fluid and begin to coat the body of the emerging fetus, and even to enter the baby's digestive tract.

The inner ecosystem will determine the effectiveness of the baby's future immunological defenses and his or her ability to digest nutrients and remain free of toxins.

Unfortunately, many babies born today are exposed to pathogens from the birth canal, and mothers unsuspectingly pass these on to their newborn children. In fact, millions of childbearing women today will culture positive for yeast (candidiasis), virus (HPV), and bacterial (group B strep) vaginal infections.

In addition, many infants begin life with another disadvantage—they inherit poor prenatal *jing* from their parents (see Chapter 3). This means they will have very little constitutional energy throughout their lives. Weakened adrenals and thyroid are a widespread problem in babies today. Their pathways of detoxification often do not work well because of this inadequate energy, poor peristaltic movement in the intestines, and congested livers.

As many babies are commonly fed formula, these factors are often compounded by a lack of colostrum at birth; colostrum is necessary for building the immune system so that the baby can combat any pathogens in its environment and be able to fight fungal and viral infections inherited from its mother. Because these events occur "invisibly," no one pays much attention to them.

Physicians and nurses are more concerned about how well the mother is doing and if the baby has all its fingers and toes than they are about establishing the unseen world of the baby's inner ecosystem. *Yet it is this inner ecosystem that will determine the effectiveness of the baby's future immunological defenses and his or her ability to digest nutrients and remain free of toxins. In other words, it is integral to quality and length of life.*

Microflora have incredible survival and adaptive power, which allows them to recognize and overcome pathogenic bacteria, transforming themselves to fight and to flourish.

I remember a time when newborns were treated very delicately. Because so many infants and children died from infectious diseases in the generations before us, most mothers understood how very vulnerable the baby was during the first six months of life. Parents didn't allow many visitors; only the immediate family was permitted to hold the newborn, who was kept indoors and protected from exposure to germs and extremes in climate.

Sadly, this is not true today. The first few weeks are a time to "show off" the infant to as many people as possible. I've often seen newborns exposed to extreme temperatures and stresses at shopping malls and friends' homes so that parents won't be inconvenienced and can resume their busy lives. Parents will hold and play with their babies even if they have bad colds and coughs. We've forgotten about the dangers of infection today, because we feel that we have these medical "safeguards" called antibiotics to always protect us. But antibiotics often do as much harm as they do good.

Because a baby's defenses simply aren't in place yet, and its natural abilities to defend itself against toxins are significantly lower or nonexistent, we should be even more vigilant about establishing the inner ecosystem and protecting the baby from environmental threats.

Early vaccination during this time is *dangerous*. In fact, during this time nature is already hard at work to "vaccinate" us with a highly intelligent immune system—one that can resist ever-mutating pathogens.

Microflora . . . They're Not Just Beneficial . . . They're Brilliant

As mentioned in the last chapter, we have been indoctrinated to believe that all bacteria and yeast are harmful and must be destroyed. We don't understand that when nature is in balance, she provides natural defenses—good bacteria and beneficial yeast that destroy the bad.

Because most of us believe that all bacteria are the enemy, we have come to rely on antibiotics to destroy them. But this is rather like throwing out the baby with the bathwater . . . because, in destroying the good bacteria, antibiotics also kill the bacteria that keep us alive. I liken this to "friendly fire" in times of war. We're not just killing the enemy; we're killing our fellow soldiers and comrades on the battlefield.

The other very important thing to remember about beneficial microflora is that *they are highly intelligent*. They have incredible survival and adaptive power, which allows them to recognize and overcome pathogenic bacteria, transforming themselves to fight and to flourish.

Your Gut—the Primal Brain

Have you ever used the expression "I have this gut feeling"? Believe it or not, your gut (also called the enteric nervous system) thinks and communicates in a highly sophisticated and orchestrated manner. It has more than one billion sensory and motor neurons; and it utilizes information-processing circuits (neurotransmitters) such as dopamine, serotonin, nitric oxide, and norepinephrine to transmit and receive messages. In other words, it *communicates.*

We at Body Ecology refer to this enteric nervous system as the "primal brain." The next time you run away from a stressful situation, ask yourself if it was your brain in your head or the primal brain in your gut that got you moving! Nausea, abdominal pain, the urge to vomit, feelings of satiation, butterflies in the stomach, and so on are the gut brain's way of warning us of danger from ingested food, infectious pathogens, or unpleasant stressors.[2]

It makes sense that a highly intelligent gut would have highly intelligent ways of communicating. Scientists now know that in addition to being able to communicate with members of their own species, many bacteria can also "talk" to members of other species using a universal chemical language (see sidebar at the end of the chapter). Individual bacteria secrete signaling molecules called *autoinducers* into their environments, and as the number of bacteria in a colony increases, so does the concentration of the signaling molecules. Once a critical mass—or *quorum*—of bacteria and autoinducers is reached, specific behaviors can be initiated. This process in the gut is called *quorum sensing,* and it allows bacteria to coordinate their behavior on a global scale and to act like enormous multicellular organisms.[3]

As environmental conditions inside your intestines and all throughout your body change rapidly, microflora need to respond quickly in order to survive. These responses include adaptation to nutrients and avoidance of toxins. For *pathogenic* (bad) bacteria to survive, they must coordinate their efforts (join forces to become stronger) in order to penetrate the immune response of the host.

Healthy bacteria, on the other hand, communicate in very beneficial ways. One of the functions of healthy gut flora is to help erect an "electric fence" to protect the environment in our intestines from pathogens.

THE BABY BOOMER DIET

Healthy vs. Unhealthy Microflora—
Fermentation vs. Putrefaction

With all this activity taking place inside your gut, it should now seem quite logical that your small and large intestines are the hub or power center of your well-being. Both disease and health have potential there. And what will you, as the master of your inner garden, allow to grow there? Will you allow "weeds" such as pathogens (parasites and yeast) to grow there; or useful fruits, vegetables, and lovely flowers (beneficial microflora)?

What does it mean to have an intestinal garden that is balanced and productive? Well, *everything!*

Microflora are responsible for:

- Hormone production
- Immune-system effectiveness
- Vitamin production and assimilation
- Cholesterol metabolism and synthesis
- Controlled glucose levels
- Normal bowel functioning and protein synthesis
- Youthfulness and protection against the degenerative diseases of aging

But when healthy intestinal flora are exposed to a toxic environment, they can be transformed into dangerous microbial bacteria that attack, rather than support and maintain, our organs. These are just a few of the health challenges that are linked to putrefaction and a compromised inner ecosystem:

- Leaky, inflamed, and wounded gut syndrome
- Adrenal fatigue
- Obesity
- Heart disease
- Arthritis
- Infections such as candida and herpes

off

86

The Signs of Aging

Beneficial bacteria and yeast have long been thought to slow down the aging process. Their use has been advocated by some pretty impressive innovators who had the courage to sidestep the conventional thinking of their day. Élie Metchnikoff, a Russian microbiologist and a contemporary of Pasteur, developed the very radical theory (at the time) that certain white blood cells could engulf and destroy harmful bodies such as bacteria.

Driven to desperation by the deaths of his two wives (one from tuberculosis and the other from typhoid), Metchnikoff made the study of microbes and the role they play in the immune system his life's work. His theories about white blood cells were scorned by the "microbe hunters," such as Pasteur and German bacteriologist Emil von Behring, but Metchnikoff was later vindicated, winning the Nobel Prize in 1908.[4]

Metchnikoff lived to the age of 71, unusual for his day. He believed that lactic acid could prolong life, and drank sour milk every day to prove it! He is one of our earliest probiotic pioneers and practitioners!

As for Looking Younger . . .

Bacteria affect us in cosmetic ways as well. Bad bacteria cause fine lines on the skin, freckles, and age spots. That's why skin-care companies are now putting probiotics into their creams and lotions. But beautiful skin cannot be purchased in a jar. It is the result of being clean from deep within ourselves. This can only be accomplished by removing dangerous substances from our bodies and putting back in the finest nutrients and purest water. Fortunately, Body Ecology has a highly effective methodology for doing this. We are finally returning to the knowledge and discoveries of people like Metchnikoff, whose work was often dismissed or obscured by others. Now we must reeducate our bodies as well as our minds.

Like the womb, our inner ecosystem has been an unseen mystery. Most of us have very little awareness of what goes on inside our wounded inner garden—our colon and small intestine.

In the sections ahead, you will discover how to get to know your body ecology and what it needs. I'll explain how to make sure the space inside your digestive tract is reserved for beneficial yeast and bacteria that work *for* your body rather than *against* it. You'll learn practical guidelines on how to properly cleanse, the benefits and pleasures of a probiotic diet, and some eating principles and practices that will reestablish your vital connection to the earth and transport you back to the Eden-like garden you lost so long ago.

From the Physician's Desk

"What's going on in the gut could be made into a Spielberg movie."

The amazing thing about bacteria is that they do exactly what we humans do. They communicate. They are social. We even refer to them as "cultures," the same way we refer to the French or American or Spanish culture. Bonnie Bassler, Ph.D., who is a medical investigator and a professor of molecular biology at the Howard Hughes Medical Institute, said it best: "We scientists were all wrong thinking that bacteria live asocial, reclusive lives. There isn't any way they could accomplish the terrible and the wonderful things they do on earth acting as individuals."[i]

Bassler contends that bacteria are gregarious by nature, preferring to crowd together in complex, multispecies communities. Most humans want to be where the action is. We move to big cities because there is a richer culture and a more multicultural environment available to us. We flourish in complex, often competitive situations. And we have intricate and meaningful ways of communicating. So do bacteria.

Bacteria communicate with each other through a method called quorum sensing. What this means, simply, is that bacteria release chemicals from inside their cells known as *autoinducers,* or "signaling molecules." These signaling molecules give bacteria a way to "count" one another. When they reach a critical number, they come together in the same way a voting quorum comes together to pass a referendum. As a quorum, bacteria are able to share resources and information with each other. They can also form bridges among one another and create opportune communication networks. It takes a quorum to make what Bassler calls "a population-wide alternation of gene expression." In other words, it truly does take a village to create systemic change.

As a single individual, a bacterium doesn't have a particularly strong voice. But as a group or "working conglomerate," they have great impact. It's like the sound of one solitary instrument versus the entire Boston Philharmonic.

This rather astounding and complex process is replicated on our teeth every morning. There are 600 species of bacteria on our teeth every night when we go to bed. When we wake up, they are in exactly the same organization as the night before. How do they maintain this blueprint or "biofilm"? They do so by communicating with each other, knowing what other cells are out there and using the information to function collectively. Bacteria have to behave in this way because their environment changes so rapidly. They must respond quickly in order to survive.

So how does this relate to our inner ecosystem, our gut?

There are at least 500 to 600 species of bacteria in our gut, and they are all competing for space and food. They have to respond in a variety of ways: they need to adapt to the availability of nutrients; defend against other microorganisms, which may be competing with them for the same nutrients; and avoid toxic compounds that are potentially dangerous to them. In fact, what's going on inside our gut would make a very frightening but fascinating Spielberg movie. Bacteria feed themselves from the food we take into our bodies.

While beneficial bacteria help us digest our food and make several B vitamins and vitamin K, pathogenic bacteria can turn food into a poison by oxidizing the essential fats we eat, and turning nitrates into cancer-producing nitrosamines.

To ensure we get sick and stay sick, pathogenic bacteria need to join forces and coordinate their virulence in order to escape the immune response of the host (us!) and establish a successful infection. Creating an antibiotic-resistant biofilm, they then take up residence and feast on us for their benefit, leaving us with a nasty infection. To make matters worse, many of the antibiotics we take to heal ourselves of infection may have little effect, if pathogenic bacteria and their biofilms have overwhelmed the intestinal tract with the force and intelligence of their numbers.

This is the real genius behind the Body Ecology system. It ensures that greater numbers of beneficial bacteria have taken up residence and created cities (biofilms) in the gut and are talking to each other. This "cross-talk" between bacteria and the intestinal ecosystem is the key to health. It promotes the proper utilization of nutrients and defends against sickness. The dietary and lifestyle choices in the Body Ecology system, particularly the use of fermented foods and probiotics, are some of the best ways I know to prevent illness.

— *Leonard Smith, M.D.*

---

[i]Bonnie Bassler, "Microbial Chatter: How Bacteria Talk to Each Other," New York Academy of Sciences, delivered in a speech at Princeton University, Howard Hughes Medical Institute, reported by Marcia Stone in the *Academy eBriefings,* August 23, 2006.

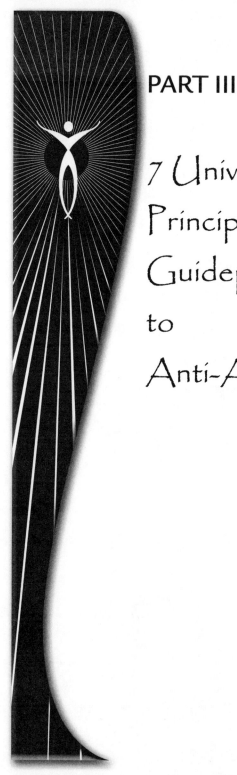

PART III

7 Universal Principles— Guideposts to Anti-Aging

Chapter 8

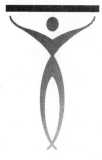

The Principle of Uniqueness: Knowing Yourself

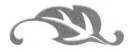

We Baby Boomers share collective experiences that formed our unique generational identity. But it is an identity built on individuality, transformation, self-exploration, and reinvention.

Renewing by Honoring Who We Are

The first of the 7 Universal Principles, the *Principle of Uniqueness,* states that you are a singular, one-of-a-kind individual. That's it: you're *unique.* Yes, we have most of the same pieces and parts: a heart that beats, lungs that breathe, eyes that see, and a brain that thinks. And as Baby Boomers, we share many of the same formative experiences that forged our generational identity. We were encouraged to test limits and explore our world. We share a history and a community. We've watched Presidents come and go, suffered through pain and loss, and felt ourselves change—physically, emotionally, socially, and financially—with each passing year. We know where we were the day President Kennedy was shot. We remember the moon walk, the march on Montgomery, Watergate, and

Vietnam. But while we might be similar in many ways, we are clearly more different than alike, and it is these differences that really matter. We have diverging needs; childhood experiences; and ways of thinking, learning, and being. These differences give us identity and individuality—and we Boomers love that!

Some of us are more active than others. We may enjoy the outdoors or prefer to curl up indoors with a good book. Some of us have rich social lives full of family, friends, acquaintances, and a calendar stocked with events. Others keep things simple, preferring to interact with a very small circle of intimates. Some of us live in the country, soaking up the sunshine, plants, and fresh air; while others crave the hustle and flow of city life, reassured by the sounds of traffic.

For some of us, years of stress, toxins, and poor lifestyle choices may start to surface in midlife as unpleasant reminders of aging. We may be experiencing weight problems, sleep difficulties, or pains in the places where we used to play, to paraphrase '60s singer Leonard Cohen. We are even seeing how "sex, drugs, and rock 'n' roll" may have led to health problems we had never considered during our more reckless teen years.

AARP magazine recently reported that some physicians believe that past marijuana smoking may increase the risk for head and neck cancers. About four million Americans—many of them over 45—are estimated to be harboring hepatitis C, a sometimes deadly souvenir of heroin use. And speed, often the first drug of choice among experimenting Baby Boomers, assaults the brain's dopamine system, making things slow down, just as aging makes things slow down.

Alcohol abuse has also ranked high among Boomers, and in 2002, 38 percent of younger Baby Boomers (ages 35 to 44) and 31 percent of older Boomers (ages 45 to 54) were current users of some form of tobacco. Loud music from high-voltage rock concerts may also have left its mark. Whereas hearing loss used to begin to plague 60- and 70-year-olds, it is now showing up in 40- and 50-year-olds. Postponing pregnancy, as many women of our generation did, also increased the use of fertility drugs, which can raise the risk of ovarian cancer in some women.

The sexual freedom of the '60s also resulted in an increase in sexually transmitted diseases (STDs). For example, women who contracted the human papilloma virus (HPV) are at higher risk for developing cervical cancer, which strikes some 12,800

Anti-Aging Application

*T*he Principle of Uniqueness is all about aging gracefully. This means adapting our diet and our lifestyle to our emotional and physical needs at each new stage of life. Baby Boomers are masters of reinvention, so this principle is especially suited to our flexibility and openness to learning new ways of being. Staying young in our attitudes and in our spirits will be critical to our longevity.

women a year. This disease often develops when women are between the ages of 40 and 60.[1]

This is by no means intended to be alarmist, as there are many Baby Boomers who did not explore these paths, who experimented lightly, or who emerged unscathed. It is important, however, to point out some of the possible health consequences from our generation's "youthful indiscretions."

Boomer Differences

During each decade of our lives, we have different and constantly changing needs. What was important to us at 20 is less so now; and hopefully we will feel better in our 50s, 60s, and 70s than we did in our youth.

Think that's myth and hyperbole?

Think again! I have been living the Body Ecology Way for more than a decade now, and I feel better than I did when I was in my 20s or 30s. Why? Because in many ways my body is healthier. And today I have a much better understanding of who I am and of my own unique needs. I'm more authentically me.

And these are exciting times! Never before in the thousands of years of human history have we ever known so much about the workings of the body and the brain. Scientific knowledge is advancing so rapidly that attaining a more prolonged state of youthfulness is right here, right now.

I think something happens to us when we start to feel as if we've reached a level of personal satisfaction. Besides still focusing on reaching our personal goals, we also begin to act more altruistically . . . turning our attention to the world around us. My children are grown, and I can now better prioritize my vitality and vigor, and put my newfound energy to good use by leaving the planet a better place than I found it.

How to Know What Your Body Needs

The beauty of the Principle of Uniqueness is that we all respond to and digest every morsel—be it of food or information—differently. Depending on your personality type, you are either reading these words with a healthy dose of skepticism or a hopeful kind of flutter in your heart . . . or are finding it hard to read at all because you're jumping up and down with unbridled eagerness to get started. Your uniqueness will bring its own properties to this diet, and I am simply a guide to help you embark on your own path to anti-aging.

The journey begins with honest self-evaluation: where are you, right now, today; and how prepared are you to take that very first step?

Thankfully, we can look to the past and see what we have done to our bodies. This can be measured through a series of simple, effective, and inexpensive tests that give us a clear snapshot of our current health status.

Six Valuable Tests for Self-Analysis

The following six valuable tests can show you where your deficiencies are so that you can correct them with lifestyle choices and a healing, yet delicious, eating plan. All six are easily obtained from your holistically oriented doctor, who can interpret the results for you. Fortunately, they also come with a summary so that you can read these results yourself without medical training.

1. Hormones: A complete hormone panel would include DHEA, testosterone, progesterone, estrogen, pregnenolone, and cortisol. You'll also want to test for other key hormones, especially those associated with the thyroid (for men *and* women). Growth-hormone levels also decline dramatically starting in our mid-30s. This hormone was thought to only be necessary for children who were growing, but it is one of the most important to keep us forever young.

It is not in the scope of this book to discuss hormones in depth, but diet, exercise, and Chinese tonic herbs are essential to any hormone-rebalancing program. In fact, often these three are all that is needed to correct hormone deficiencies. Eliminating stress is also key, as it destroys the life of the adrenals, where most of these hormones are manufactured.

This book will outline the foods to eat to help restore your hormones to their original youthful levels. In fact, I often recommend a three-month change in lifestyle, focusing on diet, herbs, exercise, and anti-aging therapies . . . like acupuncture . . . *before* you even have your hormones tested. Then you'll obtain a more accurate reading of what your body can really do on its own. Oftentimes, these natural methods may be all that is needed.

2. Fatty acids: This simple profile determines the amount—and kinds—of fatty acids present in your blood. Such acids denote the presence of cholesterol, and levels thereof, and are important as we age in order to determine such risks as heart disease and cancer.

3. Minerals: Minerals and toxins can affect the immune system, sexual and cardiovascular functions, mental wellness, and more. A typical laboratory mineral test uses a hair sample to measure levels of 11 essential minerals and nine toxins.

4. Infections: Caused by yeast and viruses, infections can be detected with live-blood-cell analysis.

5. Heavy metals: There are many ways to test for heavy metals—for instance, by a hair analysis, urine test (DMSA challenge), stool test, and blood test.

6. Blood type: We should all know our blood type, as each specific type holds some valuable clues to anti-aging (see the next section).

What about Allergy Tests?

You may wonder why allergy testing is not on my list. For years people have sent me their allergy tests, and I usually glance at them and then set them aside. I know that once they are on the right diet with fermented foods and certain lifestyle changes, these allergies will quickly disappear.

Your Blood Type Provides More Clues to Halt Early Aging

First, let me say that blood typing is just one means we have of assessing personality and physical and nutritional requirements. There are many others. Knowing that blood relays the most fundamental nourishment for our bodies, it seemed to me that different blood types might react differently to certain substances in food. While there is not a lot of "hard science" to date on diet and blood type, it makes a lot of common sense to look further into this theory. Blood carries the nutrients of foods into our cells, and clearly not all blood is exactly the same.

In Japan extensive research on blood type and personality began more than 60 years ago, and today it is even more common to hear the Japanese ask your blood type than it is for Americans to ask for your astrological sign.

I have a special relationship with Japan. I lived there from the ages of 12 to 15. As I mentioned, I also studied with Lima Ohsawa, who developed macrobiotics with her husband, George. During my years of travel and study in Japan, I had an opportunity to learn firsthand the ways in which the Japanese used blood types; and it immediately caught my attention—especially because several years earlier I had also become fascinated with the work of Dr. James D'Adamo.

After meeting Dr. D'Adamo and reading his book *One Man's Food . . . Is Someone Else's Poison,* I began to question everyone about his or her blood type in an attempt to verify if it could indeed provide clues to our individual uniqueness, as well as indicate the foods and lifestyle choices most compatible for a specific type.

While Dr. James D'Adamo's theories were based on patient observation, his son Peter D'Adamo has tried to use a more scientific approach by studying the activity of lectins (proteins found in food). Peter found that eating the wrong lectins for your blood type could cause weight gain, early aging, and immune problems.

I have blended the research from Japan and much of the research of both James and Peter D'Adamo with my own observations. After 26 years of working with people of all ages, I want to present you with a summary of my own current thoughts only to inspire you to continue to look more deeply into this subject. Blood type is simply another example of how we are not all the same. (For more on how each blood type should eat, see *The Body Ecology Diet*.)

Blood Type and Personality

There are four blood types: *A, B, AB,* and *O.* See if you can recognize yourself. . . .

- **Blood type A:** Type A individuals tend to be cooperative, sensitive, clever, passionate, and smart. Often bottling up anxiety in order to get along with others, they may hold in their emotions until they explode. Many are tense, impatient, and unable to sleep well. While they are capable of leadership positions, they may not choose professions that cause too much stress for their tightly wired systems. In Japan many A's are involved in research related to science, economics, manufacturing, and so forth; or they are teachers. Their uncompromising minds are always discovering more about the world and refining their expertise. The research by A's on microflora and other areas of medicine is some of the best and most meticulous in the world. They are perfectionists.

- **Blood type B:** Type B individuals tend to be balanced. They are thoughtful like A's, yet ambitious like O's. Highly empathetic, they are understanding of others and opposing points of view, yet often hesitant to challenge or confront. Chameleonlike and flexible, they make patient and objective friends.

- **Blood type AB:** These individuals tend to be very charming and popular. They don't sweat the small stuff and can be seen as spiritual and even at times a bit "flaky." Only about 2 to 5 percent of the population are blood type AB. There is never a dull moment in an AB's life, so if you find one for a friend, consider yourself lucky! You'll enjoy some exciting times together! Sometimes it is difficult to be an AB. Even they are confused about who they are. Plus, they're often changing their minds. AB's don't like to fit in anyone else's "box." If they feel too confined, they'll break out of that box and do things their own way.

- **Blood type O:** O blood types tend to be loners or leaders; and are intuitive, focused, self-reliant, and daring. They handle stress better than other blood types and have strong immune systems, a well-developed physique, and a physically active nature. Since O's handle stressful situations with a certain level of detachment, they make good leaders. This hardy blood type is frequently not aware, however, that the foods they eat and their lifestyle choices are harmful. They often are not as "tuned in to" their physical and emotional needs as A's are. They can abuse themselves for a long time and then suddenly find themselves falling apart.[2, 3]

Taking Matters into Our Own Hands

One of the wonderful things about growing older is that we come to a better understanding of who we are—how much we share in common with others, and what makes us special. Because we've tried and abandoned many things along the way, we have now settled into ourselves more, and we find that we have less to prove. We can be more authentically who we were always meant to be.

And today there are many resources for self-discovery that our parents and grandparents never dreamed of. There are many excellent books on almost every subject, and the Internet is literally at our fingertips. A wider array of supplements and alternative therapies are readily available to us. However, it can be challenging to decipher all this information, and once we've decided what works best for us, we may not know how to start. The next chapter discusses Step by Step, a principle that is very useful as we begin to implement new healthy choices in our lives.

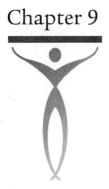

Chapter 9

The Principle of Step by Step: Knowing Where and How to Begin

The health challenges now facing Baby Boomers didn't happen overnight. They were created in the same way they must be confronted—step by step.

To Everything There Is a Season

The Principle of Step by Step is a universal law and is not unique to the Baby Boomer Diet. It can be seen throughout nature and in hundreds of activities we complete each day. Every tree that matures does so in an orderly fashion, adhering to an imprinted set of steps it has followed for hundreds or thousands of years. A simple seed is planted in the ground, watered, tended, fed, and given sunlight; and eventually it grows to tower over the forest that nurtured and protected it. It does so day after day, month after month, year after year. Time-lapse photography collapses this progressive evolution, making the gradual, methodical process of growth seem quick and dramatic. In reality, though, it takes time to learn, to change, and to see the fruits of our efforts.

One of the loveliest gifts that comes with the passing of years is a deeper appreciation and understanding of this process. Most of us would never give up the wisdom we have gained over time . . . step by step . . . even if we were allowed to start our lives over again. Without this wisdom, we'd simply make the same mistakes again anyway. It's how we learn . . . step by step.

The Principle of Step by Step also tells us that we can't do everything we would like to do all at once. If we try, we will surely fail.

By the time you have finished reading this book, you will have learned many tools to help you reverse aging. But please, don't try to pick up all of them right away. You can't. If you take a minute to tune in to your intuition, certain tools will seem more appealing and easier for you to use. It will seem more urgent for you to adopt some, and your intuition will tell you to try these first. A few of the tools in this book may be ones you've been using for years, while others are the missing pieces that will excite you with new possibilities and inspire you to take action. Still, new tools are best introduced step by step; master one or two, and then add another when you are ready to do so.

Taking the Time to Heal

The step-by-step concept is one of the most important healing concepts to embrace. Yet we often take it for granted and overlook it due to its simplicity. However, this universal law answers important questions: (1) *How long will it take to rejuvenate and heal?* and (2) *Where do I start, and what steps do I take first?*

Let's answer the first question first, because part of the Step by Step Principle is about time—taking the time to heal.

The seasons of the year have an order. We cannot violate this order—we cannot go from winter directly to summer without first having spring. In spiritual traditions, this is the principle of dawning: dawn occurs little by little in the transition from night to day, and so it goes for all things in nature.

Unfortunately, we often spurn the Step by Step Principle, and our health suffers as a result. An example of this is when we are unwilling to take the time to get over a cold or the flu and reach for medicine and antibiotics as a "quick cure." This

Anti-Aging Application

*T*he Principle of Step by Step, with its emphasis on conquering infection and building energy, has clear anti-aging benefits. Infections in the body cause inflammation, the build-up of free radicals, hormone imbalances, and nutritional deficiencies, all of which are key factors in why we age.

suppresses our immune system and weakens our vital life forces. A strong, hardy body will naturally *cleanse* . . . pushing out toxins. Taking unnecessary drugs only drives these toxins back into the cells and makes our blood even more acidic. Drugs stop the cleansing process, which the body uses to get rid of illness. Disease is driven deeper into the body, giving the potential for an even more serious illness later. In taking drugs, we halt the body's self-regulating effort to eliminate its toxins step by step. If we allow nature to take its course, cleansing and healing will take place, also step by step. (Please note that cessation of medication should be undertaken with your doctor's supervision.)

Our unwillingness to take time got us into trouble when we replaced home-cooked meals with fast foods. Unlike previous generations, few of us take the time to learn which foods are best for us—to plan menus, shop, and prepare them. Fast-food meals have allowed us to skip over these steps, resulting in diets that satisfy our taste buds and cravings but not our nutritional needs. We've aged as a result of toxins found in these foods and the lack of nutrients our bodies have needed to stay young.

How We Got to Where We Are Today

The last chapter talked about how each one of us is unique, but there is one thing that is true for all of us: *we have built up a lifetime of toxins that are gradually breaking down our bodies.* This breakdown has been occurring step by step—in fact, the increments often were so small that we didn't even notice them.

Accumulation of toxins, nutrient deficiencies, chronic infections, deteriorating organs, poor lifestyle habits, and genetic tendencies toward certain imbalances are now beginning to show. That unexpected appearance of a heart problem, cancer, bulging veins, hair loss, or yeast overgrowth didn't happen "all of a sudden." These conditions are the result of many assaults on your body over a long period of time. The good news is that healing also takes place in a step-by-step sequence, and all you have to do is start.

This book holds exciting answers for what to do, but please be realistic and know that for the remainder of our lives we Baby Boomers will be reversing the "follies of our youth."

So where do we start? What steps do we take first?

The rest of the chapter contains a simple formula that will provide you with a step-by-step road map for your journey's start toward reaching the Fountain of Youth.

I've often been amazed by how no one has quite understood or followed this formula before now. Even the brightest and best holistic doctors don't truly understand or adhere to this part of the Principle of Step by Step. Consequently, they have not been able to help us when we go to them for advice.

You have most likely heard the expression that "a journey of a thousand miles begins with a single step." Where do you begin "stepping," however, when you want to become young again?

The *first* step to regaining your youth and your health begins with four simple yet profound actions that you will focus on each day until you master them. While each is a separate action, they must all be accomplished together. That is not really difficult to do, as the four steps are related and intertwined; one supports the other. This is the most effective way to begin implementing the Body Ecology system of health and healing, and you can go at your own pace in customizing these steps to your unique needs.

Let's explore each one:

1. Create Energy

First and foremost, create energy. Nothing else can happen until this initial step has been taken. Most of us Baby Boomers began experiencing loss of our prenatal jing energy by our 40s. It may first manifest itself in joint and muscle pain or a general feeling of life seeming kind of flat.

But there are other signs. Do you feel spacey and forgetful at times? Suffer hormonal imbalances? Are you losing muscle tone? Often constipated? Are you no longer sleeping well? These are just some of the many symptoms that show that your vital prenatal *jing* and your daily *chi* energy have been compromised.

The most important first step we can take as we begin to reverse aging is to restore our original energy. Baby Boomers must be particularly sensitive to this. We are a generation of overachievers. We tend to keep very busy and to feel that we aren't really "living" unless we're "doing." We've never learned how to relax. Too many things compete for our time and our energy—the Internet, cell phones, television—filling our world with incessant chatter. We may not even be aware of how much the static has increased over the years.

> *I can certainly see a time coming soon when Baby Boomers begin to form support groups and live in health-based communities where the focus is on educating and encouraging people to slow down and build relaxation into their daily routines.*

Now, as many of us begin to experience "empty-nest syndrome," where we feel less "useful," or encounter new stresses such as having to take care of our parents, we must begin to learn how to conserve our energy and find ways to nourish ourselves.

I can certainly see a time coming soon when Baby Boomers begin to form support groups and live in health-based communities where the focus is on educating and encouraging people to slow down and build relaxation into their daily routines. Take a few moments to consider the things that are draining *you* of vital energy: Not enough sleep? Too many commitments? Toxic relationships? The amazing superfoods and anti-aging therapies found later in this book will provide you with excellent solutions to begin renewing your energy day after day . . . step by step.

2. Conquer Infections

During the course of your lifetime thus far, how many different drugs have you taken? Vaccinated often as children and given frequent rounds of antibiotics, ours is the first generation to reap the rewards and the devastating effects of pharmaceutical-driven medical care. Birth-control pills were taken by most of the women in our generation, and many of us used and still use recreational drugs. Alcohol has played an important role in our social life, and we are the first generation to have so much sugar abundantly available whenever we want it.

Well, today eight out of ten Americans suffer from candidiasis. The drugs, alcohol, stress, and sweet foods so available to us have accelerated this yeast/fungal problem (which you are most likely experiencing right now). The life we lead gives fungi even more opportunity to thrive. This serious chronic infection will only become more acute as our immunity diminishes with age, and this sets the stage for cancer.

The Body Ecology system of health and healing ("The Diet") originally began as a way to conquer yeast infections. It is the most complete and comprehensive antifungal diet available. The Diet and its 7 Principles are just as effective for preventing and reversing aging as well. Infections cause inflammation, which then causes us to age, and diagnosing and conquering them all is essential to any anti-aging program.

When infections like candida are corrected through the Body Ecology approach, energy automatically goes up, and susceptibility to disease goes down. Other common infections most of us are struggling with include viral herpes; bacterial infections in the gums; low-grade, chronic bacterial infections in the bladder; and *H. pylori* bacterial infection in the stomach, causing ulcers.

These all deplete the body of energy. When they are conquered, the energy to rejuvenate and to stay young becomes yours.

3. Correct Digestion

When the digestive tract doesn't work well, nothing works well. As a Boomer, you may be experiencing some of the signs of a compromised digestive tract, such as constipation, diarrhea, inflammation in the gut, irritable bowel syndrome, and flatulence. It is essential that you heal the gut lining and establish a healthy inner ecosystem, repopulating the intestinal tract with friendly microflora.

When first starting The Diet, during the first five to ten days, many people with an inflamed mucosal lining will want to "rest" the gut by eating primarily soft or liquid foods—broths, purees, and green smoothies—and also lightly steamed leafy-green and ocean vegetables.

4. Cleanse from Toxins

We must actively remove the toxins from our bodies. These toxins are in our organs and in our cells. They come to us from nutritionally deficient, poorly digested, and poorly combined foods. They are in the water, in the air, and even in our self-destructive feelings. They are in drug residues and ingested metals, such as lead, aluminum, and cadmium. We have inherited toxins from our parents, and passed them on to our own children. Toxins snuff out our spiritual power and our intuition. When they are removed from our lives, boundless energy is created.

(The concept of cleansing will be covered in greater detail in the next chapter, as it is the third principle of the Baby Boomer Diet.)

Making Progress

Taking a step-by-step approach to healing doesn't mean that your progress has to be slow. You can choose how quickly you embrace the steps, and you may experience immediate improvements in energy and vitality. On the other hand, you might need to go at a more moderate pace. Be realistic. Don't take on more than you can handle. When you feel comfortable with one step, move on to another.

For example, when you first start the Baby Boomer Diet, you may have very uncomfortable symptoms of "die-off." This is because you're beginning to create more energy, and your body wants to eliminate all those toxins stored in your cells. As it dispels them, unpleasant symptoms occur. You will soon learn how to deal with this "cleansing," but if you absolutely can't stand it or if you need to feel better for work, you can slow down the cleansing by transitioning slowly into The Diet little by little . . . step by step. You choose.

Here are four simple steps you can take in the beginning that can make an enormous difference in your goal to regain your youthful energy and appearance:

1. Cut back on or eliminate sugar and high-carb sweets. Even those so-called energy bars are loaded with sugar, depleting your essential prenatal life force. Instead, you will be introduced to several alternative sweeteners that will allow you to still enjoy the sweet

taste without the damaging and aging effects of sugars . . . even honey and the "healthy" sugars.

2. Change the oils you are currently eating to the extra-virgin, unrefined fats and oils of The Diet. Later in this book you'll be provided with a delicious array of fats and oils to keep you looking and feeling great. They also make eating more pleasurable.

3. Add some fermented foods to your diet, such as young coconut kefir (see Chapter 15). This is perhaps the most important step of all, as you'll soon learn.

4. Pay attention to cleansing your colon. You might consider trying your first colonic, if you've never had one before (see Chapter 25). Cells also need to eliminate their toxic waste. When you're constipated, your cells are, too. They also feel toxic, sluggish, and irritable. Actively cleansing with diet, herbs, colonics, and home enemas will soon become commonplace once our generation understands that we must purify our bodies to reclaim our youth. We have no choice, really.

Success comes step by step. That's why you must be very determined to stick with The Diet until you master it. Advance according to your own personal pace, the one that supports you the best. Persevere. When you have a setback—an old symptom or reaction—take only the next step that allows you to get back on track. The beauty of this program is that if you do stay with it, you will have victory; you will successfully reverse the aging process and return to the youth and vitality you've been longing for.

As you begin to implement The Diet, I hope you will treat your body as an evolving experiment in self-awareness. Unlike other dietary approaches, the Body Ecology Way is not a short-term "fix," but rather an ongoing journey of personal discovery and adaptation.

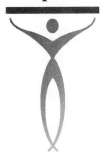

Chapter 10

The Principle of Cleansing: Knowing How to Purify from the Inside Out

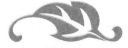

Brainwashed as children by TV commercials that encouraged us to conquer nature rather than cooperate with it, we Baby Boomers have become disconnected from our built-in capacity to heal ourselves.

Purify to Create a New You

The Principle of Cleansing is certainly the least appreciated and most often misunderstood of the 7 Principles. Yet cleansing plays a vital role in anti-aging. It is nature's way of allowing the body to get rid of unwanted toxins, waste, and foreign substances. Aging cells are constantly being replaced with new ones and new tissue. If we are to remain forever young, toxins must come out of the cells in our organs. Cleansing is the process that accomplishes this—carrying away cellular debris.

A speck of dust gets in your eye, and you blink and tear up—to cleanse out the dust so it won't hurt you. A similar thing happens when a virus invades your system and you get a fever; it's your immune system working to purify your body of that toxin.

Many of the signs and symptoms of aging are a direct result of the vast amounts of toxins we've accumulated since conception. They are stored in the liver, causing it to be congested; our joints ache, our skin wrinkles, and our eyes develop macular degeneration. Toxins devastate our sensitive endocrine system, which produces anti-aging hormones, such as HGH, melatonin, DHEA, progesterone, and testosterone. When we peel back the layers of this mostly unintentional damage, we begin to feel, and certainly look, years younger.

What most of us don't realize is that our bodies are constantly working on our behalf to purify and cleanse us of these toxins. In fact, the ability to purge toxins out of each cell is really quite remarkable. (We pay extra for ovens that are self-cleaning, yet our bodies do it for us for free!)

But over time, our cleansing organs begin to wear down. For example, the liver—that miraculous and overburdened organ of detoxification—shrinks as we age. By the age of 70, it will likely have decreased to 81 percent of its original size. It will not only receive a smaller blood supply, but it will also be less able to do its important job of cleansing. If we choose to use drugs, they will no longer be eliminated as efficiently, predisposing many of us to overdose. A better solution is to follow the

One of the secrets to remaining forever young is to never lose the ability to purge toxins and waste. Instead, welcome and assist your body in this natural process.

recommendations for foods, supplements, and cleansing therapies in Body Ecology's Baby Boomer Diet . . . fermented foods, healthy fats, enzymes, and colon cleansing.

The Toxic Buildup

Every child born today—including our very own grandchildren—has inherited a long list of serious toxins as a premature (and quite unwanted) "birthday present." According to the

Environmental Working Group (EWG), laboratory tests of the umbilical-cord blood of ten newborns found that the samples contained an average of 200 chemicals that can cause cancer, brain damage, birth defects, and other health ailments. Sonya Lunder, a scientist with the EWG, explains: "This is conclusive evidence that babies are being exposed to hundreds of industrial chemicals throughout pregnancy. The placenta isn't a magic shield."[1]

When we're young, our cells have walls that are soft and pliable. As the body begins to fill with more and more free radicals, these walls, made of a fatty membrane, become hardened. (To get a better idea of what happens to your cells as you age, place a lemon on the counter and watch how the skin hardens from the oxygen.)

If cell walls remain soft and pliable (from antioxidant-rich foods), nutrients carried in your bloodstream enter your cells, while waste products are sent back out into the bloodstream, where they are eliminated in a variety of ways. Examples of how the body eliminates toxins are: bowel movements, urination, skin eruptions, sweating from a fever or the summer heat, tears, vomiting, coughing up mucus, and (special to women) the monthly menstrual "cleansing."

Unfortunately, we have been taught that cleansings are "bad" and need to be *suppressed,* so we pop a few pills, keep on working, and try to pretend they're not really happening to us. Indeed, while we were growing up, we Baby Boomers (and our parents, who believed so strongly in the miracles of modern medicine) were brainwashed to *stop* the cleansing.

Our Bodies Were Created to Remain Young!

As we get closer to death, we will begin to lose the ability to purify unless we choose (with strong intention) to change this natural course of events.

If you had or still have strong prenatal *jing,* you will also have a strong ability to cleanse. One of the secrets to remaining forever young is to never lose this ability to purge toxins and waste. Instead, welcome—and assist your body in—this natural process.

If you're someone who proudly boasts, "I never get sick," I don't want to burst your bubble, but ask yourself, *Do I have the vital energy to cleanse?* As you change your diet and create more energy, please *expect* to do so.

This is certainly not to suggest that you welcome an *infectious* disease like tuberculosis, AIDS, or pneumonia. These, along with chronic viral and fungal *infections,* are *not* cleansings. Indeed, the aim of this book is to show you how to build a stronger immune system to protect yourself against infectious disease, and give you the tools to heal these chronic infections.

But every Baby Boomer should feel the gratitude and joy that comes with realizing that our bodies were created with this amazing function embedded within us—this ability to purify *in order to heal and stay young.*

Modern Drugs Often Suppress Cleansing

Thousands of years ago, ancient Chinese healers knew the dangers of suppressing the body's natural healing process. Their work—designed to restore prenatal *jing* energy and enhance daily *chi* energy—included the use of natural foods and herbs that activated the energy of the cleansing organs so that they could do the job they were created to do.

Medicines used by modern Western science today stop, close down, or interfere with the "pushing out" process of cleansing. When was the last time someone congratulated you for having a cold? We are simply not taught to look at cleansings in this way. We regard colds and fevers as *a body in rebellion,* so we beat it back into submission with drugs and denial.

We look upon *symptoms* such as skin eruptions, mucous discharge, sore throat, headaches, aches and pains, depression, lethargy, increased fatigue, and fevers as illnesses, so we suppress the symptoms with drugs. In fact, turn on your television

Anti-Aging Application

*T*he Principle of Cleansing has special relevance to the DNA theory of aging (see Chapter 3), which suggests that we have a fixed genetic predisposition toward certain symptoms of aging and age-related diseases. But a body that frequently rids itself of toxins can ultimately take a detour from many of these "predetermined" genetic paths, such as breast cancer or Alzheimer's.

set almost any evening and you'll find a drug commercial promising to cure any one of these.

And what can you expect from continual use of drugs that are only suppressing the symptoms? Imagine this: If every time a young man called a woman for a date and was pushed away with a nasty reply, he'd eventually stop calling. The same is true for the body. Although your body is amazingly "persistent," it will gradually become more out of balance and acidic, and at last concede defeat.

Since the drugs are also not correcting the *source* of the problem, the toxins and nutritional deficiencies remain, and the immune system weakens with each onslaught of drugs, losing its life force. We age early and die sooner.

Dismantling and Rebuilding

As you follow the Baby Boomer Diet, you will at times experience healing and a renewed sense of vitality. You'll feel and look great. However, do expect, and welcome, the times of cleansing when you ache, feel tired, feverish, or even ill, knowing that when you arrive on the other side of the cleansing, you'll be free of damaging toxins.

Often the flu-like, depressed, and exhausted feelings are also caused by the die-off of the pathogenic yeast causing the infection candidiasis. This is called the *Herxheimer die-off reaction*. As the yeast die off and exit through normal body channels, they release toxins that cause these symptoms to occur. Please be assured that this die-off is normal. Toxins wreak havoc when they first enter your body; it makes sense they would also cause some disquiet on the way out.

"Is This How I'm *Supposed* to Feel?"

Cleansing looks like a disturbance to the entire system. Think of it as a little like spring-cleaning. When you decide to clean your living room, you begin dusting, vacuuming, washing the windows, and moving things around. The dirt and grime start to fly, furniture is rearranged, garbage bags are filled, and it may look as if order couldn't possibly come out of such disarray. If someone arrived in the middle of this process, your living room would look pretty disrupted and possibly worse than it did before you began! But if you stick to the plan and keep at it, in the end it will look much better and feel more livable than it did before.

The greater the die-off reaction, the more uncomfortable you may feel. A home enema or a visit to your colon therapist at the first sign of cleansing will greatly help in this regard. It's extremely important to adhere to The Diet strictly during this time, to give yourself the maximum opportunity to heal. It's easy to get discouraged when you believe yourself to be just as "sick" as before, but have faith that when this healing period ends, you will have taken an important step toward your goal of a longer, healthier life.

We don't just cleanse physically; we also do so emotionally. As your body cleanses, you may feel inexplicably weepy, on edge, fearful, full of doubt, and angry. Without warning, you may feel like lashing out at someone verbally or even physically. This is all part of the elimination of stored-up *emotional* toxins connected to your *physical* organs. Just know that these feelings are normal, and it's beneficial to release them in a safe environment.

It may help you to bear in mind that nature is kept eternally young and renewed by the constant cleansings of storms, hurricanes, tidal waves, floods, ice, and snow. Think of how fresh and clean spring feels after the wet and snowy cleansings of winter or after a major spring storm . . . how fresh and pure the air has become.

Don't be afraid to cleanse—your body has the wisdom to only do so when it is strong enough and ready to handle this process. When you're cleansing, do what is recommended when you come down with a cold: flush the colon, rest, keep warm, and drink lots of fluids. You do want to keep your energy up during your cleanse: eat warm broths and soups (such as miso soup), and alkalize your bloodstream with a green drink and a green smoothie (some recipes are included in this book). Probiotic liquids will also build your immunity and energy.

How Long Will It Take?

Cleansing is a continuing, step-by-step phenomenon. When you're healthy, you will find that it is ongoing. Your most significant period of cleansing may occur during your first three months, and especially during the first few days and weeks, on the Baby Boomer Diet. This is a time of great healing.

The length of cleansings is different for everybody, and it depends on how long the toxins have been in your body and how deeply embedded they are. For some, it takes three months to a year to feel the positive effects of anti-aging through cleansing. Most people feel a lot better after only two weeks on The Diet.

While cleansing symptoms do clear up (usually within three to ten days), you can shorten their duration and "minimize discomfort" by cleansing your colon with an enema or a colonic. (For more information on colon therapy as an anti-aging strategy, see Chapter 25.)

You Call the Shots

The Baby Boomer Diet works because it supports your body in doing what it was designed to do: cleanse itself and restore inner balance. While you can't *stop* cleansing, nor would you want to, you might be reassured to know that you have some control over the process.

How quickly do you want to cleanse? Well, if you were climbing a mountain, and you knew that everything you ever desired was waiting for you at the top, how fast would you move to get there? Conquering the adverse effects of aging is like climbing a challenging mountain. You'll have to go step by step, using special tools to make the job easier, but it's *you* who will decide how fast to go.

Helpful Tips for Cleansing

- Avoid the following acidic foods: sugar, fats and oils, salt, grains, animal proteins, nuts, and seeds.

- Cleanse the colon as soon as possible.

- Get plenty of rest, and reserve your energy for healing. Do not exercise at this time.

- Alkalize your body with a green drink, a green smoothie, or a spoonful of apple-cider vinegar added to a glass of water.

- Drink alkaline, mineral-rich water.

- Nourish your body with raw and cooked alkaline vegetables from the land and ocean.

- Build your immunity with fermented vegetables and liquids.

- Eat warming, soft foods, along with soups and broths (try natto and miso).

- Call a friend who can gently remind you that you are just cleansing, and to stay the course.

- Practice gratitude for this gift embedded within, and visualize a younger you!

To paraphrase the wisdom of a biblical verse: "Be like a child to enter the gates of heaven." As we begin the process of returning our bodies to a childlike state of nontoxicity, youth, and vitality, living here in this dimension will seem more like heaven. Rewarded with the wisdom of 40 to 60 years, we Baby Boomers can now clearly visualize what we want and can use our talents—acquired over a lifetime—to create heaven for ourselves and for those we love: our children and grandchildren.

In the next chapter, we will explore one of the most important lessons of life: *finding and creating balance.*

Chapter 11

The Principle of Balance: Knowing the Dance of Yin and Yang

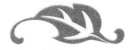

As Baby Boomers age, the excesses of the past start to catch up with us, and we see that we must adopt a different approach in the second half of our lives. How do we achieve balance after years of full-throttle intensity?

Baby Boomers who practice yoga are probably familiar with the famous "Tree Pose," also called *Vrksasana*. This beautiful pose, where you stand on one leg while reaching toward the ceiling with your arms, requires both a focused muscular energy and a calm, easy grace. Many people find it much more challenging than they expected. If you hold yourself too loose and forget to concentrate, you'll topple over. If you hold yourself too tight and forget to breathe, you'll miss the wonderful feeling of openness and extension this pose can bring. When done correctly, the Tree Pose makes you feel rooted and strong, just like the trunk of a tree connected deeply in the earth, but it also makes you feel free and dynamic, the way branches release and reach to the sky. In short, this pose requires *balance.*

Like most yoga poses, the Tree Pose embodies *yin* and *yang,* a careful harmony of contractive and expansive energy. Yin and yang are complementary opposites, two interdependent and creative forces of change that are always seeking equilibrium.

These universal Chinese principles have been essential to helping humans classify and understand the natural world. Yin and yang energy has been applied to the use of herbs and to food as well. Even disorders within the body can be better understood and brought into balance when these two opposing energies are utilized skillfully.

Yang energy is outward, activating, drying, and warm or hot. These words may stimulate thoughts of the sun and of fire.

Yin energy is inward, stored energy. It is nourishing, moistening, cooling, and anti-inflammatory. These words may remind you of water or of the moon.

Yin and yang are only relative terms. For example, women are thought to be more yin (receptive and nurturing) and men more yang (protective, forward, and aggressive). In reality, however, a woman can have so much yang energy that she is more yang than many men. But because yin and yang are never static, this very yang woman may have a yin, sensitive, nurturing side as well.

These two terms are fascinating and fun if you are a seeker of the truth. And this concept of yin and yang is amazingly useful in reversing aging.

Know Yourself

Supposedly inscribed over the entrance to the ancient temple at Delphi were the words KNOW THYSELF. An extended version of this is sometimes cited as: "Know thyself—and thou shall know all the mysteries of the gods and of the universe."

One of the great gifts in growing older is to finally have a better understanding of who you are—your strengths, weaknesses, desires, and needs. But have you given much thought to whether you've inherited a yang or a yin constitution?

If you are more yang, you have larger bones, may be sexually aggressive, and have higher levels of testosterone. You might be more outgoing and hot-tempered, and you could anger easily.

You may rarely become tired or ill, but when you do, illness comes on suddenly and can be quite intense.

If you are more yin, on the other hand, you may be more reflective and quiet; have a smaller frame; be sexually passive and estrogen dominant; and be more cautious, anxious, and sometimes even fearful. You may have fragile health and suffer from lifelong chronic problems.

Aging and Disease vs. Body Ecology Foods and Supplements

How might the principles of yin and yang apply to disease? Well, an earlier chapter discussed how illness and disease are caused by imbalances. These imbalances can occur when either yin or yang dominates in the body.

Yang illness emerges when there is too much fire energy (inflammation) or when we are too stressed-out (uptight, with pulses racing). Yin illness occurs when we are too depleted (fragile, exhausted, and anxious).

Yang problems show up in a dramatic way. An example might be sudden pneumonia. Yin problems are more elusive and mysterious. A low-grade viral infection that comes and goes is an example of a yin condition.

As we age, we have traditionally become too yin (weak and depleted). This weakness allows inflammation (too much heat or yang energy) to thrive in our bodies. The right foods and supplements help us build the foundation to reverse the signs and symptoms of aging.

Remember, one of the primary anti-aging goals of the Baby Boomer Diet is to create more *daily chi energy* and to restore our *prenatal jing energy*. Both can be accumulated or stored for later use, or exhausted or used up entirely. The foods on the Baby Boomer Diet will create the foundation we need to rejuvenate and store energy.

Balance in Our Foods

The principles of yin and yang are also embodied in what we eat, so it makes sense that food would become a powerful agent of change and rejuvenation. What follows is a brief explanation of the yin/yang Principle of Balance and diet. But please know that you do not have to fully understand this principle. Indeed, it is far too complex to master quickly. It is, however, inherent in the Baby Boomer Diet and is one of the reasons why The Diet works so well.

Foods can be classified as too contracting, too expansive, or naturally balanced. Salt, for example, is considered very contracting and can even "shrink" the fluid in our cells. When our foods are too salty, we become edgy, even irritable. We might even suffer from a "yang" headache. Other examples of yang foods are eggs and animal proteins. Animals contain salt in their blood, making this food more contracting. When we eat too much animal protein and salty cheeses, we can become tense and closed, resulting in constipation.

Conversely, sugar is considered an overly expansive food. The bloodstream quickly absorbs it and produces quick energy (most people reach for a candy bar, alcohol, and even tobacco when they are too constricted with stress, because these are expansive substances . . . they relax us and produce a calming effect). An excess of sugar from substances such as coffee, alcohol, and chocolate; and from refined carbs such as breads, can create an imbalance in the blood, resulting in a hyperactive and overly kinetic ADHD state.

What this means for your diet is that you need to constantly be aware of balancing expansive and contracting foods. Too many contracting foods

One of the great gifts in growing older is to finally have a better understanding of who you are—your strengths, weaknesses, desires, and needs. But have you given much thought to whether you've inherited a yang or a yin constitution?

create a desire for expansive food, and vice versa. There's a reason most nightclubs and bars include bowls of salty peanuts and pretzels on the tables. The constricting salt creates a craving for something more expansive and sugary (alcohol). Alcohol, in turn, creates a need for something more contracting and salty (peanuts). This forms a vicious cycle that leaves the

Anti-Aging Application

*C*ombine sugar with stress, and you've got a recipe for cellular death—the bubonic plague of modern times. In the Middle Ages, it was called the Black Death. Today's plague might be called the "White Death." This is how devastating long-term use of processed sugars and refined carbs can be to our health and longevity. (See the mitochondrial-decline theory of aging in Chapter 3.)

body swinging back and forth in an attempt to stay balanced.

Some foods have built-in or inherent properties of balance and harmony: green land vegetables, sea vegetables, grain-like seeds such as quinoa and millet, and red-skin potatoes fall in the middle between contractive and expansive. These foods provide the most balanced and most healing energy for your body.

On the next page, you'll find a chart that shows you the continuum of expansive and contracting foods. It can help you plan meals that leave you feeling balanced and satisfied.

A Few Final Thoughts on Balance

Balance is not just about food, and it is a process rather than a final destination. We at Body Ecology regard the quest for balance and moderation in our lives as an ongoing awareness and conscientious effort. It's a practice and a principle that pervades every aspect of our lives—from our relationships, to how we manage our time, to the effort we give to healing ourselves.

The last section of this book will provide you with some proven anti-aging methods for reducing stress and achieving balance and well-being in your life. Next, we'll look at an important area of balance in the diet: acid and alkaline.

The Expansion/Contraction Continuum

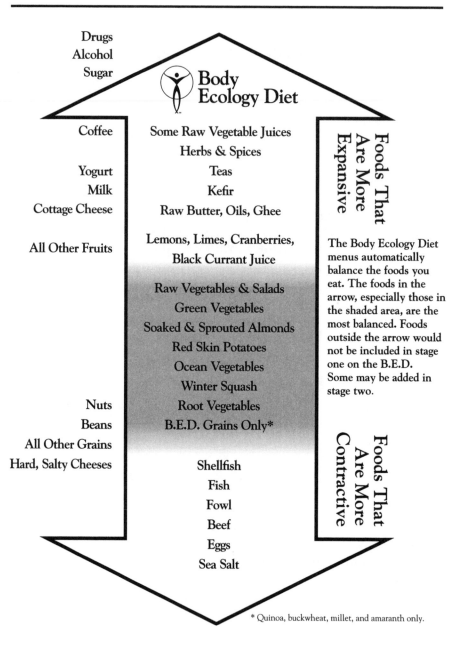

Drugs
Alcohol
Sugar

Body Ecology Diet

Coffee

Some Raw Vegetable Juices
Herbs & Spices

Yogurt

Teas

Milk

Kefir

Cottage Cheese

Raw Butter, Oils, Ghee

All Other Fruits

Lemons, Limes, Cranberries,
Black Currant Juice

Raw Vegetables & Salads
Green Vegetables
Soaked & Sprouted Almonds
Red Skin Potatoes
Ocean Vegetables
Winter Squash

Nuts

Root Vegetables

Beans

B.E.D. Grains Only*

All Other Grains

Hard, Salty Cheeses

Shellfish
Fish
Fowl
Beef
Eggs
Sea Salt

Foods That Are More Expansive

The Body Ecology Diet menus automatically balance the foods you eat. The foods in the arrow, especially those in the shaded area, are the most balanced. Foods outside the arrow would not be included in stage one on the B.E.D. Some may be added in stage two.

Foods That Are More Contractive

* Quinoa, buckwheat, millet, and amaranth only.

122

Chapter 12

The Principle of Acid and Alkaline: Knowing How to Choose Your Foods

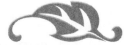

Most of us Baby Boomers are eager to slow down the aging process, and we want to get started right away! When the acidity in our diets is reduced, cells remain alive and healthy much longer. We age more slowly.

Homeostasis: Built-in Mechanisms for Achieving Balance

One of the most amazing features of the human body is its ability to keep body temperature, blood volume, and oxygen levels relatively constant, even when the environment around us is in constant change. This marvelous capacity for self-regulation and stability is called *homeostasis,* and it should be very reassuring to us. It shows us that our bodies constantly exert themselves on our behalf to maintain balance. In short, our bodies are working *for* us, not *against* us!

We shiver when we're cold, which increases heat production through muscle activity. We sweat when we're hot, which encourages heat loss by opening more blood vessels in the skin. We blink to protect our senses when the light is too bright or there is pollen in the air.

The pH, or balance between acid and alkaline, of our blood, saliva, and urine is also carefully regulated within a narrow range. The ideal pH of blood should be 7.36 to 7.44; if it drops below 7.2, it has become dangerously acidic and we can die. An even *slightly acidic decline* in pH, however, allows infections and disease and even cancer to develop inside us. It's vital that we maintain our blood close to the ideal of 7.4, especially if we want to reverse and prevent aging.

If you feel that you're aging too quickly, you must pay special attention to this Principle of Acid and Alkaline. Indeed, one of the main reasons we age is because the body becomes acidic. Do you have excess-blood-sugar problems—that is, insulin resistance or diabetes? Both are conditions that create acidity. This means that you will age sooner if your blood sugar is not brought into a healthy, normal range.

To keep your body more alkaline, your diet should consist of foods mostly from the plant kingdom—especially vegetables from the land and the sea. The more color, the better: dark green, leafy vegetables and dark—even black—ocean veggies, properly prepared so that you can digest them, are excellent examples of alkaline foods that keep your body within that ideal pH range.

When our bodies are too acidic, our cells hold onto toxins, and even if we try to stimulate the cells to cleanse and release these toxins so that we can stop aging, they cannot.

But Why Are Our Bodies So Acidic?

Perhaps for many of us, stress is the number one cause of acidity. Stress raises cortisol, and then sugar levels skyrocket. Because many of us in our generation are so in love with life and always on the go, we deal with constant stress, much of it of our own choosing. These elevated levels of cortisol and sugar keep the body very acidic. The only way we can change this is to intentionally create moments of peace and relaxation for ourselves. Practicing the art of gratitude for everything, even the challenges of life, helps tremendously, too.

And then there is diet. . . .

The Sweet Life . . . Not So Sweet

According to the U.S. Department of Agriculture (USDA), each American consumes 133 pounds of added sugar every year. A full one-third of our calories is obtained from junk food, soft drinks, sweets, alcohol, and salty snacks. This is one of the key reasons why the body of the typical American is heavily acidic rather than alkaline.

But there are other factors that contribute to this overly acidic condition:

- Carbohydrates
- Constipation (this is a really big one)
- Poor filtering from the liver and kidneys
- Improper food combining
- Drugs (both medicinal and recreational)
- Fatigue
- Negative thoughts such as worry and anger

When your body is too acidic, this means that it is losing and craving valuable alkaline minerals, such as sodium, calcium, potassium, and magnesium. Imbalances that result in too much acidity can lead to conditions such as arthritis, allergies, cancer, infectious diseases such as viruses, overproduction of yeast, obesity, bone loss, gout, adrenal malfunction, heart disease, depression, aggression, macular degeneration, and more. The only way to correct this imbalance is by reducing acidity and increasing alkaline levels; and you can do this best with Body Ecology's amazing probiotic diet, with stress-relieving herbs and therapies, and with the lifestyle changes you will discover in Part IV.

How Chronic Infections Play a
Role in Keeping Our Bodies Too Acidic

When we have low-grade infections in our bloodstream, such as herpes (a viral infection) or candida (a fungal infection), these pathogens literally eat minerals from our blood for their own needs. This loss of minerals continues to keep the body acidic. It also ensures that the pathogens have the perfect environment in which to continue to grow and multiply. We are in a vicious cycle that never ends and causes us to age. Obviously, these chronic infections must be brought under control, and this can be done the Body Ecology Way. When we alkalize our bodies with mineral-rich foods, these pathogens will die off. You can see why an alkaline diet is so essential.

When our bodies are acidic, our cells hold on to toxins, and even if we try to stimulate the cells to cleanse and release these toxins so that we can stop aging, they cannot. Why? Cells were created in such a way that they are not allowed to dump their poisons into the bloodstream when it is already too toxic. But when we take cleansing herbs, eat cleansing foods, and do colonics, our cells will then let their toxins out.

Here's an analogy: Let's say you live in New York City and the garbage collectors go on strike. After several weeks of everyone putting their trash out on the streets, the accumulation of garbage would force the mayor to announce that all inhabitants must retain their trash in their homes until the strike ends. Well, your cells are in a similar situation. They know it won't do any good to dump more toxins into the bloodstream, only to have them reabsorbed.

Anti-Aging Application

When our blood becomes too acidic, it will actually trigger genetic markers for disease. It also sucks important minerals from the blood, which can impact our hormone levels and weaken the respiratory system, meaning there is less oxygen for our cells.

(See hormonal- and mitochondrial-decline theories of aging in Chapter 3.)

The solution is to first alkalize your blood and begin to use cleansing techniques, such as colonics, and herbs that encourage the toxins to come out. Switch to a mineral-rich, probiotic-rich, sugar-free diet.

Alkalizing Your Body Through Diet

There are certain foods you will want to avoid and certain foods you will want as a mainstay of your diet if your goal is to combat aging. Think *minerals* when it comes to alkalizing, and this will help you choose wisely. Avoid the foods that deplete minerals from your blood and bones. *Eat the foods that replenish them and store them in your bones.*

Acidic foods to avoid:

- Sugar, candy, and soft drinks
- Alcohol (wine, beer, and hard liquor)
- Flour products
- Beans, soybean products, and tofu
- Processed foods and preservatives
- Dairy foods with sugar, such as commercial ice cream
- Rice, hemp, and almond milk (contain sugar)
- Soy milk and soy cheeses
- Dried fruit
- Artificial sweeteners (Splenda, NutraSweet, saccharin, and Equal)
- Commercial refined vinegar

There are some acidic foods that are okay to eat on the Baby Boomer Diet.

These should be consumed in limited quantities and should be of the highest quality available. Keep the proportion of these items down to 20 percent of your meal, and include them only if they are right for your body.

Acceptable acidic foods:

- Animal protein (beef, poultry, eggs, fish, and shellfish)
- Buckwheat

- Organic, unrefined oils (olive, pumpkin seed, and coconut)

- Nuts and nut butter (except almond butter, which is more alkaline)

- Fermented dairy kefir and yogurt (from cow, sheep, or goat milk)

- Fermented cheeses

- Stevia or Lakanto sweeteners

Healthy *alkalizing* foods should make up the largest portion of your diet.

Eighty percent of your meal should be alkaline-forming foods. These include the following:

- Green drinks

- Most land vegetables

- Ocean vegetables

- Cultured vegetables

- Millet, quinoa, and amaranth

- Sea salt

- Herbs and herbal teas

- Seeds (except sesame)

- Mineral water

- Raw apple-cider vinegar

- Young coconut kefir

- Probiotic liquids (InnergyBiotic, Dong Quai, and CocoBiotic [available from **www.bodyecology.com**])

- Soaked and sprouted almonds

- Sour fruits (lemons, limes, unsweetened cranberries and black currants, and pomegranates)

There are also neutral foods, which do not add to an acidic condition. These include raw butter, ghee, and cream.

*P*H paper is an easy and convenient way to check your level of acidity. Inexpensive pH strips can be purchased in your local health-food store and come with instructions and a color chart. You simply hold the pH paper under your urine stream several times a day and compare it to the chart enclosed in the package. Your first morning urine-test paper should be yellow to light green, indicating acid production from the previous day, but as the day goes on, the urine should become more alkaline—that is, if you're eating 80 to 90 percent plant-based food. Your saliva can be used as well, but this simple test is a good way to calculate your food needs.

No More "Senior Moments"!

Are you forgetful and distracted? Do you have problems with focus and organization? This doesn't have to be a *fait accompli* of getting older. You can begin reversing these frightening and frustrating symptoms simply by "alkalizing" your blood now.

The Baby Boomer Diet can have a direct impact on your mental functioning and memory. One of the most obvious signs of an acidic body is an inability to stay focused. You may also find that you're less disciplined or that your willpower is slipping. Excess acidity depletes your adrenals of the large amounts of minerals they require to be healthy. DHEA (often called the "youth hormone") is made in these glands and is important for healthy memory. For example, a person with Alzheimer's has low levels of DHEA.

In Chinese medicine, the adrenals are paired with the kidney, bladder, brain, sexual organs, and skeleton. Mineral-deficient, acidic blood affects all these parts of the body. And what are the possible consequences? Our skeletons develop osteoporosis, we lose control of our bladders, and we begin to forget those we love the most.

The Principle of Acid and Alkaline demonstrates that premature aging is optional and preventable. It is a very important one to master if you want to stay forever young. The next chapter will cover two more principles that can help structure your diet, and are effective methods for restricting calories and improving digestion.

Chapter 13

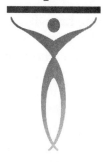

The Principle of Food Combining & the Principle of 80/20: Knowing How to Eat

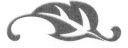

The "Battle of the Bulge" that hits Baby Boomers in midlife can be more like a minor skirmish—with these little-known secrets to weight loss and healthy digestion.

Many of us Baby Boomers have been plagued with digestive problems for decades. Even those of us who were fortunate enough to eat, digest, and absorb anything we wanted when we were younger are now most likely experiencing bloating, gas, acid indigestion, stomach pain, undigested food in our stools, diarrhea, constipation, and fatigue after meals. The billions of dollars' worth of drugs prescribed each year for digestive problems make it clear that digestion is truly one of our most serious health problems.

Even though we are spending a lot of money on drugs to address these problems, research shows that our generation is not comfortable taking them. Fortunately for us, poor digestion can be prevented and corrected without the need for expensive drugs with negative side effects.

Today we have the advantage of solid scientific knowledge that gives us a precise understanding of how our digestive tracts function. We know about the essential enzymes that must be produced in each of our digestive organs to break down every kind of food we eat . . . proteins, sugars, and fats. And, if we are lacking in any of them, they are available as supplements.

Digestive enzymes taken consistently with meals will help us maintain the youthful levels that we need in order to delay aging. But there are three other important tools we have at our disposal in the Baby Boomer Diet to enhance our ability to digest food:

1. Fermented foods

2. The Principle of Food Combining

3. The Principle of 80/20

In Chapter 15, you will learn more about fermented foods, and in this chapter you will learn how to apply the simple rules of food combining and 80/20 that will allow your digestive tract to do its job more efficiently . . . without a lot of extra effort.

The Principle of Food Combining

Food combining means to deliberately eat certain foods with other foods. Why do we do this?

- **Because foods that are not compatible in the stomach digest poorly and prevent us from obtaining the nutrients in those foods.** This is why we eat . . . to obtain nutrients to nourish the cells in our bodies so we have energy.

- **Because when foods digest easily, there is less bloating and gas in the digestive tract.** This gas is not only uncomfortable and embarrassing, but it is also often a frequent cause of constipation. Gas pockets in the colon literally stop the flow of material through the digestive tract.

Anti-Aging Application

*T*he Principle of Food Combining and the Principle of 80/20 are directly related to one of the most proven methods of life extension we know of today—calorie restriction. Because food combining improves the way we digest what we eat, making the nutrients and minerals more available to us, we can eat much less.

- **Because incompatible foods can cause an over-production of alcohol and sugars.** Pathogens such as yeast feed off these sugars and multiply more rapidly in these prime conditions, creating more toxins and more acidity in the body.

- **Because people today tend to have low stomach acid.** Hydrochloric acid (HCl), produced in the stomach, triggers the other enzymes to go to work and digest our foods. Without this acid, we become protein-malnourished and even more deficient in minerals . . . aging rapidly. As we age, almost all of us become deficient in HCl. When we properly combine our food, focus on alkalizing our bodies, and even use supplemental enzymes with HCl, efficient digestion can occur. In other words, give your stomach a break; don't force it to do what it can no longer do.

The Benefits of Food Combining

It allows for excellent utilization of nutrients. Even if you eat the healthiest foods on the planet, if they are poorly digested, the nutrients in them are not absorbed. Most of the degenerative conditions facing us today (especially cancer) are ones where the body is literally wasting away. When our bodies lack nutrients, we lose muscle tone, the elasticity of our veins, our vision, the minerals in our bones, our hair's color and thickness, our youthful hormones, our mental abilities, and more. Proper food combining greatly assists in the absorption of nutrients.

133

It causes us to look and feel younger. Poorly digested foods are toxic foods. As they travel to our intestines, undigested proteins, fats, and carbohydrates turn into dangerous poisons and gases. These toxins affect our thinking, behavior, and mood. Toxic people *look* toxic—their bodies are often bloated, and their complexion is dull in color. The toxins stemming from our digestive tract are definitely affecting how quickly we age.

> *Properly combined food is assimilated and metabolized better, reducing the likelihood that it will be stored as fat. Why haven't weight-loss "experts" caught on to this?*

It helps us maintain metabolic enzymes. Besides the *digestive* enzymes in the stomach and small intestine that break down food into nutrients, we also have *metabolic* enzymes in every cell of our bodies. Metabolic enzymes produced by the liver, pancreas, gallbladder, and other organs are catalysts that speed up the chemical reaction within our cells, helping create energy. They also help the cells detoxify. We could not see, hear, feel, or think without them. *How is this related to aging?* In a nutshell, you want to retain your metabolic enzymes close to the same level they were when you were a child. If you combine your food in such a way that each meal digests well, and if you consume enzyme-rich fermented foods and also use high-quality digestive enzymes, you will *retain* more of these precious metabolic enzymes. This is a powerful yet simple tool you can use to regain your vitality, while keeping yourself from aging.

It reduces gas and other signs of indigestion. Another plus to food combining is the elimination of embarrassing flatulence. Gas and stomach gurgling will be minimized or disappear.

It helps us maintain our ideal weight. By utilizing the Principle of Food Combining, you'll also have discovered a "best-kept secret" to keeping the weight off. This is because properly combined food is assimilated and metabolized better, reducing the likelihood that it will be stored as fat. I have always been amazed that the companies that sell products that promote weight loss haven't caught on to this valuable tool.

Six Rules of Food Combining

Food combining always seems so complicated to people, yet it is actually one of the easiest of the principles to implement. In fact, if you practice it for one week, it will become second nature to you. There are six simple rules to food combining:

Rule #1: Eat *animal protein* with nonstarchy vegetables.
Why? Simply put, when you eat animal-protein foods such as eggs and meat, your stomach produces hydrochloric acid and an enzyme called pepsin. When you eat a starch such as a potato or rice, an enzyme called ptyalin is secreted, creating an alkaline condition. Put the two together, such as chicken and rice, and the acid and alkaline conditions neutralize each other, inhibiting effective digestion.

- **No!** Chicken and rice
- **Yes!** Fish with stir-fried or steamed vegetables

Rule #2: Eat *grains* and *grain-like seeds* (that is, quinoa, millet, buckwheat, and amaranth) with starchy and nonstarchy vegetables.
Why? This combination is the easiest of all meals to digest. On the Body Ecology program, grain-like seeds are preferred over grains because they are gluten free and lack sugar, yet are higher in vegetarian protein. When you're practicing calorie restriction with optimal nutrition, "less is more." Your goal is to eat a smaller portion of a food yet obtain more nutrients (more protein). (Additional information on grain-like seeds can be found in Chapter 20.)

- **No!** Chicken and rice, beef hamburger on a wheat bun, or pizza crust with cheese and salami
- **Yes!** Rice stir-fried with onions, garlic, broccoli, yellow squash, and red pepper
- **Yes!** Potatoes with quinoa

Rule #3: Eat *fruit* alone and at least 30 minutes before any other meal, or combined with a protein/fat (see below). Or eat *acidic fruit* combined with leafy-green salads.

Why? Because fruits pass through the digestive tract very quickly. When they are eaten with animal-protein foods (such as eggs and bacon) or starchy vegetables (such as potatoes or winter squashes) or grains (such as toast), they become trapped with these other foods. Then the fruit sugars cause fermentation; bloating; and gas, which can remain in the digestive tract for hours—and even days—causing discomfort, embarrassment, and constipation.

Most fruits are not encouraged on the Baby Boomer Diet, especially in the earliest stage, because they are too sweet. When you eat very sweet fruits (bananas, dates, or figs, for example), especially in the morning, this weakens your adrenals, thus lowering your energy for starting the day. *Sweet* fruits also contribute to a systemic yeast overgrowth. Once your inner ecosystem is well established from consuming fermented foods and liquids in your diet, and your body becomes more alkaline, you can add in members of the sour-fruit family, such as berries or grapefruit, and combine them with milk kefir and nuts and seeds.

- **No!** Traditional breakfast of eggs, orange juice, toast, and bananas
- **Yes!** Bowl of blueberries combined with milk kefir and walnuts
- **Yes!** Blueberries with raw cream
- **Yes!** Grapefruit with avocado (a protein/fat) on lettuce leaf
- **Yes!** Glass of fermented young-coconut juice with any chosen fruit
- **Yes!** Tomato (an acid fruit) in a leafy-green salad

Fermented foods eaten with fruit contain beneficial microflora that eat up the sugars in the fruit. Fats, like butter, ghee, and raw cream, help slow down the absorption of the sugars in the fruit.

Rule #4: Combine *fats* and *oils* with animal protein, grains, grain-like seeds, and starchy or nonstarchy vegetables. They can be enjoyed in a meal *with protein* and *with the recommended grain-like seeds.*

Why? Nature seems to put fats and oils in many foods naturally. On the Body Ecology program, cooking with ghee, coconut oil, and red-palm oil is preferred because their fatty acids can take a higher heat before losing their nutritional value. Raw, extra-virgin oils can be used on top of, in, or with our foods. Nature seems to have created fats in such a way that they go with everything we eat. They are an important anti-aging nutrient. (See Chapter 17.)

- **Yes!** Salmon in a leafy-green salad with other raw veggies and an extra-virgin-oil dressing

- **Yes!** Baked potato or acorn squash with raw, organic butter

- **Yes!** Quinoa tabouli salad with an extra-virgin-oil dressing

Rule #5: Combine *protein/fats* with other protein/fats. (Protein/fats are foods that contain both protein and fat.) Avocado, dairy foods (milk and milk kefir, yogurt, and cheese), and nuts and seeds are all protein/fats and are easily digested when eaten together. Protein/fats also combine well with fruits from the acid-fruit family. If you have "strong digestive fire," you may find that you can also eat them with animal-protein foods. (For many, nuts and seeds are difficult to digest.)

Why? These foods combine well because they are alike in nature. Sometimes the fat is of vegetarian origin (as in an avocado), and sometimes it is from an animal protein (like the fat in dairy foods), but all seem to be quite compatible.

- **No!** Milk kefir (a protein/fat) with toast (a starch)
- **Yes!** Diced organic chicken (a protein) in a leafy-green salad with finely chopped walnuts (a protein/fat)
- **Yes!** Leafy-green salad with avocado, roasted pumpkin seeds, and raw veggies
- **Yes!** Milk kefir (a protein/fat) with blueberries (an acid fruit) on top
- **Yes!** A leafy-green salad with avocado, walnuts, and raspberries tossed with a milk-kefir dressing

Rule #6: Combine *protein/starches* with nonstarchy vegetables from the land and ocean.

Protein/starches contain mostly starch but also some protein. Beans (also called pulses) are both protein *and* starch. Remember that proteins and starches don't combine well, so these foods are naturally more difficult to digest.

Why? Since these foods are innately difficult to digest (and are acidic), combining them with an easily digested, alkaline food (vegetables) works best.

- **No!** Black beans with rice
- **Yes!** Black beans with onions, garlic, celery, and kale
- **Yes!** Garbanzo beans in a leafy-green salad

The Principle of 80/20

The Principle of 80/20 works well in conjunction with that of Food Combining, as both are about correcting and improving digestion. Many of us have "eyes that are bigger than our stomachs." We eat huge portions, consuming not only to the point of satiation, but usually well beyond that. This puts far too much stress on our already-overtaxed digestive tracts and slows down the digestive process, which in turn creates an environment where yeast can flourish.

Earlier I talked about how the foods on the Baby Boomer Diet emphasize *quality* over *quantity;* they are so satisfying and nourishing that you will need less food in order to feel content. So, while you are on The Diet, you may find yourself applying the 80/20 Principle quite unconsciously and with little effort. It has three simple rules:

1. Eat until your stomach is 80 percent full, leaving 20 percent available for digestion.

2. Eighty percent of the food on your plate should be land and/or ocean vegetables, with the remaining 20 percent reserved for a meat protein, grain, or starchy vegetable.

3. Approximately 80 percent of the foods on your plate should be alkaline forming, and 20 percent should be acid forming.

Rule #1: Leave more room

Leave a little room in your stomach (approximately 20 percent) for the digestive juices to do their job. This means leaving the table before your stomach is *full*. Come back later if desired and eat again. If you're malnourished, you may need to eat more often; six smaller meals a day are preferable to two or three large, "overstuffed" meals. This is practicing *calorie restriction with optimal nutrition,* because the foods on The Diet will be excellent-*quality* foods. Also, once you introduce fermented foods and liquids into your diet, you will find that your digestion improves so dramatically that eating less will really be eating more. More nutrients will be absorbed and enter your cells, leaving you satisfied with less food.

Rule #2: Eat more vegetables

The second part of the 80/20 Principle relates to food combining. In addition to eating too much, most Americans eat meals with a preponderance of acid-forming foods (animal proteins, pasta, bread, and rice) and a deficiency of alkaline-forming foods, such as nonstarchy vegetables. So, the second 80/20 rule suggests that at least 80 percent of the food on your plate be land or ocean vegetables. The remaining 20 percent can be:

*   Animal protein, such as fish, poultry, lamb, or eggs

*   A nut or seed pâté

*   A starchy vegetable, such as a potato, artichoke, or butternut squash

Although this rule may seem a bit daunting at first, you will immediately begin to experience its benefits. No more after-meal fatigue or bloating. No more acid indigestion or feelings of anxiety. Instead, you will leave the table calm and satisfied. You will also be digesting a superior level and quality of nutrients, which will give you the energy that seems to have gone out the door along with your Grateful Dead records.

Rule #3: Eat more alkaline-forming foods

A preponderance of acid-forming foods in the American diet makes it especially important to eat more alkaline-forming ones, creating a healthy ratio in the body. For more on how to create the proper acid/alkaline balance, see Chapter 12.

Master Food Combining Step by Step

This is a new way of eating, so be kind to yourself and give yourself a month or so to become a master of these rules. Break up each part into steps. For example, plan just one meal with your favorite protein food. Broiled salmon, perhaps? Then serve the fish with a leafy-green salad and two other nonstarchy vegetables. Maybe asparagus? Broccoli? Yellow squash sautéed with onions? A serving of cultured veggies (see Chapter 15) would also complete your perfectly combined meal.

Keep the food-combining chart (on the facing page) on your refrigerator, and refer to it often in the beginning. Before you know it, these rules will become a part of how you eat quite naturally. I can promise you that if you forget them or choose to "cheat," you'll quickly see how effectively they work.

B.E.D. Food-Combining Chart

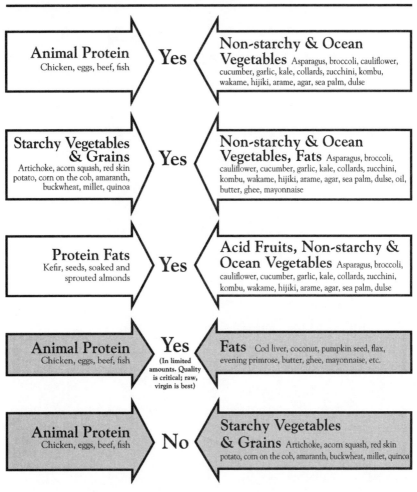

Animal Protein Chicken, eggs, beef, fish	**Yes**	**Non-starchy & Ocean Vegetables** Asparagus, broccoli, cauliflower, cucumber, garlic, kale, collards, zucchini, kombu, wakame, hijiki, arame, agar, sea palm, dulse
Starchy Vegetables & Grains Artichoke, acorn squash, red skin potato, corn on the cob, amaranth, buckwheat, millet, quinoa	**Yes**	**Non-starchy & Ocean Vegetables, Fats** Asparagus, broccoli, cauliflower, cucumber, garlic, kale, collards, zucchini, kombu, wakame, hijiki, arame, agar, sea palm, dulse, oil, butter, ghee, mayonnaise
Protein Fats Kefir, seeds, soaked and sprouted almonds	**Yes**	**Acid Fruits, Non-starchy & Ocean Vegetables** Asparagus, broccoli, cauliflower, cucumber, garlic, kale, collards, zucchini, kombu, wakame, hijiki, arame, agar, sea palm, dulse
Animal Protein Chicken, eggs, beef, fish	**Yes** (In limited amounts. Quality is critical; raw, virgin is best)	**Fats** Cod liver, coconut, pumpkin seed, flax, evening primrose, butter, ghee, mayonnaise, etc.
Animal Protein Chicken, eggs, beef, fish	**No**	**Starchy Vegetables & Grains** Artichoke, acorn squash, red skin potato, corn on the cob, amaranth, buckwheat, millet, quinoa

NOTES: All fruits should be eaten alone (30 minutes before or 3 hours after eating) with exception of the acid fruits, which may be eaten with protein fats. Only very sour acid fruits are on the B.E.D. (lemons, limes, cranberries, and black currant juice).
SUGAR–Not on B.E.D., but should be eaten alone (30 minutes before or 3 hours after eating). Does not combine well with any other foods.
DAIRY–Not on B.E.D. If introduced later, ferment and eat alone (30 minutes before or 3 hours after eating) or with raw salads, acid fruits, or seeds and nuts.
PROTEIN STARCHES–Dried peas, soybeans, and beans are not initially on B.E.D. If introduced later, they should then be eaten with non-starchy vegetables and cultured veggies.

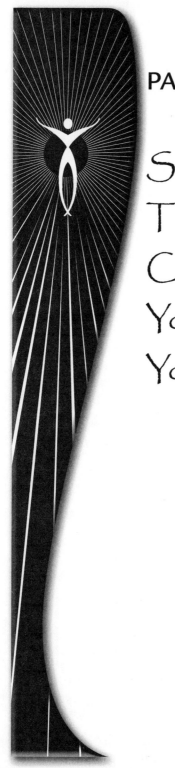

PART IV

Superfoods
That
Create a
Younger
You

Chapter 14

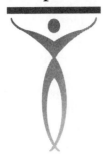

The Art of Eating: A Social and Soulful Path to Nourishment

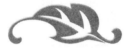

Most of us completely underestimate the power of food. Foods are far more effective in restoring energy and modulating oxidative stress than any supplement or drug on the market today. *Along with our positive thoughts and intentions, food offers us the greatest potential to reverse the aging process.*

Food is never boring or one-dimensional. It can be contractive or expansive, aggressive or calming, dry or mucus forming, heat producing or cooling, acidic or alkaline . . . the list goes on and on.

Food as Energy

Food affects us emotionally and spiritually. It has an intrinsic energy and intelligence that it communicates to us on a cellular level (see sidebar on next page). This energy can actually alter our behavior, performance, and appearance. I've seen many lives elevated—renewed and healed—through the power of wholesome, nutritious food.

Because of its healing potential and spiritual energy, food should be sacred to us—prepared with reverence and consumed with gratitude. But alas, even though the passing decades have brought us more insight and wisdom, many of us still make our food choices based on our taste buds and our desire for immediate gratification.

Every time we eat, we must now be asking ourselves, "What does my body *need,* not just *want?* How can I nourish and heal myself with the food I put on my plate today?"

As we make our eating choices, we must also reflect on how the food was grown or raised, how it was slaughtered and transported to us, and so forth. These choices not only impact us on an individual level, but have global implications as well.

Research shows that Baby Boomers will remain quite active and busy as the decades pass. We will still need plenty of energizing nutrients (protein, minerals, vitamins, antioxidants, enzymes, and small amounts of high-quality fats and oils) to sustain our dynamic lifestyles. But because our bodies won't

Our Very Cells Recognize Food as Friend or Foe

*E*very piece of food we consume comes into contact with our cell surfaces, which are loaded with receptors that identify it as positive, neutral, or negative. Our cells recognize something as a "friendly food" or an "unfriendly food." There is a whole field of science devoted to this, called *nutrigenomics,* or the way food as information speaks to our genes. Food elements contact cell surface receptors, which pass the information to cell messengers called *kinases, chemokines,* and *cytokines.* These messengers take the information to the nucleus and give it to the genes. This process is called *signal transduction.*

Our genes respond positively to organic, natural foods. In other words, a mostly plant-based diet, including properly prepared grain-like seeds, land and ocean vegetables, fermented foods, and a modest amount of organic animal products. The genes in our cells respond positively when they receive messages from a simple piece of broccoli, containing myriad molecules with names like *indoles, carotenoids, lutein, glucosinolates, isothiocyanates, sulforaphanes,* and many more.

be as efficient at digesting foods, we will need to find ways of preparing them so that we can utilize the nutrients more effectively.

Eating less but also eating foods of higher nutrient density are two of our most important tools for keeping youthful, disease free, and fit. We can bring our thoughts and intentions to *how* we eat as well; and mealtimes can be wonderful opportunities to practice developing our hearts, minds, and wills.

Food Is a Medicine That Speaks to Our Souls

Unlike more traditional cultures, we are never taught to think of food as a tool for healing. But it is really much more than a remedy for what ails us; indeed, it is food for the *soul*.

In his book *The Yoga of Nutrition*, Omraam Mikkael Aivanhov, a spiritual master from France, writes: "Food is a love letter sent to us by our Creator, and we must learn to read it. It is the most eloquent, the most potent of love letters, for it says, I love you and I am giving you life and strength."[1]

Food is full of sunlight, flavor, color, shape, and texture. How sad that we swallow it without reading the love letter carefully.

Aivanhov continues: "Food is condensed, concentrated Light and sound. Light sings: Light is music, it speaks; Light is the voice of God."[2]

Mindful Eating

Do you eat unconsciously or quickly so you can get on with the really important things in life? Instead of enjoying a meal quietly and consciously, are your daily cares and stresses churning about in your stomach? Do you leave the table feeling sluggish and sleepy?

It's little wonder many of us don't digest our foods properly. The *way* we eat is every bit as important as *what* we eat.

Many spiritual traditions practice mindful eating, which simply means to slow down and truly experience the aromas, flavors, and textures of the food. Chewing it slowly and well, and enjoying it in a quiet setting—rather than being rushed, agitated, and halfway out the door—is an essential part of this practice.

Ideally, we should treat the body as if it is a sacred laboratory where each day we experiment with delicious foods and herbs while carefully observing how it responds.

Part of the stress and anxiety so many of us feel today is because we have lost our connection with nature and our gratitude for her amazing gifts to us. When we eat with gratitude, we reestablish that vital link to the natural world around us. We must learn to have a deeper appreciation for those who make our meals possible; and, if we've prepared them ourselves, we do so with a listening spirit, allowing our intuition to take over so that we are tuned in to what our bodies are asking for in that moment. We come to learn the difference between eating until we are overfed and doing so until we are satisfied.

Ideally, we should treat the body as if it is a sacred laboratory where each day we experiment with delicious foods and herbs while carefully observing how it responds.

What else is involved in mindful eating? Preparing our meals deliberately and thoughtfully so that everything we need is easily at hand . . . setting a beautiful table . . . taking time to breathe deeply throughout the meal . . . designating a space and time that's quiet and uninterrupted—all these are ways we make eating a kind of spiritual practice, a sacred rite where food is transformed into strength, energy, love, and light.

Inside the Body Ecology Foods

Body Ecology foods are replete with fortifying *chi* energy—ideal for anyone who wants to feel more vigorous and vital.

Body Ecology foods are *probiotic*—ideal for creating a strong, disease-free body. The word *probiotic* might be a new one to you. It means literally "for life." Probiotics are living microorganisms that have a beneficial effect on the body because of the way they function in the digestive tract. Most probiotics contain *Lactobacillus* or *Bifidobacterium,* which are beneficial bacteria. All of the probiotic foods and supplements recommended on The Diet are safe, effective, and designed to enhance intestinal health

Probiotics have many documented health benefits:

- They enhance immune function.

- They help reduce the risk of intestinal illnesses.

- They assist lactose-intolerant people with lactose digestion.

- They provide protection against infections.

- They replenish the gut with healthy bacteria after the use of antibiotics.

- They may reduce the risk of allergies if given to children early enough in life.

- Recent research suggests that they may help in the management of inflammatory bowel disease and decrease the risk of certain cancers.

Body Ecology foods offer a perfect balance of proteins, carbohydrates, and healthy fats—ideal for people who have suffered through exclusionary, nutritionally lopsided diets.

Body Ecology foods are antifungal—ideal for people with yeast infections.

Body Ecology foods are gluten and casein free—ideal for people with allergies to wheat or milk protein.

Body Ecology foods are low in sugars—ideal for people with weight issues, candida, or adrenal fatigue.

Body Ecology foods have the greatest bioavailability, meaning they are quickly and efficiently accessed by the body—ideal for people with low energy and weakened digestive systems.

Body Ecology foods are nutrient-dense—ideal for anyone who wants to look and feel better!

Some Things You Might Experience on The Diet

New Tastes and Textures

Humans have six basic tastes—*sweet, salty, bitter, savory, pungent,* and *sour.* Probiotic foods provide the sour taste, which may be one that is less developed in you than the others. A wide variety of tastes and colors is essential to obtaining all the nutrients that food has to offer. Some of the Body Ecology fermented foods, such as young coconut kefir and milk kefir or cultured vegetables, may be a new taste sensation to you. Try to keep an open mind as you explore foods outside your comfort zone.

The idea of eating sea vegetables may make you wrinkle your nose . . . or you may be someone who won't skip a beat when confronting these new additions to your food arsenal. If at first you're a bit skittish about some of the foods, that's okay.

Remember the Principle of Step by Step? It's okay to take your time. You'll soon find yourself adding sea vegetables to soups and stews and salads and stir-fries because they have so many flavors and are so fortifying that you miss them when they're not there. Their high mineral content is very important to aging Baby Boomers, because as we advance in years, our bodies become deficient in these minerals.

If you are more accustomed to traditional high-calorie grains, such as rice or pasta, some of Body Ecology's recommended grain-like seeds, such as quinoa and millet, may be a bit different. I think, however, you'll find that they are quite full of flavor and offer a refreshing variety to your daily fare. Body Ecology grain-like seeds are some of the most nutritious foods in the world. Eat them often but especially later in the day, as they are calming and conducive to sleep.

Over time your body has acquired a "memory" for the foods it thinks it wants, even if they are unhealthy! It will take a little time to "reeducate" your palate. After you've been on the Baby Boomer Diet for a few days, you'll begin to experience the more robust and potent flavors of pure, whole, well-combined ingredients. As your body acquires new food memories, the result will be a greater appreciation for the essence and aromas of truly healthy, satisfying foods. Time to reawaken your palate!

Intestinal Discomfort

If you're not accustomed to eating fermented foods, at first you could experience some indigestion (gas and bloating). This is because the mighty microflora are busy changing their environment (your intestines) into a much more pleasant place. They want to survive, colonize, and thrive. In a week or so, this phase will pass; however, this is a good time to drink plenty of springwater (away from meals), make sure your bowels are eliminating well, and do enemas and colonics (see Chapter 25) to cleanse yourself of the toxic material that is making you age way before your time.

Share What You're Learning!

I encourage you to experiment and explore! Find those foods that suit your tastes and needs the best. Getting to know these new foods and how to prepare them in fun and interesting ways is one of the joys of The Diet. As a matter of fact, we welcome new recipes and discoveries. Please feel free to e-mail Body Ecology so we can share your recipe with others on our website: **recipes@bodyecology.com**.

In the pages that follow, you will learn about new foods, new ways of preparing them, and how to maximize their benefits for optimal health and healing.

From the Physician's Desk

"Many of the foods we eat today are new to our genetic code, and our genes respond to them in often-negative ways."

For too long we have underestimated the impact of food on the body. Over the course of 70-plus years on the planet, our bodies take in 20 to 25 tons of food. The gut lining, like the lungs and the skin, is one of the most absorbent areas in the body, and as we know, three-quarters of the immune system is located there. Our greatest exposure to foreign material is through the food we eat, and this food provides critical information that is interpreted by the immune system.

The gut lining reads food like a book, and it recognizes what it likes and doesn't like, and whether the food is friend or foe. Food is not some undifferentiated substance that passes benignly through our systems and is never heard from again. It has qualitative differences. Until very recently, for example, we thought all protein was the same. Thirty grams of protein were deemed to be the same all across the spectrum, whether in the form of beef, legumes, nuts, or fish. Now there's been a paradigm shift; and we know that just as with carbs, there are good, bad, and neutral proteins. We have finally begun to recognize that food consists not just of fat, protein, and carbohydrates, but of infinitely subtle messengers that communicate information to our bodies in profound ways.

High-quality food—rich in antioxidants, enzymes, and minerals, with the right kinds of natural carbs that are slowly absorbed—speaks to our genetic code in a way that keeps our bodies healthy and happy. On the other hand, poor-quality food causes our cells to go into a defense mode and up-regulate our immunity. Once food gets into the blood, it starts affecting receptors on our cells.

Before going further, some simple definitions with regard to cells are in order. A cell consists of three general areas:

1. **Cell membrane**—surrounds, protects, and contains the contents of the cell. It is the site of all receptors that take information from outside to inside the cell.

2. **Cytoplasm**—contains the cell's vital machinery for making materials such as proteins (endoplasmic reticulum, or ER); managing cell energy (mitochondria); and breaking down old, worn-out proteins (proteosomes)—as well as hundreds of other types of machinery with various functions.

3. **Nucleus**—contains the genetic code (23 pairs of chromosomes, which contain thousands of genes). These are protected by the *epigenome,* a series of enzymes and complex molecules surrounding the genes. The epigenome responds to information brought to it through the cytoplasm by carriers called *protein kinases.* The epigenome then opens in a controlled manner to allow some genes to be expressed and others to be silenced.

This is how our cells "read" the food we eat:

• Once digested food gets into the blood, it begins interacting with cell surface receptors that take the information about the food and send it to the inside of the cell (the cytoplasm).

• Inside the cell, specialized cell messengers interact with the molecules of food entering the cytoplasm, and take the information of the food into the nucleus at the center of the cell.

• The genes in the nucleus are covered by the epigenome, much like a book is enclosed by its cover. The epigenome responds to the electrochemical messages it receives from the protein kinases.

• This allows the epigenome (book cover) to selectively open some genes (pages), which will be "read," while others will remain closed.

• The genes that are read (gene expression) send messages back to the cytoplasm, which contains protein-making factories.

• Proteins will be manufactured to maintain the health of the cell or to alert it to foreign invaders. In the latter case, protein messengers (pro-inflammatory cytokines) sound the alarm within the cell and send the message to all surrounding ones that something of danger is present.

- This reaction can be very minor and undetectable except by sensitive blood tests, or it can manifest as sinus congestion, abdominal bloating, or a headache. In severe cases, such as peanut allergy, it can be instantly life threatening.

Not even a hundred years ago, our diet was confined mostly to meat, dairy, eggs, seeds, nuts, legumes, and vegetables. We didn't have manufactured and processed foods. They are new to our epigenetic and genetic code. Our codes have to respond to these new entities in some way, and unfortunately, it is often negative. However, it is only our beautifully formed body following its ancient codes (or blueprints)—and trying to protect itself—that causes the immune challenges.

The power of the Body Ecology foods is that they are in synchronization with our ancient codes. Therefore, on The Diet, the immune system will most likely stay in balance. This is important because there are many other factors, such as physical and emotional stresses, that can overactivate and/ or dysregulate (impair) the immune system, especially in the presence of poor diet and environmental choices. I have seen many healthy young people do very well until they face college finals and follow them up with a wild night of unhealthy foods, alcohol, and partying. They may then find themselves sick for days, weeks, or months thereafter.

— *Leonard Smith, M.D.*

Chapter 15

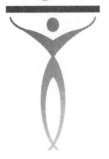

Fermented Foods:
Anti-Aging Miracles

As ancient as the great Flood of Noah,
fermented foods are becoming the new "stars"
of the natural-foods world.

Modern science is now confirming that fermented foods are the quintessential anti-aging foods. They are essential to restoring our prenatal jing and are the true "superstars" of the natural-foods world. At Body Ecology, we are pleased to be able to teach you how to use them to reverse biological aging.

The focus on these ancient . . . yet new-to-you . . . foods is what makes the Body Ecology Way stand out above all other "diets" being promoted today. It works! In fact, it makes the other ways of eating obsolete. This chapter shows you why you really *must* include fermented foods daily to regain the vitality of your youth.

What Are Fermented Foods?

By the time Baby Boomers were born, the refrigerator was an essential appliance in the home. Although we take it for granted, it is a relatively young technology. Even our parents might recall the iceman bringing frozen blocks to a wooden icebox that was lined with tin. So how did people survive without refrigeration for thousands of years? They ate foods fresh from the fields and dried, smoked, and fermented them.

In some parts of the world, fermented foods are believed to be the food of Noah's ark, when the world was covered with water. They were certainly included in the diets of American Indians, who preserved their meats and fish by fermenting and smoking them. To ensure that they had vegetables through the long winter months, they fermented and then buried them in earthenware containers.

Probiotic-rich fermented foods may seem either foreign or familiar, depending upon your cultural heritage. All traditions still have their own versions of cultured foods, which are staples in the diet. In Germany, a significant percentage of fermented foods and beverages are consumed today in the form of beer, wine, sourdough breads, sauerkraut, kefir, and *kvass*. The Germans and Portuguese enjoy a regional raw, fermented sausage, called *rohwurst* and *chourico*, respectively.

In Russia, children are offered a glass of kefir (fermented milk) at school on a regular basis. In China, the government distributes cabbage to the population each fall to ferment and store through the cold winter months. Indonesians eat *tempeh*, a fermented soybean cake; and in Japan, fermented foods from both soybeans and dairy lead sales in the natural-foods arena, spurred on by a tremendous amount of research by doctors, food companies, universities, and medical schools.

American Baby Boomers grew up with cheese, sauerkraut, yogurt, soy sauce, and dill pickles—foods that are traditionally fermented. Unfortunately, the mass-produced versions found in our supermarkets are not real food. If you read the labels on these items, you'll notice that most of the brands on the market are pasteurized and contain added refined vinegar and poor-quality salt. Pasteurization by high heat destroys precious enzymes and beneficial microflora, and the addition of refined salt has contributed to many of the health problems we face today. These products are nothing like the live, enzyme-

and microflora-rich fermented foods and beverages you're encouraged to eat and drink each day on The Diet.

Benefits of Fermented Foods

As we age, our nutritional requirements do not change, but the number of calories we consume ideally should be reduced, especially in our 40s.

As you now know, limiting the amount of food you eat per day . . . or calorie restriction while optimizing nutrition . . . is the one sure way that researchers agree slows and even reverses biological aging.

Well, it is a fact that you can't effectively or safely practice calorie restriction with optimal nutrition without having fermented foods in your diet.

Calorie restriction is only effective when you both limit calories and *increase the quality* of what you eat and digest. The fermented foods and liquids you're learning about in this book will allow you to do just this. But they also have a host of other benefits:

— **Fermented foods create a healthy inner ecosystem.** Fermented foods lay the foundation for our internal garden of microflora: the "Missing Piece" that must be inside of us, supplying energy for everyday life. Fermented foods contain the microorganisms essential to the nourishment and health of our intestines. With every meal containing these foods, our inner garden renews itself.

— **Fermented foods are a must for immunity.** Up to 80 percent of the immune system resides in the gut-associated lymph tissue in our intestines. The microflora living there play a key role in keeping that region healthy and free of pathogenic (bad) bacteria, and *us* well nourished and immunologically hardy.

Immune senescence is a recently coined term that refers to the biological changes that take place in our immune systems as we age. Simply put, as each decade passes, the immune system becomes significantly weaker and less able to protect us, making us more prone to infections such as the flu and to cancers. There's no point in living longer only to die from preventable diseases. However, administering potentially harmful flu shots to the elderly is not the Baby Boomer way. I predict that instead, delicious fermented foods will become much more appealing as a "protective tool" once more of us understand their power to keep our immune systems hardy.

— **Fermented foods act as alchemists.** The beneficial microflora found in fermented foods and drinks perform chemical magic by manufacturing B vitamins deep down inside you, where they are easily assimilated through your gut wall. They also make vitamin K_2 *(menaquinone),* now positively linked to cardiovascular and bone health. Recent studies also show that vitamin K_2 helps reduce the symptoms of diabetes.

— **Fermented foods and beverages can be more potent than probiotic supplements.** That's because the microflora obtained from organic foods grown in the ground form powerful synergistic relationships with one another that ensure that they flourish. They must survive in nature versus being grown in a lab. The microflora travel down your digestive tract, escorted along by the foods and liquids that they grew in. This helps them survive stomach acid and digestive enzymes so they colonize in greater numbers. While probiotic-supplement companies keep offering ever-increasing numbers of bacteria per capsule, *probiotic foods contain hardier microflora than those found in these supplements,* which actually work better when you also have *fermented foods* and *liquids* in your diet.

— **Fermented foods provide more nutrients.** The microflora abundant in unpasteurized, fermented foods provide additional enzymes to properly process nutrients, markedly increasing their availability.

— **Fermented foods improve digestion.** The microflora in fermented foods help protect the gut lining. They also increase the bioavailability of each meal so you can better absorb nutrients, allowing deficiencies to be corrected.

As the years go by, our digestive tracts tend to show signs of wear and tear. The mucosal lining of our intestines becomes less efficient, and absorption decreases. Often an increase in intestinal permeability occurs, which may allow toxins to pass through more easily and poison us. Our lessening ability to smell and taste foods can make the very act of eating less appealing. Enzyme production also decreases.

In addition, there may be impaired absorption of vitamins, particularly B_{12}, B_6, and folate, as well as minerals such as calcium, magnesium, zinc, and iron, due to low stomach-acid production. Motility and peristaltic contractions weaken, and we become constipated. Constipation also contributes to diverticulosis (small pockets in the colonic lining). A weakened gag reflex increases the risk of choking. Hemorrhoids, reflux, heartburn, peptic ulcers . . . the list goes on and on.

— **Fermented foods are raw . . . but more than raw.** Raw foods may be difficult to digest, especially as we age. Many are very rich in sugars, which make our bodies too acidic, feeding yeast, viruses, and other pathogens. Fermented foods have all the benefits of raw foods . . . including enzymes, antioxidants, and cell messengers such as polyphenols and catechins . . . yet none of the disadvantages.

— **Fermented foods control cravings.** Carbohydrates, sugar, and alcohol leach minerals from our bones, making our blood more acidic, so avoiding them is essential for restoring our prenatal energy. However, since they are addictive, many people do not have the willpower to resist these cravings. With two related epidemics—obesity and diabetes—threatening to take the lives of many Baby Boomers sooner than we'd like, fermented foods and drinks (such as cultured vegetables and young coconut kefir) become a godsend.

— **Fermented foods allow us to enjoy mildly sweet foods found in nature.** Microflora eat the sugars in foods and shield us from damage that sugar can often cause. However, too much sugar can disrupt the balance of the beneficial flora. The amount found in natural foods is conducive to their growth. How perfect that we can enjoy the sweet taste of a carrot while our microflora benefit from the sugar.

— **Fermented foods are detoxifiers.** Due to planetary toxicity, now more than ever we need to put these microflora to work on cleaning up our environment.

Microflora ingest toxins, like pesticides and the mercury found in fish, as well as other harmful materials, and remove them through colonic elimination. (At least 70 percent or more of the weight of the bowel movement is bacteria.)

Most often red and green cabbage, kale, and collards are used in combination with other vegetables to make "cultured vegetables." These are members of the cruciferous family that contain glucosinolates and other active molecules, such as indole-3-carbinol (I3C) and di-indolylmethane (DIM), which can alter detoxification of estrogen in the liver. With these in the diet, estrogen can be converted into safer pathways that decrease the risk of ovarian, uterine, and breast cancer, as well as help with inflammatory conditions, like premenstrual syndrome.

— **Fermented foods make a healthy "fast food."** These foods and beverages are healthy alternatives to fast food. They are filling, nutrient rich, and easy to digest. Additionally, their high liquid content makes them ideal fast breakfast foods. A smoothie made with fermented milk kefir is a perfect way to start the day for the many Baby Boomers who digest dairy well. A nondairy smoothie made with young coconut kefir is great for those who don't.

— **Fermented foods restore acid/alkaline balance.** Fermented foods are excellent for helping restore the best possible acid/alkaline balance. Because the microflora are so efficient in promoting colonic absorption of minerals such as calcium and magnesium, our blood can pick up the minerals and carry them out to our cells. With the correct mineral balance, the body remains in a healthy alkaline range. Cancer, diabetes, yeast, and viruses can't grow in an optimal alkaline environment.

— **Fermented foods provide a sour taste for improved digestion.** The sourness of fermented foods (due to the lactic acid produced by the microflora) stimulates peristaltic movement so that our intestines eliminate properly. To be well balanced, according to Ayurvedic medicine, a great meal should have as many of the six tastes (sweet, sour, salty, bitter, pungent, and astringent) as possible, in the right balance.

Given the healing benefits of fermented foods, it's never too late to start reinforcing your inner ecosystem—and rebuilding your health.

Find the Fermented Foods That Work for You

Fortunately, there are a growing number of options for enjoying fermented foods, and you can choose according to convenience and your own unique palate.

Once again, these are quintessential anti-aging foods. Yes, they are new to many of us and involve a bit of a learning curve, but these fermented foods and drinks are so critical to our vitality and longevity that they are well worth seeking out. In fact, they may be our number one ally in our quest to age "youthfully" and healthfully.

Remember, when fermented, a food or liquid becomes sour. Many of us are not familiar with this taste and only enjoy the sweet and salty tastes. But please eat and drink these sour foods for a week and you'll soon be "hooked." Visit Body Ecology's website (**www.bodyecology.com**) for more articles on fermented foods, and discover how they can help prevent or reverse many health conditions and add many more years to your life.

The following sections feature three especially amazing fermented foods: *cultured vegetables, cultured vegetable juice,* and *young coconut kefir.*

Cultured Vegetables

Cultured or fermented vegetables have been around for thousands of years. Captain Cook took barrels with him on his long voyages to the South Pacific. They protected his crew from developing, and dying from, scurvy.

Indeed, they have been survival foods for many cultures, and we humans might not be here if we hadn't learned how to ferment vegetables as a way to preserve them, providing us with nutrients through long winters. You may be familiar with kimchi, a cultured-vegetable product from Korea consisting of bok choy cabbage, carrots, green onions, ginger, garlic, and hot peppers. And certainly, most of us are familiar with sauerkraut, coined by the Austrians from the German *sauer* (sour) and *Kraut* (greens or plants).

Cultured veggies are raw, cut, and shredded vegetables that have been left to ferment at room temperature. This allows the naturally present lactobacilli and enzymes to proliferate, creating a vitamin-, mineral-, and enzyme-rich superfood.

Keeping in mind that microflora act as alchemists, fermenting vegetables not only increases their nutrient value, but also negates the adverse effects some have on our bodies. For example, cabbage, kale, and collards have a thyroid-suppressing effect when eaten raw . . . something to be aware of in this day and age when many of us have issues with low thyroid. However, when we ferment them, we still get the benefits of the enzymes found in raw foods, but without the thyroid-suppressing effects.

Certain sweet vegetables—like sweet potatoes and beets—are very rich in sugar; and when they are cooked, they become even sweeter, a problem for many people with conditions such as candida and diabetes. Fermenting allows us to benefit from their nutrients while the microflora feed on their natural sugars.

If you prepare your cultured vegetables using the Body Ecology Culture Starter (available at **www.bodyecology.com**) . . . you will have a food that is rich in a special bacteria called *L. plantarum*.

Today, many people suffer from irritable bowel syndrome (IBS). *L. plantarum* has been shown to help repair the damaged intestinal mucosa implicated in IBS. In fact, one study found that regardless of how it was administered, *L. plantarum* lasted for up to ten days in the digestive tract of mice with no unwanted side effects, making these bacteria an ideal probiotic for inflammatory conditions, like IBS and colitis.[1]

A study from Sweden found that *L. plantarum is just as effective as a conventional antiseptic in preventing the most common cause of ventilator-associated pneumonia (VAP) in hospitals.*[2] And a number of researchers have shown its effectiveness at breaking down bile acids and lowering blood-serum cholesterol.[3]

This is a hardy microbe. It is antiviral and is resistant to bile acid and to antibiotics. It's comforting to know that if you must use an antibiotic, these bacteria will remain in your intestines, preventing an overgrowth of yeast/fungus.

Recipe for Cultured Veggie Juice

1. Fill a blender with chopped green or red cabbage.

2. Add springwater until blender is 2/3 full.

3. Blend at high speed for 2 minutes.

4. Add package of *L. plantarum* starter culture.

5. Pour mixture into a glass jar with a tight-fitting lid.

6. Let sit at room temperature for 3 days.

7. Strain and place in refrigerator.

8. For a second batch, simply add 1/2 cup of the first batch to the second, and it will be ready in 24 hours.

Drink 1-1/2 cups of cultured vegetable juice per day . . . divided throughout the day. We suggest drinking a small juice glass with each meal, as it greatly assists digestion. Several ounces upon waking and at bedtime when the stomach is empty are also wise.

Cultured Vegetable Juices

A small juice glass of cultured veggie juice is perfect with any meal. It provides the sour taste to stimulate digestion, as well as peristalsis to ensure that food moves through your digestive tract with ease. At Body Ecology, we love cultured veggie juice so much that years ago we began to recommend that parents give it to their newborns to help prevent colic, autism, and other childhood disorders. A baby may make funny faces at this strange sour taste when given tiny spoonfuls soon after birth, but it helps with digestion of milk and builds a stronger immune system. (With a strong immune system, a child is less likely to become "infected" by a vaccination and develop autism.) Another nice plus: When babies are introduced to the sour taste early in life, they don't develop a "sweet tooth." They grow up feeling quite satisfied with the sweetness in a carrot or a berry.

Please share the value of fermented foods and drinks with your children and grandchildren as they see you enjoying several glasses of cultured veggie juice each day. Remember, the secrets to health and long life were traditionally passed from generation to generation through explanation and example. Fermented foods are the answer to the childhood-obesity epidemic.

Young Coconut Kefir (YCK)

The Story

One of my deepest passions is to use food to heal and save our children. When I first started to hear about autism and the rising numbers of children affected by this alarming worldwide pandemic, I wondered what I could do to help. I lived in Atlanta at the time, and to my amazement, I found a flyer in a local market promoting a Defeat Autism Now (DAN) conference that very weekend.

I attended that first DAN conference in 2001 and was impressed by the doctors who were speaking. They seemed to have an accurate diagnosis of what was physically wrong with the autistic kids (heavy-metal toxicity, yeast infections, digestive disorders, addiction to carbs, mineral deficiencies, sleep problems, and so on); but at that point there seemed to be a dearth of real, promising solutions. I immediately noticed some startling parallels between the symptoms of the children and those of many people I had worked with over the years. I truly thought I could offer some solutions . . . at least with respect to diet.

A "Feel-Good" Tonic

*K*efir means "feel good" in Turkish. Milk kefir has been called "nature's tranquilizer" or "nature's Prozac" because of its calming effect. It contains *tryptophan*, an essential amino acid that when combined with calcium and magnesium helps calm the nervous system. In fact, the body converts tryptophan into serotonin—a neurotransmitter, or chemical messenger in the brain allowing for communication between nerve cells. Serotonin, also referred to as 5-HT, is known to modulate emotions, mood, memory and learning, temperature regulation, behavior, cardiovascular function, muscle contraction, endocrine regulation, sleep, and appetite. This makes it especially helpful for people who are depressed, high-strung, or nervous; or who have trouble sleeping (serotonin converts to the sleep hormone melatonin)—not to mention for those wishing to improve memory.

Around that time, circumstances suddenly forced me to move to Los Angeles, where I met a man named Don Kidson who introduced me to young coconuts from Thailand. Knowing it was too sugary for people on the Body Ecology Diet but impressed that the water had such cleansing properties, it suddenly occurred to me that we might ferment it with Body Ecology Kefir Starter. Don and two other friends helped me create the very first batches of young coconut kefir. Once Don and I began to share this new discovery with others, word spread like wildfire. *This water in its fermented form seemed to have magical benefits.*

As we know, "all is in Divine order," so right on time, in 2002, my first autistic child walked into my life. Or his mother, Diane, did. . . . She called me one fateful afternoon to talk about her son Thomas, who had been diagnosed with autism at the age of three.

With my guidance, Diane immediately put Thomas on the Body Ecology Diet, and to my amazement, she was actually able to find young Thai coconuts in Charleston, South Carolina, where she lived. Diane's clever and creative efforts, combined with her strong intention to heal her son, resulted in a full recovery for Thomas. He has been healthy for more than eight years now.

Diane and I went on to create BEDROK, a support community for families struggling with autism. Years later, we continue to see amazing success with the Body Ecology protocol. (If you know of someone with an autistic child, please send them to **bedrokcommunity.org**, where they will receive amazing information and support.)

Today, more and more people are discovering the benefits of coconut water. While DAN conferences have slowly morphed into more of a pharmaceutical resource for physicians and parents, many of the orginal DAN doctors have moved away, preferring to offer a more successful and caring approach. They know diet is more important than drugs, for example. They recommend cultured vegetables, coconut kefir, and the Body Ecology Diet to their patients and have enjoyed remarkable results. In fact, if you want a great doctor, find one who is successfully treating children with autism.

I believe that an antifungal diet, along with Body Ecology recommended foods such as young coconut kefir, is not only invaluable in the *treatment* of autism, but also the key to *prevention*.

To date, because our BEDROK moms know how to prevent autism, siblings born later are totally free of this devastating illness. We feel this stands as testament to the importance of fermented foods while a fetus is forming in the womb and immediately after birth. In fact, fermented foods and drinks and the Body Ecology Way of Life should be a part of a child's diet from conception (via his mother) until the day he draws his last breath.

Young Coconut Kefir's Benefits

Most people are familiar with coconut meat and water from the mature (brown, hairy) coconut. A green coconut is the same food, but younger. The liquid inside is much more like sweet water and is different from prepared coconut milk. Please don't confuse *coconut water* with *coconut milk,* which is actually made from warm water and the meat of the mature coconut. *Coconut water* is the liquid found naturally inside the young coconut. It is full of B vitamins and minerals, especially potassium and sodium—two important minerals for heart and adrenal health. This water has been known for centuries to have a cleansing effect on the liver, kidneys, and heart.

While unfermented coconut water makes a delicious drink on its own, it is too sweet to be *medicinal.* Drinking it will make your body too acidic and encourage the growth of pathogens (viruses and yeast) and tumors. You can still obtain the benefits of this superfood, however, by *fermenting* the young coconut water, making young coconut kefir (YCK)—a bubbly, champagne-like drink.

It is much easier to obtain fresh coconut water in health-food stores today than it once was. Thai coconuts have the sweetest water in the world, which is best for fermenting. Body Ecology has begun to import fresh, frozen *organic* coconut water from Thailand. Many Whole Foods Markets and other health-food stores are carrying it in their frozen-food section. (If you have any difficulty finding it locally, please visit the Body Ecology website.) Not only is coconut water in cans or aseptic packages pasteurized, but it isn't sweet enough to ferment.

From the Physician's Desk

"We have at least 10 trillion cells in our bodies and 100 trillion microbes in the form of bacteria, parasites, and fungi. Managing these microbes should be a top priority."

We shall not cease from exploration / And the end of all our exploring / Will be to arrive where we started / And know the place for the first time.

This excerpt from T. S. Eliot's poem "Little Gidding" is just an elegant way of saying "history is destined to repeat itself." I think this is particularly true of our emerging awareness of how beneficial bacteria and fermented foods balance our inner ecosystem. Pioneers like Donna Gates are really revivers of ideas we've known for thousands of years, but which have been lying dormant and largely ignored.

There is evidence, for example, that 2,500 years ago fermented dairy was used in Iraq, and just 100 years ago, people such as Nobel Prize winner Dr. Élie Metchnikov talked and wrote about the anti-aging benefits of fermented foods. Fortunately, we are once again beginning to realize the importance of this overlooked area of health. However, there are parts of the world that have always routinely used fermented foods. When I was traveling with my wife in Denmark and Sweden, there would be jars of fermented yogurt on the table to take with meals. It was simply a natural part of the diet. In fact, fermented foods have been used for thousands of years in many regions of the world, ranging from Europe, Africa, and the Middle East to India, China, and Japan, where they depended upon bacterial cultures long before refrigeration was available.

Certainly, refrigeration has been a wonderful addition to life—and has saved a lot of lives—but we've also lost something vital in the process by forgetting about the value of culturing foods. Once again, we are now revisiting this most valuable technology as a cornerstone of health.

There is another major reason why cultured foods should be a part of every meal. Every year 70 million people in the United States check into the ER due to food poisoning, regardless of whether they eat at home or in restaurants.

This problem can be diminished with the regular use of fermented foods, or *probiotics*. Science has shown that fermented vegetables and drinks fill the gut with beneficial bacteria. These probiotic-laden foods make their own biofilms and antibiotics *(bacteriocins)*, which kill, disable, and crowd out pathogenic bacteria.

Beneficial microflora are basically an excellent insurance policy. In healthy people, the percentage of pathogenic bacteria in the body is much lower than the amounts of neutral and beneficial bacteria. When we become sick or get out of balance in some way, then the pathogenic bacteria can start multiplying, and literally take on a life of their own. Unless we are proactive, these pathogens disrupt the microfloral balance, leading to often-permanent degenerative diseases.

In conclusion, let's remember we have at least 10 trillion cells in our bodies and 100 trillion microbes, mostly in the form of bacteria, with some fungi, parasites, and viruses. The necessity of managing these microbes to the degree we can should be obvious. Yet most of us have little or no notion of friendly bacteria or how to culture our foods.

I believe that if you were going to make only one beneficial change in your lifestyle and health in the next year, it should be to begin integrating fermented foods into your diet. Most health programs talk about the importance of healthy carbs, exercise, getting your omega-3s, and so forth. The Body Ecology program, however, is one of the few to address the importance of the inner ecosystem and bacteria management through fermented foods.

— *Leonard Smith, M.D.*

Chapter 16

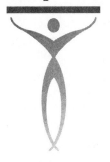

Sugar: How Sweet It Isn't

Even in the 1940s, enlightened health professionals were implicating sugar as a dangerous poison and major culprit in aging. How can we satisfy our taste for sugar without harming ourselves?

The Sugar Scourge

During World War II, just prior to the births of the first Baby Boomers, sugar and sweetened dairy products such as ice cream were rationed. Indeed, they were thought to be luxury items . . . rarely obtained. Once the war ended, the restriction was lifted, and sugar consumption increased dramatically. Suddenly, highly sweetened foods—including refined, puffy, sweetened cereals and a number of brands of soda pop—began hitting America's supermarket shelves. The switch from farm-grown foods to processed ones, where sugar was often used as a preservative and "flavor enhancer," further shoved consumers down the high-sugar path . . . coinciding with a continual decline in our health.

Coincidentally (or was it?), polio suddenly emerged as an "epidemic" and became a serious threat to America's Baby

Boomer generation. From 1945 to 1949, an average of more than 20,000 cases of polio were reported per year.

In 1951, a medical book entitled *Diet Prevents Polio* was published by Benjamin P. Sandler, M.D., a noted authority on nutrition who lived and practiced in North Carolina. Despite its unassuming cover and title, this little blue book would generate a storm of controversy.

Dr. Sandler wrote:

> Specifically, I suspected that children and adults contracted polio because of low blood sugar (hypoglycemia) brought on by a diet containing sugar and starch. I reasoned that the poliovirus was able to cross tissue barriers, reach the brain and spinal cord, invade the nerve cells, damage or destroy them and cause paralysis. And I further reasoned that if the blood sugar never fell below 80 mg, polio could never result. I suspected that during a polio epidemic only those children and adults who experienced periods of low blood sugar would contract the disease and that those individuals who were in actual contact with the virus but who maintained normal blood sugar levels would not contract the disease.[1]

Dr. Sandler began to teach his patients that low blood sugar—caused, paradoxically, by eating high-sugar foods such as soft drinks; fruit juices; ice cream; cakes; canned and preserved fruits; and starches, including bread, potatoes, and grits—led to hypoglycemia, a lowering of immunity, and a susceptibility to polio. By increasing "protective proteins" (that is, eggs, fish, poultry, beef, milk, and cream); eating lots of vegetables (for example, string beans, cucumbers, greens, lettuce, turnips, carrots, red beets, cabbage, and onions); and even limiting fresh fruits in the diet, Sandler believed one could protect oneself against the disease during an epidemic.

As early as 1948, in an interview in *The Asheville Citizen,* Sandler is quoted as saying:

> The crisis is here and hours have become precious. . . . I have been impelled to bring this directly to the newspapers because of my profound conviction that, through community cooperation and general acceptance of a diet low in sugars and starches, this epidemic can be got under control in about two weeks' time. . . . I am willing to state without reserve that such a diet, strictly observed, can build up in 24 hours' time

a resistance in the human body sufficiently strong to combat the disease successfully. The answer lies in maintaining a normal blood sugar."[2]

Today it is well accepted that when we eat *dietary* sugar, it causes a yo-yo effect on our *blood* sugar. Dietary sugar creates a temporary *spike* in our glucose, followed by a dramatic *drop* in glucose, causing our energy to plummet. To regain energy, we crave and then eat another sweet-tasting food or drink that will send it soaring once again.

Sandler was right on target in his understanding that maintaining healthy blood sugar (and, I would add, the right pH balance of the body) made one susceptible to polio. His recommendations to avoid sugar had a dramatic and immediate impact in the form of a reduction of polio cases in North Carolina . . . but only temporarily. Unfortunately, his work was mocked by his colleagues and ignored by most of the public. The marketing efforts of companies such as Rockefeller Milk Trust and Coca-Cola, coupled with our enthusiasm to eat whatever we desired, saw sugar consumption returning to previous levels. Soon, polio statistics would also climb to as high as 58,000 cases by 1952.

Sandler's warnings that sugar consumption was the underlying cause of a life-threatening health epidemic were also frighteningly prophetic. We Baby Boomers have been addicted to sugar since infancy, and now as we age, we are once again experiencing multiple *epidemics* of poor health, including obesity, diabetes, Alzheimer's, cancer, and digestive diseases such as Crohn's. Obviously, to reverse the aging process, we must stop the madness and avoid the consumption of sugars. We must do so for our own well-being and, especially, for the well-being of our children and grandchildren, because autism, obesity, diabetes, and cancer have now become *their* epidemics.

When you think about how much sugar is found in processed foods today, it's pretty scary. Statistics say that more than 20 percent of the total calories we consume each day are from refined sugars. Sugar is hidden in our foods under the guise of *sucrose, dextrose, maltose, sorbitol, turbinado*—and more. In fact, the average person consumes his or her body weight in these empty, dangerous calories, plus more than 20 pounds of corn syrup, in one year.

Death by Spoonful

Sugar may "help the medicine go down," but it definitely also depletes us of our prenatal life force, our *jing*. And, unfortunately, death by sugar is usually slow and can be *physically* painful. As my friend Dr. Joe Mercola stated on his popular health website (**www.mercola.com**): "The health dangers ingested sugar creates when habitually imposed upon human physiology are certain. Simple sugars have been observed to aggravate asthma, muster mental illness, move mood swings, provoke personality changes, nourish nervous disorders, hurry heart disease, deliver diabetes, grow gallstones, hasten hypertension, add arthritis, and on top of all of that . . . it will kill you!"[3]

Sugar hardens, weakens, and poisons every system in the body including the endocrine system. As powerful as any drug, it lifts us up, only to knock us right back down.

If Joe's words of warning that sugar is slowly but surely killing us may seem a bit too dramatic to you, there is much research to support his statements. Recent cell-metabolism experiments suggest that when worms were fed glucose as part of their diets, they lived for a *shorter* amount of time than those that *never consumed* it, according to researchers from the University of Jena, Germany.[4] If these findings in worms hold for humans, then even in healthy people, the breakdown of sugar into glucose has detrimental effects on life span.

Sugar consumption may not only shorten our lives, it may make the quality of our final years quite a bit bleaker as well. A study conducted by the American Society for Biochemistry and Molecular Biology showed that high sugar consumption in an otherwise-normal diet could affect the progression of Alzheimer's disease. Using a genetic mouse model, researchers found that mice that were given 10 percent sugar water showed poorer learning and memory retention than the control group, and their brains contained more than twice as many amyloid plaque deposits, which play a major role in the destruction of nerve cells and are an anatomical hallmark of Alzheimer's.[5] The connection between diabetes and Alzheimer's has long been known. In fact, some scientists even refer to Alzheimer's as "type 3 diabetes."

And Sugar Makes You Look and Feel Really Old, Too

Dietary-sugar molecules bond to protein molecules and create "cross-linked proteins," meaning that proteins start bonding to each other. This is called glycosylation (see Chapter 3 and the glycation theory of aging). Basically, tissues stiffen and do not function efficiently. Cataracts are an example of stiffening of our eye lenses, and we lose our sight. Stiffening skin tissue becomes tough, yellow, and leathery. You can imagine what it looks like to see the results of cross-linked proteins accumulating in cartilage, lung tissue, arteries, and tendons.

Sugar hardens, weakens, and poisons every system in the body, including the endocrine system. As hormone production

Artificial Sweeteners . . . On Their Way Out!

While it may have seemed smart at one point to turn to artificial sweeteners such as aspartame (NutraSweet and Equal) and sucralose (Splenda), we now know that these alternatives are a double-edged sword. The average American consumes more than 50 pounds of artificial sweetener per year, often unwittingly, in snacks and soda pop. Aspartame has been found to create side effects such as memory loss, blurry vision, and headaches.

Even if you were to risk these side effects in exchange for weight loss, evidence is now showing that aspartame actually contributes to obesity. One of its ingredients, the amino acid *phenylalanine,* blocks serotonin, which plays a role in controlling cravings. The effect on your body may be that you start to crave all of those high-carbohydrate, processed foods that can sabotage your dieting goals.

Sucralose has elicited similar findings, such as enlargement of the liver and kidneys, shrinking of the thymus gland (which plays a role in immunity and disease fighting), lymph atrophy, decreased red-blood-cell count, decreased fetal body weight, and diarrhea, just to name a few.

Stevia has none of these side effects, and is all natural! It has no calories, is low on the glycemic index, and produces no increase in blood-sugar levels.

slowly fades away—especially in our adrenals and the pituitary, which produces growth hormone—our sex drive diminishes, men become impotent, and energy wanes, causing us to lose our ability to cleanse out toxins. We become more and more constipated, and our intestines fill with decaying fecal material. Signs that we are poisoning ourselves are gray hair, weak fingernails, bone loss, and sarcopenia (loss of lean muscle, replaced by fat). Perhaps worst of all is that our brains literally shrink in size and develop holes.

Because sugar is devoid of vitamins, minerals, and fiber, it creates an acidic body—and one day, a checkup at the doctor's office reveals that we have cancer cells growing rapidly out of control. *As powerful as any drug, sugar lifts us up, only to knock us right back down.* It has long been known that sugar's addictive properties and withdrawal symptoms are similar to narcotics. Are we shocked, then, that most of us are sugar addicts?

It should come as no surprise that our children and grandchildren face an even grimmer future. A recent study by researchers at the Royal Veterinary College in London found that mothers who eat junk food during pregnancy and while breast-feeding may be putting their children at risk for overeating and developing obesity. The study was carried out on an animal model, in which researchers observed rats fed a diet of processed junk food during pregnancy and lactation. The rats gave birth to offspring that overate and showed a preference for foods rich in fat, sugar, and salt, compared to the offspring of rat mothers given regular feed. *The implications for humans are obvious.*[6]

In our grandchildren, we can clearly see the effects of generations of sugar consumption: early puberty, anxiety, depression, weight gain, confused minds, drug and alcohol addiction, and, sadly, increasing juvenile criminal behavior.

But statistics also show that Baby Boomers are very concerned about the amount of sugar in their diets today. They are taking greater responsibility for their own health and for their grandchildren's. They are reading labels more. They want a change.

Putting the Principles into Practice

Sugar and the Principle of Balance

The Diet is almost totally free of sugars in any form. At Body Ecology, we are committed to helping you reduce your sugar consumption dramatically. Yet, we also recognize the need that we humans have for the sweet taste. Remember that according to Ayurvedic medicine, we humans desire and even need six tastes: sweet, salty, sour, bitter, pungent, and astringent. In a well-prepared meal, the Ayurvedic cook balances the sweet taste with the other tastes on the plate. With this balance, we feel satisfied, and our organs will be receiving what they need. In other words, the sweet taste is just as important as salty, bitter, sour, and so on, so we should not feel guilty when we desire it. It has a clear purpose along with all the other tastes and senses.

In small amounts, sugar is necessary for energy, especially in demanding situations such as physical labor or exercise. It also nourishes our sense organs and promotes strength. But it is well understood that sugar "increases tissue," meaning it causes us to become larger, even obese. In addition, the character of this taste is cold, damp, and heavy on digestion. When there's too much, we create an imbalance, experiencing lethargy, mucous conditions, constipation, and a general heaviness.

Overcoming Our Cravings for and Addiction to Sugar

The first step in overcoming a serious sugar addiction is to quell our desire for it. The sour taste does just that. We can be satisfied by eating or drinking sour, fermented foods (see the previous chapter).

Once you add fermented foods and beverages to your diet, you will begin to lose much of your desire for sweet foods. In fact, you will start to really be able to taste the natural sweetness in fruits and sweet vegetables and be perfectly satisfied with these. Candy bars, pastries, and colas will become disgustingly overly sweet.

Fermented foods must become an essential part of an anti-aging diet. They allow us to eat the healthier sweets found in nature without the sugar causing us damage. This is because the microflora in these natural foods consume it and protect us. What a perfect symbiotic relationship! We enjoy the sweet taste of a carrot while the beneficial microflora thrive on the sugar present.

Have you ever noticed how, soon after a sugar binge, out of the blue you crave salty foods such as chips? Or you might suddenly begin to crave an animal-protein meal? These cravings are your body's way of trying to maintain balance. Sea salt, an alkaline food, provides valuable minerals that are lost when acidic, mineral-leaching sugars are consumed. Animal proteins also contain salt and minerals in the blood.

Adrenal fatigue becomes the norm as we age, so to get a boost of temporary energy, many of us reach for sugar and/or salty foods. We seesaw back and forth, wanting both, but those sugary snacks that give us a short-lived boost of energy drain the adrenals even further, and a vicious cycle results. Fermented foods, on the other hand, help nourish the body so efficiently that our blood sugar stays stable, minerals are extracted and retained to build our adrenals, and cravings disappear.

Dehydration

A major cause of cravings for sweets is that your body needs water. Before you succumb to a sugar craving, try this: Sit down for five or ten minutes and drink two glasses of mineral-rich water. You'll be amazed by how well this works. You can also add stevia and lemon juice to your water to satisfy your sweet tooth. Even better, add a few ounces of a probiotic liquid such as young coconut kefir or Body Ecology's CocoBiotic.

Sugar and the Principle of Acid and Alkaline

As you know, when there is too much sugar in your body, an overly acidic condition results. (See Chapter 12: The Principle of Acid and Alkaline.) An acidic body provides an ideal haven for pathogens such as viruses, fungi, and cancer cells. Viruses, for example, have been shown to create serious chronic inflammation, which is a major cause of aging. They have been linked to heart disease as well.

Sugar and the Principle of Food Combining

Sugar should always be eaten alone. When you combine it with another food, it creates gas. (See Chapter 13: The Principle of Food Combining.)

Sweets, the Body Ecology Way

There are several natural ways to sweeten your foods and beverages that are healthy for your body. You may not have heard of all of them because they don't have billion-dollar marketing budgets behind them, but they are quietly entering health-food stores or are sold on the Internet.

The Story of Stevia

*Y*ears ago, I was instrumental in bringing stevia to the United States and published a book called *Stevia: Nature's Calorie-Free Sweetener.* The story behind this is that stevia was a huge threat to the food conglomerate Monsanto, when they still had the patent for aspartame (sold under the labels of Equal and NutraSweet). Someone (no one knew for sure) petitioned the FDA to raid those tea companies that were using the green stevia leaves in their tea bags. Stevia was then banned from being imported in the U.S.

I led a grassroots movement; and soon, with the help of Drs. Robert Atkins, Andrew Weil, and Julian Whitaker, tens of thousands of people were safely using and enjoying the white powder extract. What an interesting twist of fate that Coca-Cola, Pepsi, and Cargill, which now want to use stevia extract in their beverages, have recently obtained approval from the FDA! Personally, I see this as a victory for all of us who fought to bring stevia into the U.S.

Stevia

An extraordinarily sweet herb, stevia is 200 to 300 times sweeter than sugar—and yet, it's nearly calorie free! Stevia is a member of the chrysanthemum family (closely related to chamomile and tarragon) and is totally safe.

Stevia is available as crushed green leaves; as a crude, greenish-brown syrup; as a white powder extract; and as an easy-to-use liquid concentrate prepared from the white powder extract. In its crude, unprocessed form, the stevia plant has been consumed for centuries by the Indians of South America. The Japanese, looking for a safe sweetener substitute, developed the process used to extract two primary compounds, *rebaudioside* and *stevioside,* from the plant to create a delicious white powder. Stevia has now been enjoyed and used safely in Japan for the past 30-plus years.

The crude green stevia leaves and syrup have a strong licorice-like flavor that many do not like. So while they do have medicinal value (such as helping to heal wounds and preventing dental cavities), they are not recommended as a sweetener. The white powder doesn't have this aftertaste if used sparingly.

Neither the whole plant nor the extract will raise blood sugar, making it safe for diabetics. An excellent flavor enhancer when used in very small amounts, stevia is especially tasty in dairy and with fruits.

Stevia has been tested in human and animal studies in many major countries, including Japan, Brazil, and Israel, with no negative side effects. Ironically, of the more than 9,000 complaints filed with the FDA since 1985, about 80 percent are related to NutraSweet, yet *it* is still on the market.[7] Once the patent on aspartame had expired, more and more natural alternative sweeteners began to appear on the market. Not all are safe, however. Asparatame, Acesulfame K, and Splenda are not on the Baby Boomer Diet. (See **www.mercola.com** for excellent articles on the dangers of these.)

When purchasing stevia, be aware that there are different strengths available, some of which you may like less than others. At Body Ecology, we prefer a stevia *liquid concentrate* for its convenience. The liquid form is great for those who are just starting to experiment with stevia, because you can easily control the amount you add to beverages and foods. The white powder can be more difficult to work with, resulting in oversweetening your food. Many people tell us that our own delicious stevia concentrate is the best-tasting product on the market. It is available at: **www.bodyecology.com**.

Lakanto

Lakanto has been in use in Japan since 1996 and is served in thousands of restaurants and hospitals. It is recommended (not just approved) by the Japanese minister of health as a food for special dietary uses, and it has GRAS (Generally Recognized As Safe) approval in the United States.

What is great about Lakanto is its absolutely delicious taste, and unlike stevia, you can bake with it. You use it just like you would sugar and can even sprinkle it on your food. (Stevia is too strong to "sprinkle." In fact, a tiny bit can be too much, and you will ruin the taste of your food or drink.)

Lakanto is made from a unique patented combination of erythritol and a pure extract of luo han guo, an exotic vine fruit cultivated mainly in East Asia. Erythritol is unlike any other sugar alcohol (see more on sugar alcohol on the following pages) because it is made from the process of fermentation. The sugar in corn is fermented, not the protein . . . so those sensitive to corn can tolerate Lakanto quite well. All other sugar alcohols (maltitol, sorbitol, and xylitol) are made by hydrogenation. This may explain why Lakanto does not cause the symptoms of diarrhea that some people experience when they eat a food or chew gum made with the other sugar alcohols. Luo han guo has been used in traditional Chinese medicine since ancient times to treat a variety of ailments, such as chronic cough, heat stroke, larynx infections, and constipation.

Lakanto is an excellent choice for people who want to combat age, who want to lose weight, or who are insulin resistant or diabetic. It registers "0" on the glycemic index and causes no rise in serum insulin or blood-sugar levels. It tastes similar to maple sugar or toffee, and because it is not altered by heat, it is excellent for baking and cooking. A recipe book is available online at: **www.bodyecology.com**.

Benefits of Lakanto:

- Zero calories
- Easy to digest
- 'A one-to-one correlation with sugar
- Remarkable heat resistance
- Does not elevate blood-sugar levels
- Does not cause dental cavities
- No artificial coloring or additives
- Safe for infants, pregnant or nursing mothers, and seniors
- Delicious in coffee (but coffee is not recommended on The Diet)

Xylitol and Erythritol

Xylitol and erythritol are both called "sugar alcohols." And what is a sugar alcohol?

There are two kinds of carbohydrates: (1) *available* carbohydrates, those that the body can use and metabolize; and (2) *unavailable,* also known as "non-glycemic," meaning they have no calories. These zero-calorie, non-glycemic carbs are not used as energy by the body and therefore do not raise blood-sugar levels. This means they will not conflict with your low-carb diet and will not spike blood glucose. A healthy, natural sweetener, xylitol is considered to be an "unavailable" carbohydrate sweetener and is extracted from fruits, vegetables, and birch cellulose.

Xylitol is clinically proven to fight and lessen the occurrence of inner-ear infection. It also has many benefits for teeth, making it a natural replacement for fluoride. These proven benefits include: reducing plaque, fighting cavities, reducing the secretion of plaque acids, and facilitating the re-mineralization of tooth enamel. Additionally, xylitol may help against group B strep and has been given to mothers in prenatal clinics.

Erythritol has these wonderful properties as well.

Xylitol and erythritol are low on the glycemic index, and like stevia, are safe for diabetics and hypoglycemics. They look and taste similar to sugar, with 40 percent fewer calories. You can purchase xylitol and erythritol in your health-food store. Some people are sensitive to xylitol, and excessive amounts may cause digestive issues, including diarrhea. Erythritol is made from a different process using fermentation and rarely has negative side effects.

Eliminating sugar from your diet may be the most important first step you take in impeding the aging process. It can be challenging, but by including fermented foods and beverages in your diet, you can manage and eventually get over the desire for sweets.

Sugar is not the only area of our diet where Americans have been perilously "duped." As you will see in the next chapter, we have also been misled about the importance of healthy fats and oils in a well-rounded diet.

Chapter 17

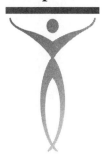

Fats: The Good, the Bad, and the Ones That Make Us Ugly

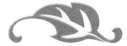

Demonized, traditional fats and unrefined extra-virgin oils are your secret weapon against many of the common diseases of aging, such as osteoporosis, macular degeneration, hormone decline, and dementia.

When it comes to progress, not all change is good. Many of the innovations of the 20th century that brought us convenience have cost us something in return. The lightbulb and computer have had both a positive and a negative impact on human health. We can add the modern-day supermarket to the list.

In 1930, Michael Cullen opened the first supermarket in Queens, New York. This seemingly progressive action would have a profoundly *negative* influence on the *quality* of foods eaten around the world.

In 1946, with a baby being born every eight minutes, more houses, hospitals, and schools were needed. Housing developments expanded farther outward from the town centers to create "suburbs." Supermarkets were one of the things that made this expansion possible.

Supermarkets liberated our mothers from the kitchen because they had to make fewer trips to the store and spent less time shopping. Before the advent of the supermarket, a clerk selected a customer's product off the shelf, weighed it, and determined its price. Supermarkets allowed our parents to inspect a product themselves and check out competitors' prices. This rivalry forced manufacturers to consider packaging their products in eye-catching ways. Jingles and slogans were born. Marketing in newspapers, magazines, and eventually television spurred fierce competition and raised prices as companies vied for our spending dollars.

But, because convenience became most important in the mind of the American consumer, other issues began to emerge. Products needed to stay on shelves for longer periods of time, and "just-picked freshness" was becoming less of a priority. Shelf stability was a problem for fats and oils because fatty acids, when exposed to heat, light, and oxygen, become damaged. The oils that contain these fatty acids turn rancid and poisonous to eat. Freshly pressed or *unrefined oils* with fragile fatty acids were not ideal for traveling great distances . . . or for sitting on supermarket shelves for lengthy periods of time. To solve this problem, "food scientists" and manufacturers of vegetable oils extended shelf life by changing or removing all of the *beneficial* fatty acids.

We were a trusting nation then. Our parents had confidence in the newly emerging miracles of modern nutritional science . . . man could improve upon nature. "Better" fats, like Crisco, became the new staple—after all . . . "Cooks who know trust Crisco." Believing in what they saw in those ads, few questioned if it was wise or healthy to eat these "plastic," nutritionally useless oils. But alas, to make foods "shelf stable," we altered and desecrated them, thumbing our noses at the "real foods" that had fueled our bodies for thousands of years. You might say we sold our bodies and souls for shelf life.

Now, 50 years later, the consequences of processing and depleting the nutrients in almost every food and drink that passes our lips, *especially altering our fats and oils,* has shaped and will continue to shape the outcome of our health for generations to come.

The Toll That Keeps on Taking

Was it only greed and convenience that set us down this dangerous path? Not entirely. The science of fats is complex. In the earlier days of our youth, scientists and nutritionists were poorly trained. Members of the media felt it was their responsibility to report to the masses what they believed was true. Our parents were young and healthy, so they wouldn't have noticed the subtle changes that were occurring in their own bodies. Unlike us, they believed that everyone has a built-in obsolescence; and conditions such as joint aches, failing eyesight, sagging skin, digestive problems, and cancer were simply a foregone conclusion.

Unfortunately, once the flaws in the bad science were uncovered, the food giants continued to suppress the truth. So, yes, it was also greed, but we must accept the role our generation has played in this. *We wanted these foods.* We wanted to feed them to our children, and today we are still "voting" for them with our dollars. Mistruths still dangle in the public's memories today, and, indeed, it's still an area of much confusion and inaccurate information.

As teens, we could eat greasy French fries and pizza and be relatively immune to their effects, but the toll of eating these bad fats and oils has been accumulating year after year. And now, as we face half a century of life, our prenatal jing has been depleted after decades of bad choices.

The good news is that Baby Boomers have the privilege of being the first aging generation to benefit from a true understanding of this complex science. While bad fats are still all around us in many of our favorite foods, for the first time we also have a superior collection of very fine fats and oils to include in our rejuvenation arsenal.

The science behind fats and oils is more complex than most of us want or need to know. Here's the solution in a nutshell:

Avoid bad fats as if the quality of your life depended on it (because it *does*), and eat the good fats that your own unique body thrives on.

This chapter will spell out the basics: why to eat fats, choosing the right ones, and learning how to use the good ones to prevent diseases of aging.

Big, Bad Saturated Fats: The Lie Lives On . . .

From the moment we were conceived, saturated fats were an important part of our prenatal diet. In the womb, saturated fat played a vital role in our brain and bone development. Because of the prevailing wisdom of the time, few of us were breast-fed. Yet healthy human milk would have supplied us with the saturated fat needed for our high energy requirements and rapidly growing bodies.

While research shows that the *amount of milk fat* varies according to a mother's diet, if you were one of the more fortunate members of our generation who was breast-fed, the *length of time* you received milk from your mother would have helped protect your prenatal jing and made you hardier.

Mothers who have been lactating for more than one year have significantly more fat in their milk. In other words, as we grow, we need *more* milk fat.

Clearly, if saturated fat is indispensable to our early infant survival, does it make sense to eliminate it from our diet now? Is the abandonment of this brain-nourishing fat and the adoption of *margarine* one of the reasons why dementia and Alzheimer's have become so prevalent in our parents' generation?

What about our aging bones—and osteopenia and osteo-porosis? Milk fat helps "drive" the minerals in milk (calcium and phosphorus) into our bones. While more than 40 percent of our bone mass is achieved between the ages of 12 and 18, we must consciously be mindful of adding minerals into our "bone bank account" throughout our lives. Saturated fat, especially from ghee and raw butter, helps us assimilate those minerals.

Blaming Saturated Fats for Heart Disease

This may surprise you, but in the early 1900s, 40 years before the first of the Baby Boomers were born, we were a nation that ate mostly saturated fats from butter, lard (rendered fat from pork), tallow (rendered fat from beef or mutton), and coconut oil. We only ate a very small amount of olive oil. *Heart disease was rare.* But then we decided to "fool Mother Nature."

In 1902, German chemist Wilhelm Normann patented the process to make hydrogenated vegetable oils. By 1911, Procter & Gamble bought the rights and made Crisco commercially available for frying and baking.[1]

By 1950, heart disease had become a leading cause of death in the U.S. Research indicated that *vegetable* oils were linked to this increase. For example, in 1957 the American Heart Association (AHA) concluded from *their* research that dietary fat did *not* correlate with heart disease. But in 1960 they issued a new statement indicating that it did . . . if it was *saturated*. For obvious economic reasons, the vegetable-oil industry—corn, soybean, and peanut—quashed the AHA research and began to attack *all saturated fats,* blaming meats, eggs, cheese, butter, and tropical oils (palm and coconut) as the heart-disease culprits. Almost five decades later, with our more sophisticated understanding of fats, the *most up-to-date research indicates that small amounts of healthy saturated fats help in preventing heart disease.*

But it is important to understand that from 1960 on, we Baby Boomers began eating a "low-fat diet" that included more *refined, hydrogenated* vegetable-based fats such as margarine made from corn, soybean, and safflower oils. This was a tragic mistake that has contributed to epidemics of obesity, eating disorders, hormone imbalances, infertility, brain disorders such as Alzheimer's, ADHD, and depression; as well as cancers, diabetes, and, ironically, *an increase in heart disease.*

We Never Lose Our Need for Saturated Fat

*A*s good as it is for us, the fat in *breast milk* is not an option for us once we grow older . . . or is it? The adult version of the saturated fat can be obtained from eating butter and ghee. And the other important fats in breast milk, which provide us with DHA and EPA fatty acids, can be found in fish oil.

Ideally, butter should be eaten raw. Ghee, also called clarified butter, is ideal for cooking. (In India, it is a tradition to place a spoonful of ghee on a baby's tongue at birth. The Tibetan monks drink as many as five cups of ghee each day for energy and warmth.) If you find that you thrive on *fermented milk products* . . . in the form of kefir, yogurt, or raw cheeses . . . you can obtain saturated milk fat in these foods as well. Although our saturated-fat needs may not be as great as an infant's, adult brains and bones can benefit immeasurably from some saturated milk fat.

The Science of Fats

The Truth about a "Low-Fat Diet"

On a low-fat diet, you can still gain weight and develop heart disease, depression, and diabetes.

To grasp why obesity has increased despite the fact that many of us have stopped eating that delicious but "bad for us" butter, we need to understand a little more about the science of fats. Please hang in there . . . it's not that complicated.

There are two types of fat (or lipids) found circulating in our bloodstream: *cholesterol* and *triglycerides*. Both of these are necessary for life. Cholesterol acts as a precursor for our sexual hormones such as estrogen and testosterone and even vitamin D (really a hormone). It is an essential part of the membrane of a cell. Triglycerides are important in the production of energy for most cells in the body (but not brain cells). They are stored in the body's fat cells until needed for energy.

Cholesterol has received far more attention in the media and will be discussed in more detail in the next chapter, on protein. The problems begin when both cholesterol and triglycerides are too high and out of balance. Obesity, heart disease, diabetes, and surprisingly, even depression are linked to *elevated triglycerides*.

You can be on a low-fat diet . . . like many of us in our generation . . . and still have elevated triglycerides in your bloodstream. Why? Because inactivity, drinking alcohol, and taking drugs (including birth-control pills, steroids, and diuretics) can raise triglyceride levels. An underactive thyroid can also put you at risk, but perhaps the biggest source is all the sugar-laden foods and carbs eaten today.

When saturated fats and extra-virgin oils—all very flavorful—were eliminated . . . foods became tasteless. No one would buy them, so our "food scientists" solved this problem by increasing the amount of sugar in them. When we have a diet high in sugars (bread, pasta, cereals, doughnuts, sodas, white rice, and the like), the liver actually makes more triglycerides . . . more than we need. In other words, when *sugars* are not burned immediately as energy, they create triglycerides that lead to heart disease, diabetes, and certainly obesity . . . even in our children.

A recent connection has been discovered between high triglycerides and the obesity epidemic, which helps explain why we eat too much even when we know it shortens our life spans. Researchers at Saint Louis University discovered that high triglycerides block *leptin,* a hormone secreted by fat cells, from getting into our brains.[2] Leptin normally tells the brain to stop eating, so if triglycerides are blocking it, we'll overeat.

And, as you now know, if you're overindulging instead of limiting calories, you will most certainly age faster.

These same researchers investigated the connection between leptin and memory, finding that indeed leptin *enhances* memory. When high levels of triglycerides block leptin, they also block memory. This is an even greater argument for a sugar-free, largely plant-based, probiotic-rich diet, like Body Ecology's Baby Boomer Diet.[3]

Please Pass the Organic Butter

While Americans have been buying the low-fat lie for decades now, the ironic truth is that raw butter can help us lose weight and become more muscular. Conjugated linoleic acid (CLA) is a fatty acid found in the meat and milk of grass-fed animals. It is produced in much higher quantities (500 percent more) in *grass-fed* animals than in those that feed on *grains* and *silage.* The important thing to know about CLA is that it is a potent cancer-fighting substance; it lowers triglyceride levels, enhances immune function, and increases the rate of bone formation. It also decreases body fat, improves glucose utilization, and can reverse the symptoms of diabetes.

The Creation of the Molecular Misfits—Trans Fats

Once traditional fats were vilified, food manufacturers saw a perfect opportunity to gain control of the market. The process of *hydrogenation* allowed oils such as refined soybean, corn, and canola oil . . . normally in a liquid form . . . to be changed into a *solid* form to create margarines, spreads, and shortenings. This had to be done to replace the traditional, hard-at-room-temperature fats (butter, for instance, or palm oil) previously used in baking, confectionaries, and frying. If made with *liquid* oils, these food products would melt into a blob.

Trans-fatty acids are "molecular misfits," and this nickname says it all. They are a perfect example of how humans can never duplicate the wonderful foods that nature provides. Trans fats lower good cholesterol (HDL) and impair blood-vessel function. But trans fats can have a negative impact in other, less-expected ways. A recent study at the Harvard School of Public Health in Boston showed that women doubled their risk of ovulatory infertility when they received 2 percent of their energy intake from trans fats rather than monounsaturated fats contained in olive oil.[4]

Trans-fatty acids show up in commercially made shortenings, margarines, and fats usually called "hydrogenated vegetable oils" and "partially hydrogenated vegetable oils." We find them in French fries, chicken nuggets, breakfast cereals, crackers, doughnuts, candies, Girl Scout cookies, and every kid's favorite, macaroni and cheese . . . a synthetic cheese. You are eating them when you ask for "butter" at your local movie theater.

As you can see, these foods have been a staple of our children for decades. And then we appear puzzled about the "mysterious epidemics" of child and teen disorders such as autism, ADHD, early menses for girls, latent sexual maturity for boys, violence, depression, obesity, and diabetes. These have become the norm and are occurring in numbers never before seen in our population.

Although we have known for some time that trans fats are poisonous, members of the edible-oil industry do not want them identified. Finally, however, new labeling laws are changing this. In 2005, New York City officials announced that all 20,000 restaurants must remove trans fats from their menu. In January 2010 California became the first *state* to ban them. Major chains such as Kentucky Fried Chicken, Wendy's, and McDonald's have caved under the pressure and have stopped cooking with them. But in many cases restaurants are still using trans fats in their cooking oils, arguing that trans-fat-free

We've been eating refined oils for more than five generations here in the U.S., a legacy that now affects all generations currently living and those who are yet unborn. A more sophisticated understanding of the science behind fats and oils clearly shows that bad fats communicate bad information to our body.

oils will adversely change the taste of foods and along with it, their sales.[5] You should be aware of this when choosing to dine out.

Buyer Beware . . . the New Kid on the Block

But take heed: read labels carefully to avoid the latest human-made fat to hit the market—"interestified" fats. These will replace trans fats in our favorite junk foods, suggesting that they are safe. Just like hydrogenated oils, interestified fats use oils (such as refined soybean oil) to create fats that are solid, are less likely to go rancid, and are suitable for frying. The oil cannot be metabolized. Yes, interestified fats are not trans-fatty acids, but they are still unnatural and chemically modified.

A 2007 study published in *Nutrition and Metabolism* reports that these latest fake vegetable-oil spreads increase the risk for heart-disease factors. K. C. Hayes, a researcher and professor at Brandeis University, has found that interestified fats *reduce HDL cholesterol* (the good one that you want to be high) and *raise blood sugar*. Early research indicates that interestified fats pose serious health risks, perhaps of a greater magnitude than trans fats, so they must be carefully avoided as we age.[6]

And . . . Don't Forget about Fried Foods

Fried foods also contribute to the diseases of aging. When oils are heated to high temperatures—as in frying, roasting, and baking—toxic molecules are formed. Two such molecules are *acrylamide* and *HNE*.

Acrylamide is a chemical formed when carbohydrates and starchy foods are baked, roasted, fried, or grilled. Examples would be: French fries, potato chips, cookies, and bread. Coffee and smoking tobacco also create substantial amounts of acrylamides. At high temperatures (338 degrees Fahrenheit/170 degrees Celsius), the sugar in these foods reacts with a protein and forms this neurotoxin. While some studies linking acrylamide to *cancer* to date appear inconclusive, other research shows that acrylamide can negatively affect both the male and female reproductive organs. Nevertheless, it *is* another unnatural chemical and a *neurotoxin*.

Restaurants repeatedly heat and reuse polyunsaturated vegetable oils when they fry foods. HNE, a highly toxic compound, accumulates with each heating cycle. This new information is troubling when we think about our grandchildren's future, especially if they take potato chips in their lunch boxes or eat at fast-food chains.

Be Suspicious of What You Find in Many Popular Health-Food Stores

Watch out for the oils that are simply marked "cold-pressed" or "expeller-pressed." Even if they are found in health-food stores, they do not have the same benefits as *unrefined* oils. A lot of what are being marketed as "healthy" oils, such as *refined* canola oil, lack color and flavor and are deficient in nutrients and fatty acids. Our livers are simply not designed to handle them. With the goal of extending shelf life, all of the beneficial fatty acids have been removed from these "plastic" oils, making them nutritionally useless.

Whole Foods Market has used refined canola oil and a refined olive-oil/vegetable-oil blend in most of the items sold in its "prepared cuisine" section. In the food business, where profit is key, *organic, unrefined oils are considered too expensive.* The cost of prepared foods at Whole Foods is usually quite high, yet many of the ingredients do not justify this. Fortunately, Whole Foods seems to be aware of this inconsistency in their corporate ideals. We have been told that, since 2010, they have begun to focus more on *quality* in their prepared foods.

If you are a Whole Foods shopper, please let them know of your concern. Contact them at: **www.wholefoodsmarket .com/contact**, and request that only *unrefined* fats and oils be used in their prepared foods. They do sell these high-quality fats and oils in their stores for use in your own home.

We've been eating *refined* oils for more than five generations here in the U.S., a legacy that now affects all generations currently living and those who are yet to be born. A more sophisticated understanding of the science behind fats and oils clearly shows that bad fats communicate bad information to the body. While *good fats can silence genes* that might be expressed as heart disease, Alzheimer's, and diabetes, *bad ones express or turn these genes on.*

So, now that we've learned a little of the history of America's "low-fat controversy," let's move on to the benefits of healthy fats and oils, and what foods we need to eat to obtain them.

Let's Simplify—
the Good Things Good Fat Can Do

In a nutshell, we eat fats and oils to obtain their essential fatty acids and their other important fat-soluble nutrients, including the vitamins A, D, E, and K. Fatty acids are the building blocks of fats. Fats provide energy and satiety, regulate cholesterol, create a stronger immune system, and relieve pain and arthritis. They are needed for health and certainly play a major role in how we age or don't.

Healthy, unrefined oils are actually being used in alternative medical clinics and spas around the world to fight depression, emotional disorders, ADHD, autism, and even schizophrenia. When eaten in their extra-virgin, unrefined state, fats and oils are also quite delicious, so they provide us with pleasure and enjoyment as well.

Here are just a few of the many anti-aging benefits of fats:

Beauty

Fats make us look great! They moisturize and replenish our skin, and they keep our hormone levels from declining, a main reason we begin to lose some of our youthful "sexiness." The right fats can cool down inflammation in the body, a significant factor in aging.

Vision

Fats are essential to the eye's rods and cones and are critical to many metabolic functions inside the eye. Some experts believe healthy fats in foods such as nuts may have the same positive effect on our eyes as they do on our hearts. The healthy fats in nuts may prevent total fat from clogging the "arteries" of our eyes. As macular degeneration and other diseases of the eyes, such as cataracts, are related to inflammation, a diet rich in leafy-green vegetables and omega-3 fatty foods that protect the body from free-radical damage is essential.

Brain Function

Fats make up 60 percent of the brain and are essential to brain function, including learning abilities, memory retention, and emotional equilibrium.

Bone Density

Osteoporosis affects more than 25 million Americans a year, mostly women. Although there is certainly a genetic predisposition (women whose mothers had osteoporosis are more likely to have it, also), heredity does not mean osteoporosis is a foregone conclusion. There is a clear link between a healthy diet and exercise and lowered susceptibility to osteoporosis. A diet high in a variety of healthy fats affects overall mineral density and absorption in the bones, helps the body properly utilize bone-related vitamins such as vitamin D, and reduces the chance of bone loss. In fact, certain fats (raw butter, ghee, fish oil, and the fat in egg yolk) actually contain vitamin D.

The Endocrine System—Hormone Production

Fats help regulate hormones, and with the youngest Baby Boomers reaching their mid-40s, hormone issues become a greater concern. If your diet is deficient in good-quality fats, it is also likely that your body is not producing hormones in adequate amounts. Fats are required to make hormones and hormonelike substances called *prostaglandins* found in every tissue, cell, and organ in the body. By contrast, unhealthy fats and trans fats actually interfere with healthy hormone production by blocking the pathways in your body that produce hormones.

Where to Find Fats

If you have even the slightest interest in nutrition, you are probably well aware that fats are broken down into different groupings—*saturated, polyunsaturated, monounsaturated,* and *trans fats.*

Let's take a look at each category. Not all the fats mentioned in this next section are on the Baby Boomer Diet. Fats and oils in bold/italic type are the ones you will want to eat throughout the week, but remember: purchase these only if they are labeled as *unrefined, virgin,* or *raw.*

Have Your Fatty-Acid Levels Tested

*W*e recommend regular testing once or twice a year to see if you are deficient in certain fatty acids. Genova Diagnostics has created a test for blood-cell-membrane fats, called the Essential and Metabolic Fatty Acids Analysis (EMFA), which gives the ratios of the various fats, including saturated, monosaturated, polyunsaturated, and trans. You might request this from your physician. Nursing mothers can have their breast milk tested for fat content as well, with a CMT, or creamatocrit, test, which estimates the fat concentration and energy value of human milk.

Where you will find saturated fatty acids:

- *Butter, ghee,* and *egg yolk*

- Lard from pigs; tallow and suet from cattle, sheep, and lamb

- Whole-fat milk, cream, and cheese

- Meats and meat products such as sausage; poultry such as chicken, goose, and duck

- Plant sources such as *avocado, palm oil, coconut oil, coconut milk,* and *coconut meat*

Raw butter is delicious melted on your vegetables and grain-like seeds; ghee, red-palm oil, and coconut oil are great for cooking. All four can also be taken by the spoonful as a fatty-acid supplement. Once you correct any nutritional deficiencies, you will need a lesser amount of these in your diet on a daily basis. The cholesterol in egg yolk is an important fat for both growing and aging brains.

Where you will find unsaturated fatty acids:

- Nuts and their oils—macadamia, walnut, pecan, pine nut, and almond

- Seeds and their oils—flax, hemp, pumpkin, canola (note that unrefined canola has an unpleasant aftertaste), chia, tea, sacha inchi, and sesame

Time for an Oil Change!

Looking for a super-nutritious cooking oil? Try this Body Ecology blend:

1 cup ghee
1 cup coconut oil
3 Tbsp. red-palm oil

While still in their original glass jars, set oils down into very warm water to melt them. Mix together in a clean glass jar. This multipurpose cooking oil is great for sautéing. You can also take a spoonful each day as a supplement.

Other great oils you may not have considered:

- **Ghee**—less mucus-forming than butter; contains butyric and caprylic acid; has antimicrobial properties; absorbs directly, for quick energy

- **Coconut oil**—excellent for thyroid; easily digested; has antifungal, antiviral properties

- **Pumpkin-seed oil**—nourishes the ovaries, bladder, and digestive tract; helps fight parasites and is a source of zinc, iron, and niacin

- **Red-palm oil**—contains vitamins A and E and lauric acid; has antifungal, antiviral properties

- **Borage-seed oil**—helps regulate a woman's hormones

- **Evening-primrose oil**—helps regulate hormones (Barlean's Essential Woman is a blend of evening-primrose and flax oil: **www.barleans.com**)

- **Flaxseed oil**—a vegetarian source of omega-3s

- **Cod-liver oil**—great to take in colder months for omega-3s and vitamins A and D

- **Avocado oil** (unrefined)

- **Walnut oil** (available from **www.florahealth.com** and **www.lanogalerawalnutoil.com**)

- **Salmon oil**—rich in omega-3s; great for weight control (available from **www.vitalchoice.com**)

- **Marine-lipid oils**—includes anchovy, sardine, and krill oil (to learn much more about krill oil, visit: **www.mercola.com**)

- **Green-lipped-mussel oil** from New Zealand

- **Hemp-seed oil**—contains a good ratio of omega-3 and omega-6 (available from **www.manitobaharvest.com**)

- **Raw butter**—contains lipase, which helps digest fat; and butyric acid, for healthier intestinal microflora

There are also some flavorful oil blends:

- **Omega Nutrition** produces a blend called Essential Balance Junior—a mixture of flax oil, extra-virgin olive oil, and pumpkin-seed oil, plus flax particulate and natural butterscotch flavor. Their Garlic Chili Flax Seed Oil is also delicious (**www.omeganutrition.com**).

- **Foods Alive** produces flax oil blended with organic garlic and paprika (**www.foodsalive.com**).

- **Green Pasture** produces cinnamon-flavored cod-liver oil (**www.greenpasture.org**).

- **Barlean's** makes a wildly popular line of "swirl" oils (**www.barleans.com**). They are excellent by the spoonful for children of all ages and are also loved by adults. Use them in your green morning-smoothie recipes.

What about Salad Dressing?

A very simple blend of apple-cider vinegar and extra-virgin olive oil, salt, and pepper is an excellent everyday dressing.

For a change of pace, check out Cindy's Kitchen (**www.cindyskitchen.com**), which makes an organic dressing of creamy miso, sunflower oil, and extra-virgin olive oil. This is the only Body Ecology–approved dressing on the market so far. A dressing with *refined* sunflower oil would not have obtained our approval, but this one contains *high-oleic* sunflower oil, created by crossbreeding the sunflower plant so that the oil in the seed has a higher percentage of monounsaturated (oleic) fatty acids—similar to olive oil. High-oleic sunflower oil is also less susceptible to destruction by oxygen than regular sunflower oil, another beneficial attribute.

As for mayonnaise, the only commercially available mayo we can conditionally recommend is from Follow Your Heart, made with grape-seed oil, which is refined. To date we have not found one that is not. Yet, it is a much better choice than all the other refined oils. If you make mayo at home, you'll find it is more delicious and certainly healthier.

- Oily fish—salmon, fish eggs, cod-liver oil, and a variety of small fish, such as anchovies and sardines
- Vegetables—corn oil (not on The Diet)
- Legumes—peanut and soybean oil (not on The Diet)

Vegetable oils such as corn, soybean, and peanut oil unfortunately have permeated the Western diet and must be strictly avoided if you want to stay young. They have been refined and stripped of any valuable fatty acids. They have also been bleached and deodorized. To your liver and gallbladder, they read like plastic. To rejuvenate, you must give these organs your special attention, and a good first step would be to stop poisoning them!

All of the above oils can be obtained in their extra-virgin, unrefined state. They can be drizzled on your vegetables and grain-like seeds. They can also be taken by the spoonful as a fatty-acid supplement.

Where you will find monunsaturated fatty acids:

- Fruits such as *olives* and *olive oil, avocados* and *avocado oil,* and *tea-seed oil* (not to be confused with tea-*tree* oil)

How Much Fats to Eat

You have probably seen figures like "30 percent of the diet can come from fats," but numbers such as these are misleading and inaccurate. What if you ate 30 percent of your fat from butter but never ate fish oil, coconut oil, or seed oils. Where would you obtain lauric, caprylic, and omega-3 fatty acids?

If you are wondering exactly how *much* saturated fat from butter or ghee is recommended or if these saturated fats are right for you at all, remember that your body is unique. As there are a number of aspects to consider (see Chapter 8: The Principle of Uniqueness), I cannot suggest, as most diet books do, to eat a certain percentage of saturated fats or to avoid them completely. You must decide this for yourself (see the box earlier in the chapter for information on testing).

In a nutshell, when you follow the Body Ecology Way of Life, you can enjoy eating a delicious variety of all the recommended *organic, unrefined fats and oils* throughout the week . . . and slowly and surely watch your youthful vitality return.

Choosing the Right Ones

Only purchase oils that are *organic* and *unrefined* for the best health benefits—and choose a *variety* so that you get the full range of essential fatty acids.

If you had an intention to become the owner of a first-class baseball team, you wouldn't hire players who were only highly skilled at pitching the ball. You'd need some great catchers and some excellent batters and outfielders, too. This is true for the fats you'll want to employ to create a new and younger you. A variety of high-quality, unrefined fats and oils can play different and important roles in your body. Include this *variety* of healthy fats throughout the week since it will be difficult to include them all every day.

Therapeutically, one to three tablespoons of unrefined essential-fatty-acid oils should be taken at least once per day . . . especially in the beginning, since you will be correcting long-term nutritional deficiencies.

Omega-3s and Omega-6s

While there are hundreds of fatty acids found in nature, two unsaturated fatty acids, *omega-3* and *omega-6,* are called

---

Hemp-Seed Oil vs. Flaxseed Oil: A Better Balance

We've all heard of the health benefits of flaxseed oil, an ideal source of omega-3. Most of us are severely deficient in this fatty acid. When you first begin following the Baby Boomer Diet, it is recommended that you use flaxseed oil to get your omega-3 levels up to where they should be. But eventually you might consider switching to hemp-seed oil. Although flaxseed oil is higher in omega-3, hemp-seed oil provides the ideal ratio of fatty acids—the perfect balance of omega-3, omega-6, and omega-9. Go to **www.manitoba harvest.com** for a good source of hemp-seed oil.

---

essential fatty acids (EFAs), because it is *essential* that we obtain these from fats in our food. If the body has these two, it can manufacture the other important fatty acids it needs.

Most of us get ample amounts of omega-6. It is in the omega-3s that we are seriously deficient. Omega-3 fatty acids are especially important for rejuvenation of our prenatal jing energy and for prevention of many problems of aging. They are needed for building cells, especially the cells of the brain and nervous system, eyes, and circulatory system, including the heart. Omega-3 oils also quell inflammation.

Flax and chia seeds are vegetarian sources of omega-3s. Omega-3s can also be found in "marine lipid" oils. This simply means fish oils from salmon, anchovy, sardines, and krill.

One of our very favorite oils at Body Ecology is derived from the pristine waters of the Marlborough Sounds region of New Zealand, where the unique properties of the ozone layer and intense UV rays cause the highly prized Greenshell mussel ("green-lipped mussel") and other life-forms to develop an unparalleled combination of lipid groups and unique omega-3 polyunsaturated fatty acids—which the native Maori have thrived on for more than 700 years.

Studies show that Greenshell-mussel oil has significant anti-inflammatory properties and can benefit patients with asthma, osteoarthritis, rheumatoid arthritis, asthma, and other inflammatory conditions. Pernax, a special formulation of Greenshell-mussel oil and evening-primrose oil, has arrived just in time for Baby Boomers. Find out more about this amazing product at: **www.pernax.com/bodyecology**.

(Most people don't realize that fish don't make the omega-3s themselves but rather accumulate these oils from the microbes and microalgae they feed on in the marine environment.)

There has been some concern of late with regard to the increased demand on wild-fish stocks and fish farmers as consumers' primary source of omega-3s. Dwindling stocks, along with the risks associated with polluted fish, have encouraged the industry to explore the extraction of omega-3 from alternative sources. One of these potential sources is a noxious weed from Australia called Paterson's Curse, which contains high levels of the stearidonic acid that fish such as Atlantic salmon can convert to omega-3 oils. Companies such as Martek Biosciences are already offering algae-derived omega-3 DHA as a dietary supplement, while other companies continue to search for sustainable and pollutant-free sources of EPA and DHA.[7]

Fat Intolerance

If you have difficulty digesting fats and oils, most likely your liver and/or gallbladder are congested. It is important to begin the process of cleansing your liver. (See Chapter 24 for more on detoxification and colon cleansing.) One of our Body Ecology products, LivAmend, has been designed to increase bile flow so that toxins leave your liver more effectively. We have testimonials and lab reports from people who tell us that LivAmend has lowered their elevated LDL cholesterol levels in a short period of time. (See the Body Ecology website for more details on LivAmend.)

Most important, creating an inner ecosystem of beneficial, fat-digesting microflora is a must to help digest and assimilate the fats you consume. Fat intolerance will improve as you eat and drink fermented foods and beverages each day.

Symptoms of fat intolerance are: pains in the neck and shoulders, spasms in the large and small intestines, feeling tired just after eating, bloating, indigestion, belching, flatulence and/or nausea, upper-right abdominal discomfort, and hard stools. Fat intolerance can be confirmed by a simple urine test or by eliminating fats from your diet for a week and noting any improvement in your digestion and energy.

Fermented foods and enzymes should be taken at every meal to help with digestion of fats. The fat-digesting enzymes are: lipase, pancreatin, and ox bile.

Keep in mind that when you eat animal protein, excessive amounts of fats, even those recommended, delay the secretion of gastric juices. This means those all-American tuna, egg, and chicken salads with heaps of mayo could be contributing to your symptoms of discomfort.

A small amount of organic, unrefined coconut oil, ghee, or red-palm oil used for sautéing shouldn't cause you any discomfort, while salad dressings or heaps of butter on your foods may. (You can find a Body Ecology no-oil salad-dressing recipe on: **www.bodyecology.com**.)

Putting the Principles into Practice

Fats and the Principle of Uniqueness

The Body Ecology universal Principle of Uniqueness tells us that we should not compare our own needs for fats and oils with those of others. Each of us is unique. The *quantity* of fat and oil to consume at one time will ultimately depend on the current health of the liver and gallbladder.

And most important, you must ask yourself, "How well do I digest these fats and oil?" Yes, butter can be a valuable fat, but only if it is right for *your* unique body. You are an experiment of one. You have to find out what your body needs at this moment in time, and that need will change constantly. Seem confusing? Not really, just tune in to your body and listen. It will communicate to you through signs and symptoms if you eat foods that are *not* right for you.

You can try to determine your own individual need for fats and oils by carefully watching how your body reacts to each one, but *ideally, taking the Essential and Metabolic Fatty Acid Analysis test mentioned earlier in the chapter is best.*

The next best thing is to try one fat or oil at a time. When you have not eaten for at least three hours, take a spoonful of the fat or oil, and watch to see how it makes you feel . . . but again, testing is far more accurate in determining your immediate and individual needs.

Here are few questions to answer to help determine your unique fat needs:

— **What is your level of activity?** If you are active, you will definitely require more fats in your diet, and you will be able to consume more butter or ghee. Remember, the enzymes lipase and pancreatin can help with fat digestion.

— **Do you live in a cold climate or a hot one?** If you live in a cold climate or in a place with cold seasons, your body will need the extra fat to help you stay warm. Baby Boomers who retire to Florida or flee to exotic islands will find they can use much less. In fact, they might do best with saturated fat from plants, such as coconut oil and palm oil.

— **Are you a large, big-boned person; or are you small-boned?** Saturated fats are important for healthy bone development. Big bones need more.

— **How's your level of stress?** You may want to increase the amount of butter and ghee in your diet when you are under a lot of stress. (Probably not an issue if you are exploring a tropical island!)

— **Are you deficient in the fatty acids found in milk fat?** Have you been avoiding butter for years and been eating margarine instead? At first you may notice that you are actually craving yummy raw butter. Your body truly needs it, so enjoy! You'll soon find that this craving diminishes, and you will be satisfied with less.

— And then, finally, you must deal honestly with these questions: **What is the current condition of your organs, especially your liver and gallbladder? How well do you digest fats today?** Many of us have livers that are very congested and toxic. As we age, the liver also begins to shrink and is supplied with less blood. Ultimately, rejuvenating this organ so that you can benefit from these healthy fats and oils will be necessary.

Fats and the Principle of Balance

Fats and oils are slightly expansive and acidic, and we innately want to combine them with sea salt, because it is strongly contractive and alkaline.

To see this for yourself, make a salad dressing with extra-virgin olive oil and vinegar or lemon juice. Taste the mixture.

Boring?

Now add sea salt and *voilà*: what a difference . . . it's become a delicious topping or dressing. (Our favorite salad-dressing salt at Body Ecology is Hawaiian sea salt from **www.selinanaturally .com**.)

When you eat fats, you will also want to balance them out with other foods. Raw daikon, leafy-green salads, apple-cider vinegar, and lemon juice are great choices because they create balance by helping with the digestion of fats. Ginger, fennel, and tumeric are examples of spices that aid in their digestion as well.

Fats and the Principle of Food Combining

Fats and oils combine well with many foods: grain-like seeds, for example, or meals with animal proteins, including dairy proteins found in milk kefir. Land, ocean, starchy, and fermented vegetables are more delicious with fats and oils.

Be Creative with Your Use of Organic, Unrefined Oils

It's Not Just about Olive Oil Anymore

Many of us are limited by our imaginations when it comes to healthy oils. We may be avoiding the bad oils, such as vegetable and canola oil, but we have made olive oil the *only* one in our pantry.

While extra-virgin olive oil is an excellent choice for salads, it's not a good idea to cook with it. Why? Under high heat, it burns easily, and when it does, it turns into a toxin. There are certain oils that are better for cooking, because they withstand a higher heat before degenerating. Some we would never want to heat because they lose their *medicinal* qualities. To retain the antioxidants and vitamin E in olive oil, eat it raw.

When you follow the Body Ecology Way of Life, ghee, coconut oil, and red-palm oil are the three oils used to sauté. Raw butter, virgin olive oil, and unrefined seed and nut oils are best drizzled right onto your food or used in salad-dressing recipes. If you want, you can add these to a sauce after it has cooled down a bit or just before eating.

What if you eat out, don't cook, or aren't preparing your food at home every day? There is nothing wrong with taking your needed amount on a spoon. Fish oils also come in capsules.

Documenting the effect that bad fats and oils . . . coupled with deficiencies of the good ones . . . have had on each generation is beyond the scope of this chapter or book, but needless to say, it has been devastating. It's time to turn the fat story around and do it right. It's up to us Baby Boomers to correct a serious wrong.

Changing the fats and oils you eat is a good, yet simple, first step. The next chapter will discuss an equally controversial topic today—*protein.*

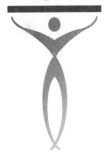

Chapter 18

Protein: Body Ecology's 7 Principles Shed Light on the Controversy

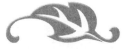

Integral to every cell in the body, protein is used to build and repair tissues, and to make enzymes and hormones. However, as we age, we must rethink our protein needs—considering type, quality, and digestibility. Body Ecology's 7 Principles can help lead the way.

I was born in Athens, Georgia, a sleepy university town. At 16, I got my first car, a Morris Minor. To me it was a rite of passage that meant freedom and independence. We Baby Boomers created the new "car culture." It was during the '50s that the first motels and drive-in banks, theaters, and restaurants emerged. Clearly, we loved our cars so much that we never wanted to leave them, not even to eat!

Bubble haircuts were in, so all day Saturday we wore big ugly rollers in our hair so that we would look "cute" for Saturday night . . . party time. We watched movies from the hoods of our cars, and drove to frat parties or to Charlie Williams's Pinecrest Lodge, where there were great bands, too much beer, and horribly unhealthy food.

It's funny how many of us associate some of the most memorable times in our lives with food. One favorite memory of mine was eating with my friends at the Varsity drive-in. The Varsity specialized in chili dogs, kraut dogs, greasy fries, and huge Coca-Colas. I especially loved the kraut dogs—perhaps an early clue to my future love affair with cultured cabbage! When I think of my teen years, I can still remember the smells and warmth of that special time.

Although they were here and gone faster than 8-track players, you might say drive-in restaurants were one of the places where our generation came of age. Did you have a Krystal burger joint or Dairy Queen in your hometown? The short-lived drive-ins of yesterday have been mostly replaced with today's far more tenacious fast-food restaurants. The greasy fries, cheap-quality burgers on spongy buns, sugary soft drinks, and sickly sweet desserts remain a permanent fixture of American culture. Now, decades later, as our grandchildren enter this world, we are beginning to glimpse the consequences of this fast-food diet.

If we had only known then what we know now!

The Beef with Beef

Our generation must begin . . . step by step . . . to undo the damage of the past. Today, there are a number of compelling reasons why we should change our eating habits with regard to animal protein. How we embrace this change on a personal level will have an impact globally. The world's total meat supply is increasing at an alarming rate. In 1961, it was estimated at 71 million tons a year. In 2007, that figure had risen to around 284 million tons. Americans continue to eat about eight ounces of meat a day, roughly twice the global average. More meat means more feed, especially corn and soy . . . which not only raises the price, but also exacts a heavy cost on our energy supplies and on our environment. In fact, nearly three-fourths of the problem we have with water quality in U.S. rivers and streams is caused by our unquenchable demand for meat.[1]

In Eric Schlosser's widely read book *Fast Food Nation,*

he talks about our poorly regulated meat industry and its potential health threats. Every day in the United States roughly 200,000 people become ill from foodborne disease. More than a quarter of the American population suffers a bout of food poisoning each year, and this is just a small fraction, as most of these illnesses are not reported.[2]

However, the problem is not with the animals, but with the way we now commercially raise them—in cruel, large-scale confinement facilities. Turning this problem around is one of the most challenging issues facing Baby Boomers; and it will take a focused effort from a healthy, energetic generation to tackle it with a compassionate heart.

So is this meant to suggest that you give up meat or other animal proteins such as fish, milk, eggs, poultry, and beef? Perhaps, but the choice will be yours to make. In this chapter you'll find exactly what you need to know to make this decision. Here are six important points to remember:

1. We need protein throughout our lives.

2. Not all proteins are alike.

3. Adequate protein can be obtained from both the animal and plant kingdoms.

4. It is not wise to obtain all your protein from animals. However, if you choose to be a vegetarian, you will have to take great care not to miss out on certain nutrients, including amino acids, minerals, fats, and vitamins found in animal products.

5. All foods have their positive and negative sides . . . including all protein foods.

6. Proper digestion is crucial to ensure that the value of high-quality protein is not lost.

What Exactly Is a Protein?

If all of the water and fat is removed from the body, 75 percent of what remains is protein. Protein consists of chains of amino acids. There are 22 amino acids that combine to form different types of proteins. Everything, from our neurotransmitters, the chemical messengers of our brains; to our organs, blood, bones, hair, and nails are composed of proteins. Nine of the 22 amino acids are called *essential,* and because our bodies can't make them, they must be obtained from the diet. We need to consume proteins or we will be deficient in these essential amino acids.

Your body expends more energy to digest protein than sugars or fats. But unlike sugars, which provide quick energy, protein provides long-lasting energy without an insulin surge (which promotes fat storage). For these reasons, protein can help keep you lean and slender.

The protein in our diets determines the amount of an important hormone in the body called *glucagon,* which helps balance insulin. While insulin can *contribute* to fat storage, glucagon helps prevent it. Body fat, especially abdominal fat, creates inflammation. And low-grade chronic inflammation leads to every disease of aging: diabetes, cardiovascular disease, cancer, Alzheimer's, rheumatoid arthritis, inflammatory bowel disease, and gum disease.

As we age, sarcopenia (muscle wasting) becomes a serious problem. The youngest of the Baby Boomers are now in their 40s, so most of us have already begun to experience a loss of muscle mass. Those of us entering our seventh decade can expect an even more rapid decline in muscle unless we make changes to our diet, digestion, and way of life. Even if we are physically active, low-grade acidosis, inflammation, and a lack of minerals in the diet will cause our muscles to disappear. Protein helps build muscles that make us look sexier and more youthful.

Sources of Animal Protein

Eggs

Contrary to popular belief, it is the egg *yolk* that is the healthiest part of the egg. Eggs yolks are great for your brain, thyroid, and hormones—they contain good fats and are an excellent source of vitamins A and D. They also contain the B vitamin *choline*—the precursor to acetylcholine, an important stimulating neurotransmitter that is deficient in the brains of those with Alzheimer's. Choline also helps convert fats into HDL, the good cholesterol.

This may surprise you if you still believe in an outdated perception that egg yolks raise cholesterol. They do, but you *want* this good cholesterol.

While it is difficult to find them, try to purchase eggs from *pasture-fed* chickens that have not been fed soybeans. In nature, chickens eat worms and bugs for their protein, not soy. They are not vegetarians. Eggs from chickens that eat their natural proteins, live cage-free lives, and are never fed hormones are the very best.

Fish & Shellfish

Oily fish, like salmon, are one of the most preferred animal-protein foods on the Body Ecology program. We recommend having fish at least two or three times per week. Avoid warm-water species, like orange roughy, because preservatives are used when they are caught. Cold-water fish are best, such as salmon, sardines, tuna, and halibut. Salmon and sardines are especially healthy because they are rich in omega-3s.

Meat & Poultry

Meat and poultry, especially from organic, hormone- and antibiotic-free animals, can be excellent sources of protein for some. While red meat has gotten bad publicity in recent years, more recent studies are coming out to debunk these myths. Beef, a complete protein, is high in minerals and B vitamins and contains heart-healthy carnitine and coenzyme Q_{10}. Lamb is also an excellent protein, strengthening to many, especially those with blood type B. The important thing to remember with regard to beef is quality and preparation.

Milk Kefir

If dairy works well in your body, this ancient food has long been thought to increase longevity. It is fun, delicious, and very easy to make with Body Ecology's Kefir Starter. Use goat, cow, or sheep milk . . . raw, if possible. Find a source at: **www.realmilk.com**. (For more on kefir, refer to Chapter 15: Fermented Foods.)

Meat in Moderation

Apart from its global impact, *excessive* consumption of red-meat protein also exacts a great toll on our health. A study of more than 500,000 middle-aged and older Americans found that those who consumed *more than four ounces of red meat a day* (the equivalent of a small hamburger) were more than 30 percent more likely to die during the ten years in which they were observed, mostly from heart disease and cancer. Sausage, cold cuts, and other processed meats also increased the risk. (See "Protein and the Principle of 80/20" later in the chapter.)

At the same time, the study revealed that those who consumed the most white meat (poultry and fish) were about 8 percent less likely to die during the study period than those who ate the least. This is because poultry contains more unsaturated fat, which improves cholesterol levels; while fish contains omega-3 fatty acids, which reduce the risk of heart disease.

Researchers stressed that the study results do not mean people should eliminate red meat from their diets entirely, but simply avoid eating it in large amounts and every day. Walter Willett, a nutrition expert at the Harvard School of Public Health, writes: "You can be very healthy being a vegetarian, but you can be very healthy being a non-vegetarian if you keep your red meat intake low."[3]

Sources of Vegetarian Proteins

Nuts & Seeds

Nuts and seeds are nutrient-dense protein/fats, best eaten after soaking 8 to 12 hours to remove the phytic acid that makes them difficult to digest. There are some good reasons not to overdo these foods. Very concentrated sources of protein, nuts, and seeds are not only acidic; they are also rich in the amino acid arginine, which often triggers viral outbreaks. If you have herpes or AIDs, avoid them or eat them in very small quantities . . . perhaps sprinkled in a salad. Take the mineral selenium and also lysine, another amino acid. Unfortunately, nuts and seeds are also rich in oxalates, which should be avoided, or at least limited, in many people's diets. (See the low-oxalate diet in Chapter 19.)

Beans

Beans are mostly a carbohydrate combined with some protein. This makes them intrinsically harder to digest. They digest best when combined with land, ocean, and fermented vegetables. To really get the benefits of the protein in beans, they must be soaked for 8 to 24 hours to remove the phytic acid. To minimize the gas-producing effect of beans, soak them for at least 8 hours, and then cook them slowly for 45 minutes in water. Pour off the water and start cooking again. This time, add a strip of the sea vegetable *kombu*. Salt can be added *after* the beans have become soft.

Eating beans only with fresh and cultured veggies in a meal is a big help when it comes to digesting them. Combining beans with a grain such as rice or with a tortilla, as is traditionally done, is not recommended. Beans can also be soaked, sprouted, cooked, and then blended up into a delicious pâté.

Fermented Soybean Foods

The best way to eat beans is to ferment them, and with soybeans, it is absolutely critical to do so. Fermented soy foods such as miso, wheat-free tamara, natto, and tempeh are definitely on The Diet and are excellent anti-aging foods.

The phytoestrogens and isoflavones in soybeans have estrogen-like activity and are structurally similar to estrogen. They bind easily to receptor sites on a cell.

While unfermented soy foods such as tofu and soy milk have been heavily promoted recently as having significant therapeutic properties for women, most of the claims (breast- and prostate-cancer prevention, reducing cholesterol, and prevention and treatment of postmenopausal symptoms and osteoporosis) have not been confirmed in well-designed clinical trials.

Instead, a more convincing body of research shows that the phytoestrogens being consumed in large quantities in popular *unfermented* soy foods (soy milk, tofu, energy bars, protein shakes, ice cream, yogurt, cheese, hot dogs, and so on) are disrupting the endocrine system. They can cause infertility and can *promote* breast cancer . . . not prevent it. Japanese researcher Hiro Watanbe, an expert in developmental biology and cancer prevention, has shown that *fermented* miso soup helps to dramatically lower the risk of breast cancer and even to reverse it.

Disturbing studies are now showing that unfermented soy foods suppress the thyroid, and tofu has been shown to negatively affect cognitive function in older people. MSG is formed during the processing of soy, and soy foods also contain high levels of aluminum.

What else is the research showing about the many negative

Natto—for Bones and Beauty

*N*atto, a traditional food of Japan, has been a staple in that country for more than a thousand years. Sometimes called "vegetable cheese," natto is simply fermented soybeans. Rich in vegetable protein and vitamin B_{12}, natto is nourishing, cooling, and antiviral. It has been linked to prevention of cancer, heart attacks, osteoporosis, and obesity. Although these health benefits are often attributed to soy, it's really the *bacteria* in natto that give it its kick. *Bacillus natto* produces various enzymes, vitamins, amino acids, and other nutrients that can only emerge during fermentation.

Under good conditions, natto bacteria can double their numbers in 30 minutes, producing various enzymes that help digestion. *Nattokinase* and *pyrazine* are two enzymes present in natto that prevent or reduce blood clotting, which obstructs the flow of blood and is often the precursor to heart attacks and strokes. Nattokinase is only produced during natto's fermentation process.

Another interesting thing to note about natto is that it has a very high amount of vitamin K, which helps in the formation of our bones. Very few foods contain naturally occurring vitamin K. People with osteoporosis tend to have low amounts, so this is an ideal natural supplement.

And finally, natto has some wonderfully "youthening" cosmetic benefits. Soybeans are high in *lecithin*, a *surfactant* (wetting agent) that balances fat and water in skin cells and on the cell surface. This may explain why Japanese women have smoother, clearer skin than Europeans and Americans. Natto is also rich in vitamin E, which helps prevent skin damage and keeps us looking young.

side effects of *unfermented* soy foods? The list is extensive and scary. It includes: high levels of phytic acid (which reduce the assimilation of calcium, magnesium, copper, iron, and zinc) and trypsin inhibitors (which interfere with the digestion of protein and may cause pancreatic disorders).

When you eat unfermented soy, your need for vitamins D and B$_{12}$ will increase. These two vitamins are seriously deficient in many people today anyway.

Note: If your sons and daughters have infants, please tell them to do their own research on the damaging effects of soy-milk formulas. Soy milk has none of the real nourishment found in breast milk. Feeding soy to a child risks permanent endocrine-system damage.

Growing in popularity since they were first introduced in 1939, soy formulas are one more factor contributing to the increasing rate of infertility in our children and grandchildren. In 1992, the Swiss health service estimated that 100 grams of soy protein provided the estrogenic equivalent of the birth-control pill.[4] Hormonal changes begin to occur after only one month on soy milk, and the large amounts of phytoestrogens present are hormone disruptors. Soy formula causes *hypothyroidism* and *autoimmune* thyroid disorders. And research shows that its phytic acid and the trypsin inhibitors stunt growth.

The soybean is difficult to ferment, and only hardy bacteria can do the job. The bacteria, working over months or even years, degrade the proteins into easily digested amino acids and the fats into fatty acids, while also reducing the starch and sugar in the beans.

If you'd like to learn more about the negative effects of soy, visit the Weston A. Price Foundation website: **westonaprice .org**. Their information is well supported by research.

Green Drinks with Algae and Cereal Grasses

Look for a whole-food green drink that contains a wide spectrum of beneficial microflora and beneficial yeast, digestive enzymes, and protein. Examples are Body Ecology's Potent Proteins and our very popular blend called Vitality SuperGreen. Knowing how important it is to alkalize the body and nourish it with easily digested nutrients that assimilate immediately, we've made sure that both of our green protein powders contain fermented ingredients to help heal the digestive tract.

Body Ecology's Grain-like Seeds

Quinoa, millet, buckwheat, and amaranth are similar to a grain and are preferred over rice, wheat, barley, oats, and rye. (See Chapter 20 for more on these important protein-rich foods.) They should be on your daily menu.

Protein Malnourishment

Perhaps you've already accepted that as the years go by your body will become less muscular. Isn't that normal with aging?

Even though we consume twice the global average of animal proteins, protein malnourishment is surprisingly quite common in America. In fact, even our children are protein deficient, yet most consume animal protein every day. *You* may have become protein deficient in childhood even if you were a big "meat eater." Why? Because even from birth, many of us have not been *digesting* the protein we eat.

Protein malnourishment elevates the amount of cortisol in our blood and causes us to feel stressed-out, sleep poorly, and age quickly. A deficiency in protein has other serious negative effects. Our organs fail; thinking, planning, and cognition go on the blink; and the immune system crashes and has difficulty fighting infections. Since our brains, bones, hair, nails, and muscles all rely on protein, they lose their vibrancy—their life force.

Clearly, protein is a vital nutrient, and *eating the right protein foods is vital for combatting aging*. But the $64 million question every Baby Boomer must now be asking is, "If my goal is to add more quality years to my life and eliminate age-related suffering, must I alter the *kind* of protein foods, as well as the *amount*, I eat?" The answer is, without a doubt, yes!

Even though we consume twice the global average of animal proteins, protein malnourishment is surprisingly quite common here in America. In fact, even our children are protein deficient, yet most consume animal protein every day. How can this be?

Putting the Principles into Practice

Over the years, I have learned that the discussion of protein is much like politics and religion . . . a provocative topic with highly charged emotions and strongly held belief systems. And, although I know to never discuss politics or religion at a dinner party, there is no way I could write a diet book and avoid this controversial area of nutrition. Wouldn't it be nice if we could let science lead us to the best answers?

Sadly, there are many hard-core scientific studies showing that we need animal protein, so there are many advocates for high-protein diets. However, there is just as much "solid science" advocating a vegetarian diet . . . especially for cancer prevention and anti-aging.

So where do you go for answers? Body Ecology can help finally put an end to this protein debate and offer something for everyone. While research on calorie restriction seems to provide significant clues, *the 7 Principles of the Body Ecology system of health and healing will once and for all clear up this confusion . . . as I find they always do.*

Protein and the Principle of 80/20
(vs. Calorie Restriction)

The word *calorie* is an unpleasant one to many of us who have been dieting for years, and *restriction* is perhaps even more objectionable to a Baby Boomer who doesn't believe in holding back when he or she wants something. Several studies actually suggest that as we age our protein intake needs to be even *higher* than what is currently recommended, and at Body Ecology we agree. We do need *"more"* protein than we are currently consuming, but not more *quantity*. In fact, the secret to pushing back Father Time is to decrease the *quantity* of protein and add more *quality*—from a *wide variety of sources,* not just animals—and to make sure we digest it better.

Thomas Jefferson probably said it best: "I have lived temperately, eating little animal food, and that not as an aliment, so much as a condiment for the vegetables which constitute my principal diet."[5] A man of many interests, Jefferson was passionate about architecture, gardening, music, wine, and food. Although he never needed to cook his own meals, it is said he frequently collected delicious recipes from chefs and shared them with his friends.

As you envision protein as a "condiment," remember the Principle of 80/20: 80 percent of your serving plate will be land and ocean vegetables; the remaining 20 percent should be animal protein. Always emphasize vegetables, with a focus on adding fermented vegetables, as this is critical to fostering vitality and a healthy inner ecosystem.

By the way, the average life span in Jefferson's day was only 45 years. Born on April 13, 1743, the third U.S. President lived to be 83, dying in 1826. Certainly this man of great intention, intuition, and wisdom had something to tell us.*

Animal proteins are potent sources of nutrition. This is one of the main reasons we don't need a large serving at a meal. Even nuts and seeds are concentrated sources of nutrition. Indeed, to truly follow what science is revealing with regard to calorie restriction, we must eat smaller amounts of very *high-quality protein*. And we must discover the proteins that are best for us!

Protein and the Principle of Balance

Animal proteins are *contractive* because of the naturally occurring salt in blood. To create balance, you will feel best if you eat them with more *expansive* foods. For example, a poached salmon or chicken fillet *(contractive)* on top of a big raw salad with a dressing of olive oil and lemon juice or vinegar, plus cultured vegetables *(more expansive),* creates a very nice balance of ingredients.

Animal protein is also acidic; and since salt, while contracting, is the most alkalizing of all foods, you might have noticed that when you eat certain acidic proteins (fish, eggs, chicken, beef, and even nuts), they taste much more delicious with sea salt. It's your natural instinct to balance the *acid* protein with the very *alkaline* salt.

Nuts and seeds are less contractive than animal proteins, as you will see if you look at the Expansion/Contraction Continuum at the end of Chapter 11. They do not naturally have the salt content of animal foods. You can salt your nuts to make them more alkaline; and they, too, will go nicely in a big raw salad with dressing, plus cultured vegetables.

Chlorella, spirulina, and blue-green algae are excellent vegetarian proteins that have become more and more popular

---

* Jefferson also said: "Every generation needs a new revolution." Ours hasn't happened yet, *and it's about time.*

today. While they are alkaline, they have an *expansive*, opening-up quality. Adding *contracting* sea salt to a drink containing algae can help create that perfect balance. I often recommend adding a pinch of sea salt to a "green veggie smoothie" in the morning, because all those expansive, raw veggies become more balanced with the more contractive sea salt.

Protein and the Principle of Acid/Alkaline

A recent study compared an acidic diet, full of acid-producing proteins and cereal grains, to a diet rich in alkaline-producing fruits and vegetables. The results indicate that metabolic acidosis from the meat-and-grain diet appears to contribute to a reduction in lean tissue mass in older adults. *The alkaline diet favored lean tissue mass.*[6]

If you choose to eat acid-forming proteins, you must balance them with alkaline-forming foods, including small amounts of sour fruits and larger amounts of vegetables from the garden and ocean. If you don't do this, you will rapidly deplete your *chi* or life force.

Protein and the Principle of Food Combining

The meat-and-potatoes meal, characteristic of the standard American diet, contributes to an inner-ecosystem imbalance. It causes you to gain weight and use up metabolic enzymes, which will age you faster. Chapter 13 covered the importance of food combining, so by now, you know that meat and potatoes (the first acid and the second alkaline) neutralize the acid in your stomach, inhibiting the first stage of digestion. When these foods enter the small intestine—where both protein and starches are digested—digestion suffers here as well. Not only that, but the door is opened to potential pathogens that would have been destroyed by the stomach acid.

To digest animal protein and maximize its benefits, always combine it with nonstarchy vegetables from the land and ocean and cultured veggies. For example, combine scrambled eggs with cultured veggies and steamed asparagus.

Nuts and seeds are a *protein/fat,* as is avocado. Dairy foods such as milk kefir and raw cheese are also protein/fats. You could drink a glass of milk kefir and eat some soaked almonds or walnuts. All protein/fats combine well with members of the acid-fruit family (such as grapefruit, strawberry, and raspberry).

All foods in this protein/fat category also can be combined with vegetables.

Examples:

- Avocado with nuts and seeds and with acid fruits.

- A salad made with romaine lettuce, avocado, soaked and dehydrated sunflower seeds, blueberries, or grapefruit sections. You could even toss in a few cubes of raw cheese (if this protein works for your body).

- A smoothie made with milk kefir, sour Granny Smith apple, celery, zucchini, and stevia to sweeten. A bit of coconut oil would be tasty, too, and a spoonful of chia seeds will add fiber and omega-3 fatty acid.

All the organic, unrefined oils combine with the proteins mentioned above. In fact, all proteins naturally contain oils. For example, salmon has salmon oil, cod liver has cod-liver oil, walnuts have walnut oil, and hemp seeds have hemp oil. Oil can even be found in algae. The brain-nourishing fatty acid DHA can be obtained from the oil in algae.

The four recommended grain-like seeds—quinoa, millet, amaranth, and buckwheat—are protein/starches. Because of the starch, most people find that these digest best when eaten as the main entrée and combined with nonstarchy vegetables. If you combine them with animal proteins and nuts and seeds, you may find that your digestion is sluggish and gassy. If you must serve a meal with animal protein and a grain, however, these grain-like seeds are a much better choice than traditional protein/grain combinations such as chicken and rice, meatballs with pasta, or eggs with toast and oatmeal.

Protein and the Principle of Uniqueness

Because the Principle of Uniqueness says that no one diet fits all, some of us may feel better and maintain more muscle mass when we eat animal protein. Some of us will feel lighter and more fit if we are vegetarians.

In other words, you will have to decide whether animal protein works in *your* unique body and how much you should be eating each day. (Or perhaps several times per week?)

The Body Ecology Way, with its 7 Universal Principles, excellent-quality fats and oils, and wide array of fermented foods and liquids, can also enhance the diet of any vegetarian or someone who is considering a non-carnivore way of life. You would then also have the benefits of a gluten-free, sugar-free diet. This will help you maintain the important anti-aging, acid/alkaline balance of your blood.

The best place to begin is by asking yourself the right questions, educating yourself, and seeking out a source for reliable testing. You might consider consulting with a Body Ecology Coach or scheduling a visit to a health-care professional who knows the Body Ecology Way.

Start paying attention to *your* body. Maybe you'll find that where you live right now requires you to eat more animal protein and fats. It's harder to eat only raw foods when you live in a cold climate, because they cool the body and provide no warmth. They work well in warmer climates, like the Southwest, Florida, Hawaii, and California, however . . . where you'll notice most raw food–ists reside.

What's your age? A growing baby will not have the same nutritional needs as someone in his or her 70s.

If you are a Baby Boomer woman, you have probably put your childbearing years behind you, but how about your daughter? Is she pregnant or nursing? Her nutritional needs change dramatically, and calorie restriction would be very wrong for her.

What's happening with your own hormones? Did you eat a lot of acidic foods such as meat, pasta, and ice cream as a child and as an adult . . . and now you are experiencing hot flashes and low libido in your 40s? An acid-forming diet will wreak havoc with your hormones, burning out your endocrine system quickly and causing you to age.

And very important, what are you *digesting* right now? Undigested food becomes another toxin in your digestive tract, so how you prepare what you eat so that you can digest it will be fundamental.

There is one commonality among everyone, regardless of age, hormones, lifestyle, activity level, and current state of health: the need for fermented foods and beverages.

Being Vegetarian or Vegan on the Baby Boomer Diet

The Baby Boomer Diet is mostly plant based but not necessarily vegetarian. Because each of us is an experiment of one, it would be violating the Principle of Uniqueness to say that everyone needs—or shouldn't have—animal foods.

Humans are the only animals on the planet that have the capability and freedom to grow and harvest a wide variety of foods. This makes living on Earth very exciting, but it has given us something else to argue about. Unfortunately, even our diet triggers strife.

Millions of us feel stronger and more grounded when we eat animal foods. We also have a powerful emotional and even genetic attachment to them, because not only have we grown up eating them every day, but also as a race we've been doing so for thousands of years, and our cells and our genes are familiar with them. They simply seem comforting and natural to us.

For many reasons, some of us prefer to be "vegetarian" while still consuming some animal products such as dairy foods and eggs. A vegetarian feels good because the animal has not been killed to provide nourishment, yet he or she is obtaining important nutrients available only in animal sources of food.

If you choose to be vegetarian or vegan, the Baby Boomer Diet can help you go about this even better.

Many of us who have tried a raw, vegan diet feel lighter and more energetic. Others of us find we cannot digest raw vegetables, but feel as if we're being judged and in the wrong if we're not eating an all-raw diet. After all, cooking kills the enzymes, right? (Chapter 19 talks more about raw versus cooked vegetables.) And, of course, raw food–ists believe that if we eat all raw, we won't age as quickly.

But the Principle of Uniqueness is infallible and cannot be ignored. You must find what is right for you. Determine your needs and know that these will change through the years.

When you embark on a vegan or raw-foods diet, you might thrive for a certain period of time . . . say, one day, one week, a month, or several years . . . on this lighter fare. This is because it is right for your *unique* body at this point in your life. But maybe you're beginning to look older, and your spine is developing a curve. Your teeth and gums have started to deteriorate, and you can't carry on a focused conversation with your accountant. These conditions can be related to protein deficiency.

It's very important to take a fish-oil supplement. Cod-liver oil, butter, ghee, and egg yolks provide vitamins A and D. Vegetarians can become deficient in B_{12} and important amino acids such as tyrosine and taurine. Full-spectrum amino-acid supplements are available but should be unnecessary if you are eating the right vegetarian protein foods and digesting them properly. Supplements are great, but there is nothing as effective as well-digested food. You might also consider adding Body Ecology's Potent Proteins powder to your diet, as this is an excellent source of B_{12}.

Always be willing to change. Your body will constantly be going in and out of balance. Your goal is to be mindful of bringing it back into balance.

Be watchful . . . and when you see symptoms of low energy, anxiety, spaciness, tooth decay, hormonal imbalances, and loss of sexual desire, it may be time to add in more grounding animal foods and/or animal fats such as butter, ghee, cod-liver oil, egg yolks, or even raw-milk kefir. Ask yourself questions such as the following:

- "What does my body need today?"
- "How active will I be today?"
- "How much energy do I need to create for my body today?"
- "My tests show that I am losing bone density; what's not working now?"

If you are less active, you may find you do best on your own unique version of a vegetarian/vegan/raw-foods diet, with occasional animal foods added in for grounding and strength.

Some of us are very active sometimes but then have quiet, restful days as well. Wake up and decide what *your* body needs for that day. It's a matter of supply and demand. You supply what *your* body demands.

How to Prepare Animal Protein for Ideal Digestion

To digest protein, you must have strong "digestive fire." This means adequate amounts of digestive enzymes in your stomach and small intestine. Hydrochloric acid (HCl), pepsin, and pancreatic enzymes (found in the small intestine) that digest protein and fats are often inadequate or nonexistent. Ironically, when you are too acidic and deficient in minerals, your stomach will not produce enough stomach acid—creating a vicious cycle: low stomach acid equals low minerals; then low minerals equal low stomach acid.

If you find you feel stronger and more grounded when you eat animal proteins but have weak digestion, then you must find ways to prepare these foods so that they are easy to digest.

Prepare as a Puree

"Blenderize" your animal proteins such as chicken or fish into a pâté (like baby food). Salmon pâté can be a tasty delicacy.

Prepare Savory Stocks

Prepare only the *broth* of the animal (fish, chicken, or lamb broth).

Dine on Rare, Raw, and Fermented Food

Indigenous people around the world instinctively knew to eat a portion of their animal protein such as fish, milk, or meat either raw or fermented. In fact, sausage is traditionally a fermented food. When you cook animal proteins, you denature the protein, and they become impossible to digest. Undigested animal protein is simply another toxin in your gut. Too much over a long time can lead to cancer.

Salmon or tuna sashimi is served in millions of Japanese homes each day. If you have not tried it yet, visit a top-notch Japanese restaurant and do your own experiment (no rice, please, only the sashimi). You will find it much easier to digest.

If you want to prepare sashimi in your own home and are concerned about parasites or bacteria, simply buy sushi-grade fish or freeze it for at least 48 hours to destroy possible parasites or bacteria. Then defrost, wash, and slice to serve.

Aid Digestion by Serving Fermented Foods and Liquids at Each Meal

Including fermented foods in your diet—especially having cultured veggies and/or young coconut kefir with your protein meals—is a must.

Cultured veggies are full of enzymes that enhance the digestion of proteins. Additionally, undigested animal protein can create toxic by-products in the intestines. The microflora in cultured veggies can negate these.

A lovely wineglass full of young coconut kefir or InnergyBiotic is a great digestive aid. Sip it slowly as you eat your meal. Young coconut kefir is a significant source of B vitamins, which are also manufactured by the friendly flora in your intestines. B vitamins are essential for proper utilization of amino acids, and neurotransmitters such as serotonin must have Bs to form properly.

Brine Poultry

Poultry should never be eaten rare or raw, but you can "brine" it to make it more tender and digestible. Also, cook it at a low temperature to make it easier to digest. To make a brine, simply put sea salt into a bowl of water and then add well-washed poultry. Let it sit for 30 to 45 minutes (to brine). Remove from water, dry, and then marinate if desired. It should be cooked at a low temperature (approximately 275° F) until the meat has turned a very pale pinkish color. Remove from the oven and cover. Let poultry sit for a few more minutes to finish cooking (meat should be white yet tender); then serve.

Take Enzymes That Digest Protein

Our ability to make digestive enzymes diminishes with age. We can live longer and are much healthier if we take supplemental digestive enzymes.

— Body Ecology created a line of three supplements to help digest the food in your stomach *and* small intestine. **ASSIST** was designed to help digest *vegetarian* protein, as well as fats and carbohydrates. (You would take these with your evening meal.) **ASSIST Protein and Dairy** is for efficient digestion of animal proteins in the stomach. (Take these with your midday animal-protein meal.) **ASSIST SI** provides powerful pancreatic enzymes that help digest proteins, fats, and carbohydrates once they reach your small intestine. (One or two taken along with all meals enhances digestion in your small intestine.)

— **Ox bile** and **lipase** are two other enzymes that may be taken when one has trouble digesting fats. Ox bile, available from Jarrow Formulas, is a must for anyone who has had his or her gallbladder removed.

More Digestive Aids

These digestive aids help maintain total body *alkalinity*, which helps balance the *acids* that are produced from proteins:

— Making **Body Ecology lemonade** by freshly squeezing the juice of one lemon (organic, if possible) into six to eight ounces of sparkling mineral water with stevia (to taste) is a great way to help digest protein. Lemon juice is acidic, and this helps your stomach become more acidic if you tend to have low stomach acid. However, when metabolized, the lemon juice becomes alkaline, creating a more balanced blood pH. Drink the lemonade 15 minutes before your meal. If you use sparkling mineral water, it, too, is acidic, but the potassium citrate in lemons actually creates a strong, overall alkaline effect *inside* your body.

— Adding one teaspoon of raw **apple-cider vinegar** to warm water and sipping it along with your protein meal is another great way to add acidity to your stomach to enhance digestion. It is also highly alkalizing once digested.

Important Note

If you don't eat a certain type of food for a while, you may find it hard to digest it at first. The intelligent microflora in your intestines work hard to digest what is sent down to them. If you are vegetarian for months and suddenly switch back to animal foods, expect temporary problems until the microflora adjust to their new food. If you have been on a high-animal-protein diet and then suddenly start to eat quinoa or millet and find you can't digest it, you now know why.

Now that you know the importance of cutting back on the amount of animal protein in your diet, while at the same time adding in much more easily digested plant proteins, what other foods will you need to embrace to restore your prenatal jing? The next chapter showcases one of the most critical food pillars in the Body Ecology program—*vegetables*.

From the Physician's Desk

"Brittle bones and muscle loss have usually been associated with people in their 70s and 80s. However, the reality is that bone loss can begin as early as our 20s. We can blame our protein-heavy, high-acid diets for this acceleration in aging."

The Price of a High-Protein Diet . . . Is It Worth It?

*I*t has been well documented that high-protein diets are a primary cause of increased loss of calcium from bones, which leads to thinning and loss of bone (osteopenia and osteoporosis). Alarming data reveal that 50 percent of women above the age of 55 have this problem.

The overconsumption of protein and other acid-producing foods, such as grains, sugars, alcohol, and salt, increases both the acid load and acid production in the body. To make matters worse, the under-consumption of alkaline-producing foods—namely, vegetables, fruits, and minerals (especially potassium, magnesium, and calcium in the citrate and bicarbonate forms)—compounds the problem, creating even more acidosis. The breakdown of calcium phosphate from bone is the body's way of correcting the acid/alkaline imbalance. So, the bones get thinner, the phosphate buffers the increased acid in the blood, and the high calcium, which leaves the body via the urine, can create kidney stones and/or greatly stress the kidneys. In addition, the higher calcium in the presence of acidosis can be deposited in areas of inflammation such as arteries, tendons, ligaments, joints, muscles, and even the brain. This is known as *ectopic calcification,* or the laying down of calcium where it doesn't belong.

A recent study showed how easily and quickly this bone-loss process can begin, even in women as young as 22 to 39. In other words, premenopausal women on a standard American high-protein diet can be putting themselves at significant risk of premature bone loss, which accumulates over time. The researchers took 39 healthy premenopausal women, consuming their typical higher-protein diet, and reduced it to .8 grams per kilogram of protein for only a two-week period. The lab tests at the end the study period showed some surprising results:

- Decreases in urine- and blood-nitrogen levels

- Decreases in renal-acid secretion

- Decreases in calcium and bone-loss markers in the urine

These data show that even in a two-week period, eating a little less protein and a lot more vegetables, fruits, and minerals can modify this chronic and dangerous problem.[i]

Another interesting point about overconsumption of protein is that the acidic environment also causes the loss of minerals, especially magnesium, in the urine. This creates many problems, including low intracellular magnesium in the endothelial cells that line the arteries. In the presence of acidosis, the intracellular calcium/magnesium ratio abnormally increases, and affects the arteries' ability to contract and relax, which often leads to hypertension. Supplementation with magnesium reduces this process of damage to the artery cells (also known as endothelial dysfunction).[ii]

In addition to bones, muscles must be considered. A recent article in *The American Journal of Clinical Nutrition* reveals that low-grade chronic metabolic acidosis promotes muscle wasting. This condition, known as *sarcopenia*, is thought to be due in part to an acid environment, and increased free radicals that damage the mitochondria (energy factories) in muscle cells. These damaged mitochondria then leak out more free radicals that damage, and may eventually kill, their own cell, leading to decreased size and strength of the muscles. Again, a diet that was high in acid foods and low in alkaline foods contributed to a reduction in lean-tissue muscle mass in older adults.[iii]

A simple formula and some examples to calculate approximate daily protein needs based on body weight appears on the following page. This general guideline will vary with individuals based on their genetics, age, and physical activity.

Attention, athletes! Your requirements may be higher, with 10 to 15 percent of calories coming from protein (or 1.2 to 1.5 grams of protein per kilogram of body weight per day).

The standard American diet (SAD) averages approximately 70–100 grams of protein daily, which is 1.1 grams (g) per kilogram (kg) of body weight per day.	This means if your body weight is 176 pounds (80 kg), your daily protein intake would be 88 g. If your body weight is 121 pounds (55 kg), your daily protein intake would be 60.5 g/day.
These numbers far exceed the U.S. recommended daily allowance (RDA) for protein, which is only 0.8 grams per kilogram of body weight each day. If one were to stick with the RDA, then:	A 176-pound person's intake would drop from 88 g/day to 64 g/day. A 121-pound person's intake would drop from 60g/day to 44 g/day.
To find your own RDA recommendation for protein:	Take your body weight in pounds, and divide by 2.2 (converts your pounds into kilograms). Next, multiply your weight in kilograms by 0.8 (yields the number of grams per day of protein that would be safe to eat on a long-term basis).

This final number would equal about 10 percent of your calories coming from protein.

However, to be safe, *everyone* should regularly check their urine and saliva acid levels (use pH paper from a health-food store) to get an idea of how much acid is being consumed and made by the body. Other factors such as dehydration, stress, genetics, overexercise, low-grade chronic infections, sedentary lifestyles with improper breathing, lung diseases, obesity, diabetes, sleep apnea, and lack of sleep may also contribute to chronic low-grade acidosis.

—Leonard Smith, M.D.

---

[i]B. Avery Ince, Ellen J. Anderson, and Robert M. Neer, "Lowering Dietary Protein to U.S. Recommended Dietary Allowance Levels Reduces Urinary Calcium Excretion and Bone Resorption in Young Women," *The Journal of Clinical Endocrinology & Metabolism,* Vol. 89, No. 8 (2004): 3801–3807.

[ii]Michael Shechter, Michael Sharir, Maura J. Paul Labrador, James Forrester, Burton Silver, and C. Noel Bairey Merz, "Oral Magnesium Therapy Improved Endothelial Function in Patients with Coronary Artery Disease," *Circulation,* 102 (2000): 2353–2358.

[iii]Bess Dawson-Hughes, Susan S. Harris, and Lisa Ceglia, "Alkaline diets favor lean tissue mass in older adults," *The American Journal of Clinical Nutrition,* Vol. 87, No. 3 (2008): 662–665.

From the Physician's Desk

"Animal protein, when in excess and overcooked, combines with fats and sugars in the diet, creating molecular monsters known as AGEs, which create active inflammation and can lead to kidney failure."

Protein and the Story of the AGEs

Advanced glycation end-products (AGEs) can do some serious damage, especially over time. An article in *The Clinical Journal of the American Society of Nephrology* makes several important points about protein and its relationship to many of the diseases of aging:

- Human studies indicate that excess dietary protein promotes progressive kidney damage by increasing the AGE burden.

- A prudent approach is to recommend that people with chronic kidney disease achieve the recommended dietary allowance of protein—0.8 g/kg per day, or about 10 percent of total caloric intake—with an emphasis on high-quality protein, low in AGEs.

- Conversely, very low dietary protein intake may lead to malnutrition, especially in those with advanced chronic kidney disease.

- The dietary AGE load can be minimized by consuming nonmeat proteins.

- There are several culinary methods that reduce AGE formation during cooking—steaming, poaching, boiling, and stewing. Frying, broiling, or grilling should be avoided, as they promote AGE formation.

- Limitation of dietary AGEs seems prudent in those with obesity, diabetes, and other risk factors for chronic kidney disease.[i]

With the gradual onset of kidney failure, acidosis again ensues and will lead to all types of inflammation and metabolic abnormalities. The preceding recommendations for how to avoid turning a meal into AGEs should become a major aging-management technology for Baby Boomers everywhere.

— *Leonard Smith, M.D.*

---

[i]Jaime Uribarri and Katherine R. Tuttle, "Advanced Glycation End Products and Nephrotoxicity of High-Protein Diets," *Clinical Journal of the American Society of Nephrology*, 1 (2006): 1293–1299.

Chapter 19

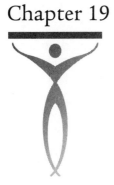

Vegetables: For Vitamins and Minerals

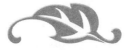

Processed foods and sweets have spoiled our taste buds, causing us to lose our instinctive fondness for natural, whole foods such as vegetables. And yet vegetables come in so many varieties, flavors, and colors—and they have so many incredible health benefits—they deserve to be billed as <u>superfoods.</u>

Most Baby Boomers can remember the famous comic-strip character Popeye the Sailor, who first surfaced in 1929 and eventually segued into a syndicated television show that aired well into the 1960s. Popeye's original creator was E. C. Segar, but the character acquired his widespread popularity when Max Fleischer, a producer at Paramount, began to release cartoon shorts in the 1930s, which became syndicated for television in the 1950s, bringing the swaggering but kindhearted sailor memorably to life for a whole new generation.[1] It was then that

Popeye's considerable strength became forever tied to his heroic consumption of spinach.

What people didn't find out until much later was that Segar had read a study published in the late 1870s that contained a misprint.[2] The article erroneously stated that spinach had ten times its actual iron content. (The real iron content is on par with most other vegetables.) But by then the Popeye mythology was well established.

During the '30s, Popeye's popularity helped boost sales of spinach nationwide, and a 33 percent increase in spinach consumption was reported. The spinach-growing community of Crystal City, Texas, actually erected a statue in tribute to the iconic hero. Popeye's love interest was Olive Oyl, and their adopted baby boy was named Swee'pea. Famous expressions like "I yam what I yam" quickly endeared Popeye to his Boomer fans. Perhaps all of these many references to produce prompted mothers everywhere to say to their offspring: "Eat your vegetables!"

Mother certainly knew best, as vegetables are nutritional powerhouses that keep us active, mentally alert, and forever young.

Vegetables Are Youth Enhancing

Vegetables from the land and the ocean might be called nature's most perfect anti-aging foods—rich in the vitamins and minerals needed to sustain and vitalize your body. A wide variety of beautifully colored vegetables should comprise 80 percent of your diet. Easy to digest, they are nutrient-dense but low in calories; and because they are alkaline, they help fight the acidic environment that causes inflammation, yeast overgrowth, and viruses, which tend to worsen as we age.

New research on vegetables and aging shows that on measures of mental sharpness, vegetables give you an edge. In a study funded by the National Institute on Aging, 2,000 Chicago-area men and women were tested at the end of a six-year period. Older people who ate more than two servings of vegetables daily appeared about five years younger at the end of the study than those who ate few or no vegetables. In addition, people who ate more than two servings of vegetables a day had about 40 percent less mental decline than those who ate few or no vegetables.

Leafy-green vegetables such as spinach, kale, collards, mustard greens, and kohlrabi appear to be especially powerful, as they contain significant amounts of minerals and the antioxidant vitamins C, A, and E. When paired with healthy fats such as olive oil, they are even more effective, as these oils help the body absorb the antioxidants. The same study also found that people who ate lots of vegetables tended to be more physically active. This in turn has a positive effect on brain acuity and memory.[3]

Vegetables Are Powerful Detoxifiers

In recent years, a lot of scrutiny has been given to the "cruciferous" family of vegetables. Cabbage, broccoli, Brussels sprouts, cauliflower, kale, collards, and bok choy are frequent favorites in our Body Ecology kitchens. They all have natural cancer-fighting substances (isothiocyanates and indoles) that help regulate and improve the 2:16 hydroxyestrone ratio, a proven predictor of hormone-related cancers such as breast and prostate. In short, a normal 2:16 ratio means less cancer risk.

Other green vegetables, including mustard greens, watercress, and Swiss chard are excellent sources of *carotenoids*, which protect against eye diseases such as macular degeneration. They are also good sources of beta-carotene, another cancer fighter.

You might not be aware of this, but healthy plants actually do defend themselves by producing a variety of bad-tasting substances that cause them to be toxic and inedible to animals and insects. Some, however, contain toxins that offer bitter or other pleasingly complex tastes that appeal to us humans. Most of these plant toxins are *phytonutrients*, important detoxifiers that help our bodies get rid of spent hormones and environmental poisons.

It's important to note that phytonutrients are more abundant in *organically grown* vegetables because, unlike

It is highly recommended that 80 percent of your diet include vegetables. Prepare them in delicious ways ... raw, fermented, steamed, sautéed, or baked—always at a low temperature. It's almost impossible to eat "too many" vegetables!

conventionally grown produce that is protected from insects by spraying with pesticides, organic cultivation preserves the natural defenses of the plant, allowing the phytonutrients to survive. Just a few of these phytonutrient-rich plants include: garlic, ginger, onions, rosemary, green tea, wasabi, and the cruciferous vegetables (as well as blueberries, black currants, and pomegranates).[4]

Land Vegetables

As you start to increase the *amount* of vegetables you eat at each meal . . . yes, even at breakfast . . . you'll also want to include a wide *variety*. There is an amazing array of vegetables available today. You'll see that their colors, textures, and shapes add excitement to any meal.

Leafy-green vegetables grow aboveground (for example, turnip greens, kale, collards, and beet greens) and are rich in chlorophyll from the sun. Not only do they help cleanse your blood, but they are also excellent sources of calcium and iron. *Eat them at least once a day.*

Root vegetables, which grow underground (for example, carrots, onions, daikon, and turnips), are slightly more contracting in nature and provide strength and winter warmth. Some root vegetables naturally contain more sugars, such as beets, parsnips, sweet potatoes and yams. If you have an inflammation-causing infection (yeast or virus) or high blood sugar, then *fermenting* these nutrient-rich root vegetables (to make cultured vegetables) is a great way to eliminate the sugar.

Low in calories and high in fiber, vegetables are excellent foods for maintaining healthy intestines and cleansing the colon.

In a nutshell, on the Baby Boomer Diet you almost can't eat "too many" vegetables. It is highly recommended that 80 percent of your diet (or about seven to ten servings per day) include vegetables—prepared in many delicious ways . . . raw, fermented, and cooked (steamed, sautéed, or baked) . . . always at a low temperature.

Recommended Nonstarchy Vegetables

Arugula

Asparagus

Bamboo shoots

Beet greens

Bok choy

Broccoli

Brussels sprouts

Burdock root

Cabbage

Carrots (if raw)

Cauliflower

Celeriac

Celery

Celery root

Chives

Collard greens

Corn (if raw)

Cucumber

Daikon

Dandelion greens

Endive

Escarole

Fennel

Garlic

Green beans

Jicama

Kale

Kohlrabi

Lamb's quarters

Leeks

Mustard greens

Okra

Onion

Parsley

Radishes (red)

Red bell pepper
   (in small quantities)

Scallions

Shallots

Spinach

Swiss chard

Turnips (and greens)

Watercress

Yellow bell pepper
   (in small quantities)

Yellow squash

Zucchini

Recommended Starchy Vegetables

Artichokes (and Jerusalem artichokes)

Carrots (mildly starchy when cooked)

Corn (fresh on or off the cob, mildly starchy when cooked)

Peas (English)

Red-skin potatoes

Shiitake and other wild mushrooms

Winter squash (acorn, butternut, or buttercup)

New Thoughts on Some Old Standbys

There are many other vegetables besides the ones recommended here that you might want to experiment with, not only for flavor, but simply for expanding your "treasure chest" of nature's gifts for reversing your biological age.

We have found that *a few vegetables are best not eaten at all* by some depending upon the health status of the individual. Examples are:

- **Cooked beets, parsnips, sweet potatoes, and yams:** These vegetables are high in natural sugars unless cultured.

- **Eggplant, bell peppers, and tomatoes:** Members of the nightshade family of vegetables, they often irritate the nervous system, and some believe they aggravate arthritis. People who are highly sensitive or hyperactive should not eat them. Others can eat them in moderation. Green bell peppers are red peppers picked at an early stage and are very difficult to digest. Our recipes only use red peppers and in small amounts. Tomatoes may be tolerated occasionally, in season, with a green salad. When cooked, they become even more acid forming than when eaten raw.

- **Russet and Yukon Gold potatoes:** These are very high in sugar. Red-skin potatoes, also called "new potatoes," are lower in sugar. Remember: Each of us is unique; and the sugars in potatoes may be fine for you, especially if you eat them in a meal with something fermented—for example, a juice glass of young coconut kefir or a serving of cultured vegetables. These fermented foods contain the microflora to digest the sugars. Potatoes also belong to the nightshade family (see above), so you may want to avoid them if they seem to cause joint stiffness and arthritic symptoms.

- **Indoor, tray-grown wheatgrass:** Really a long sprout, it is too sweet and expansive for many.

- **Mung bean and other sprouts:** Typically these have mold on them.

A cooking tip: Vegetables can be labor-intensive and time-consuming to prepare, which is why restaurants offer so few of them on their menus! But they can actually save time in the long run if you cook up larger batches so that they last for a couple of days. For example, make big pots of soups or stews that contain a variety of vegetables. Twice a week, cook dark green, leafy vegetables and ocean vegetables, but eat them all week long. Having lettuce washed and ready to go in the refrigerator will also save you time.

Oxalates—What Popeye Didn't Know

A new diet has emerged on the horizon; and it is growing in popularity, particularly among those who suffer from leaky gut syndrome, edema, autism, chronic obstructive pulmonary disease (COPD), asthma, kidney stones, vulvodynia, or have difficulty digesting fat.

For many of us, limiting oxalate-rich foods until our gut heals will be a must. The low-oxalate diet (LOD) is designed for the increasing number of people who are sensitive to *oxalates*—substances that are found naturally in the leaves, stems, and roots of many of the most nutritious foods. You may be unfamiliar with this term, but you will probably be hearing a lot more about it in the future.

Until recently, the list of valuable foods high in oxalates included strawberries, blueberries, quinoa, kale, collards, mustard greens, parsley, leeks, celery, green beans, summer squash . . . and yes, even Popeye's favorite, *spinach*. I say "until recently" because we now know that the oxalate content of food can vary considerably between plants of the same species. Differences in climate, soil quality, state of ripeness, or even the part of the plant analyzed will give a different oxalate rating, so that old list is now being reevaluated.

Our bodies always contain oxalates and routinely convert other substances, such as vitamin C, into them. They are also important for managing calcium in the body. Generally, oxalates are not harmful, because the microflora in the gut metabolize them, and they leave our bodies through our stools.

But if you have destroyed the microflora with antibiotics,

Cabbage—the Great Cancer Killer

*D*iets high in cruciferous vegetables—cabbage, kale, bok choy, and collards—result in fewer instances of certain cancers, including lung, colon, liver, breast, ovarian, and bladder. This may be because cruciferous vegetables optimize your cells' ability to detoxify and cleanse. Not only are cruciferous vegetables high in *isothiocyanates* (powerful anticarcinogens), but scientists have also found them to stimulate phase II enzymes, special liver enzymes that neutralize and dispose of toxins that cause cancer. *Cabbage is particularly beneficial.* High in anticancer compounds called *glucosinolates,* cabbage has shown very good results in lowering the risk of breast cancer.

For example, Polish women consume three times the amount of cabbage that American women do. The rate of breast cancer rose threefold when these women emigrated to the United States.[i] And when you ferment cabbage (sauerkraut), the benefits really skyrocket. Researchers have found that fermented cabbage is healthier than raw or cooked cabbage and more effective at fighting cancer.[ii]

Fermenting releases enzymes that decompose glucosinolate, breaking it down into more accessible isothiocyanates. In addition to these anticancer compounds, fermented cabbage is a good source of minerals, vitamin C, and fiber; and is easier to digest.

---

[i]Jeff Minerd, "AACR: A Diet High in Cabbage May Help Prevent Breast Cancer," University of Pennsylvania School of Medicine, October 31, 2005, **http://www.medpagetoday.com/HematologyOncology/BreastCancer/2035** (accessed 12/14/09).

[ii]Marja Tolonen, Marianne Taipale, Britta Viander, Juha-Matti Pihlava, Hannu Korhonen, and Eeva-Liisa Ryhänen, MTT Agrifood Research Finland, Food Research, FIN-31600 Jokioinen, Finland, *J. Agric. Food Chem.,* 50 (2002): 6798–6803.

with stress, or with a high-sugar diet and have never known the importance of establishing a healthy inner ecosystem, you can have oxalate issues.

Oxalates are not usually absorbed from the gut, but an inflamed, permeable, "leaky" gut lining will allow them to pass through. In the bloodstream, the oxalates bind with calcium, then crystallize. These crystals lodge in weak tissues and cause even more inflammation and pain.

This problem seems to stem from the gut. It is believed that when we become constipated and our filter organs (kidney and liver) and intestines do not work efficiently, the colon begins to absorb the oxalates rather than passing them out of the body. This leads to or intensifies many often-painful conditions, such as the formation of kidney stones.

Avoiding foods high in oxalates at least temporarily until the gut problem is solved is a must if you have any of the conditions mentioned previously. You should especially avoid some of the worst offenders—coffee, chocolate, nuts, spinach, black tea, and all wheat products.

It was once believed that dietary calcium should also be avoided. Not so. There is now plenty of research showing that calcium is actually needed when ingesting oxalate-rich foods. The calcium helps decrease the absorption of the oxalates. Prebiotics such as chicory inulin (Body Ecology's EcoBloom) will also help increase absorption of calcium from the colon.

For people sensitive to oxalates, keeping the total amount consumed per day below 40 to 60 milligrams is a must. Do not eat spinach, for example, because, when *steamed,* it contains about 697 milligrams in just a half cup . . . and even more if eaten raw. A low-oxalate food would have only 5 milligrams per serving and a medium-oxalate food would have less than 10 . . . so steamed spinach, at 697 milligrams, is not on the LOD.

(*Note:* Whenever you *boil* vegetables, a significant amount of oxalates is lost in the cooking water. *Steaming* is not as effective as boiling and, depending on the food, may or may not lower them. The cooking water or "pot liqueur" should not be eaten, as it does contain the oxalates.)

Here's some good news. Until recently it was believed that *all* green vegetables were high in oxalates. Fortunately, this is not true.

Recently, Susan Owens, who heads up an excellent website on the LOL (**www.lowoxalate.info**), began working with Liebman Lab in Wyoming to test each plant food for its oxalate content. They were quite pleased to find that not *all* greens are high in oxalates after all. After carefully testing each individual food, they learned that boiled kale (4.9 milligrams per half cup), boiled mustard greens (3.2 milligrams per half cup), and boiled collards (8.7 milligrams per half cup) were surprisingly *low* in oxalates.

So if you believe you may be sensitive to oxalates and want to avoid high-oxalate foods, it is important to obtain the most recent oxalate rating on each food (updated on Owens's website). As Owens cautions, "We can no longer make generalizations about oxalate content in foods. Research is now showing us that there are some foods in every category that are high in oxalates and plenty that are also low in oxalates."[5]

We don't want to miss out on these important foods, so what can we do if we are sensitive to oxalates?

Once again, fermentation to the rescue!

If you feel you are sensitive to oxalates—or if kidney stones, COPD, and asthma run in your family—at first limit foods high in them. But don't stop there. Keep your detoxification pathways open and working well. Do not allow yourself to become constipated. (See Chapter 24 for information on detoxification therapies.)

Ultimately, you must heal your intestines and create a vibrant, hardy inner ecosystem teeming with a variety of beneficial bacteria. Beneficial microflora in your gut not only keep it healthy, but certain strains are proving to be effective at eating up or degrading oxalates. The most effective oxalate eater is a bacterium called *Oxalobacter formigenes*. This bacterium is not currently available as a supplement, but hopefully will be someday.

However, other beneficial bacteria are proving to be effective oxalate eaters. *Bifidus infantis* (sold under the name of Life Start

It is true that cooking destroys valuable enzymes, but on the positive side, cooking can remove some harmful compounds and toxins in our food. Cooking also makes food more digestible.

by Natren) is quite effective at eating oxalates. *L. plantarum* (found abundantly in Body Ecology's cultured vegetables), and *L. breve* do so but appear to be modest eaters, and *L. acidophilus* and *L. thermophilus* were also quite good. *B. infantis* grew rapidly in the presence of oxalates, as did *L. plantarum* and *L. brevis*. This is important, as the microflora must grow well in the presence of oxalates to be useful to us.[6]

Raw vs. Cooked Vegetables

A growing number of people believe that when you cook vegetables, you destroy or minimize their nutritional content. In fact, the raw-food, vegan diet proposed by Ann Wigmore decades ago has been enjoying a resurgence in popularity for about ten years now.

However, among those in the know, this way of eating is heading out of style. It is not balanced, and nutritional deficiencies often result when only raw foods are eaten for years. Lately, some of the most well-known "thought leaders" in the raw, vegan movement are "coming out of the closet" to say that raw/vegan as a way of life (100 percent of the time, for an extended period) is *not* the way to go after all. Their courage and honesty to admit this is really admirable.

Yes, eating raw foods can be good for you . . . and has many benefits, but raw is not always the right choice. In fact, eating *all* raw can be harmful to some, as raw foods can be difficult to digest and "chilling" for the thyroid (which needs good fats, lots of minerals, and warming foods).

Putting the Principles into Practice
Vegetables and the Principle of Balance

As you learn more about the Body Ecology Way of Life and master the 7 Principles, in the end you will once again see that it all comes down to a matter of balance. (See Chapter 11: The Principle of Balance.)

The theory behind a raw diet as a way of life began with the insistence that we must eat *all* our vegetables raw because cooking destroys the enzymes needed to digest them. This is an overly simplistic way of looking at a *very complex subject*— how food handling and preparation ultimately affects nutrient content.

How Destructive Is Cooking . . . Really?

*H*ow destructive is cooking, really? If you take a deeper look into the complex topic of raw versus cooked, you'll discover that, in the end, it is really about balance.

Because everything in this wonderful world we live in has both a positive and a negative side, there is also a positive and a negative side to cooking foods. And there is a positive and negative side to eating them raw.

Well-respected food scientist Shirley Corriher provides additional insight on this subject in her excellent book *CookWise: The Hows and Whys of Successful Cooking,* where she shows how science can be applied to traditional cooking.

Here's what she had to say about cooking vegetables:

"You would expect different cooking methods to result in different losses of nutrients, and there are differences—more so with vitamins than with minerals—but not as much as you might think. The mineral loss is relatively small (5 to 10 percent) no matter how the vegetable is cooked. On the other hand, the loss of vitamins varies somewhat, but many vegetables lose only 20 percent or less no matter what the cooking method. This is not to say, however, that there isn't great variability in the nutrient content, because there are very large differences in nutrient content before cooking."

There can be a huge difference in the nutrient content of one carrot over another. The variety the carrot belongs to, the growing conditions, the time it is harvested (was it allowed to reach maturity?), and how it was cared for once it was harvested (was it refrigerated immediately?) all greatly influence the nutritional content.

For example, you can lose as much as 50 percent of your vitamin C in 24 hours by not keeping your food refrigerated. Vitamin C content will be lower if you are purchasing your food from a store with poor refrigeration.

Corriher also states that plants will have a greater amount of vitamin C and beta-carotene when they are grown in more sunlight.

Here are a few more tips to create enzyme-rich, nutrient-dense meals:

- If vegetables are cooked in water, the minerals and the water-soluble vitamins (vitamin C and some B vitamins) will be lost into the cooking water. To solve this problem, either do not cook them in water or use the broth from the vegetable water in your recipe so that you obtain those nutrients.

- If you cook your vegetables in a way that heats them to a temperature above approximately 105° F, certain nutrients such as vitamin C and thiamine are destroyed. Does this mean cooking is bad? Absolutely not. It means a wise person makes sure that the lost nutrient is supplied elsewhere in the meal.

- Lost enzymes can easily be obtained in a well-balanced Body Ecology meal. Simply sip on a small wineglass of a probiotic liquid, and of course, eat cultured veggies. For example, adding a few spoonfuls of cultured veggies made with cabbage would make up for any vitamin C lost in cooking. These fermented foods and beverages supply trillions of enzymes, enhance digestion, and provide beneficial microflora. As explained in Chapter 15, they also provide the "sour taste" that every meal should have to make it really satisfying. Sour is the taste that takes away cravings for sugar and carbs as well.

- Cooking vegetables whole, in their skin, helps prevent some nutrient loss.

May I remind you once again that meal preparation is always a matter of balance.

---

[1]Shirley O. Corriher, *CookWise: The Hows and Whys of Successful Cooking* (New York: HarperCollins Publishers, Inc., 1997): 353.

Think variety . . . and think *raw, cooked,* and *cultured* when you plan your meals. We humans have been given our creative brains and incredible intelligence to devise wonderfully nourishing, healing, and even "youthening" foods by preparing them in a variety of ways and mastering the art of balance.

Vegetables, Seasons, and the Principle of 80/20

The Baby Boomer Diet recommends that you practice the 80/20 Principle by eating 80 percent of your vegetables raw and 20 percent cooked during the hot summer months when cooked foods are less desirable, and simply reversing this during the cold winter months. If you live in a hot climate, you might want to eat more raw vegetables year-round.

Raw-Vegetable Smoothies vs. Vegetable Juices

Raw-vegetable *smoothies* . . . especially for breakfast . . . can bring outstanding nutritional qualities to your anti-aging diet. They are cleansing and healing and require less energy to digest than most foods. Regular consumption of veggie smoothies is highly recommended for all Baby Boomers.

Vegetable smoothies are preferred to vegetable *juices* on the Body Ecology program because juices don't include the vegetable *fiber.* Without it, the vegetables are assimilated into your bloodstream too quickly and make your body acidic. In a smoothie, the fiber is "blenderized" but still there, helping improve detoxification and elimination.

Vegetable smoothies are alive with enzymes and, depending on what you put in them, can be the most nutritious foods you will eat all day long. They can be an excellent source of proteins, fats, vitamins, and minerals to help rejuvenate your body.

They are also alkaline forming and mildly expansive— drink them to balance acidic, contractive conditions. When you wake up each morning after a long night's sleep, your body tends to be dehydrated, too acidic, and too contracted, so vegetable smoothies are a superior alternative to breakfast cereals. Also, consider a day of "fasting" on them to give your liver and digestive tract a rest.

Body Ecology Smoothie Tips

1. While your smoothie will have a base of filtered water, I suggest that approximately 50 to 70 percent of the total vegetable content be celery. This is a rich source of natural sodium, ideal for recharging and building your adrenals. Zucchini, romaine lettuce, a few sprigs of cilantro and mint, and cucumber are some favorites to include in your starter base. Then add any of the other ingredients mentioned below:

2. A small *sour* apple, such as a Granny Smith, or other *sour* fruit or juice—pomegranate, unsweetened açaí, cranberry, or black currant—works well in a green smoothie to make it more delicious. However, very sweet vegetables such as carrots, beets, and fennel are best avoided.

3. Smoothies should be consumed alone on an empty stomach, allowing about 30 to 45 minutes to digest before eating solid foods. They are very filling.

4. Organic, unrefined fats and oils can be added to your smoothie recipe. Examples are: hemp-, pumpkin-, and flaxseed oil; macadamia, walnut, and pine-nut oil; coconut and avocado oil; and raw cream.

5. "Chewing" your smoothie by holding it in your mouth and mixing it with saliva allows the digestion process to begin, which makes a big difference.

6. Chia seeds can add even more fiber. Body Ecology's EcoBloom is both a fiber and a prebiotic that helps feed the friendly microflora to help them grow stronger and colonize more effectively. It also helps with absorption of calcium.

7. Blend in extra proteins from one of the following: un-denatured whey-protein concentrate; milk kefir; yogurt; coconut milk; Body Ecology's Vitality SuperGreen, Potent Proteins, or Fermented Protein powder; or a scoop of raw nut or seed butter.

8. Vanilla flavoring and noncaloric sweeteners such as stevia or Lakanto (see Chapter 16) are nice additions if you like your smoothie on the sweet side. A pinch of sea salt helps create balance. I love potassium-rich Hawaiian sea salt.

9. And please don't forget a splash of your favorite probiotic. Add either a probiotic powder or a probiotic liquid, such as Body Ecology's Young Coconut Kefir, InnergyBiotic, Dong Quai, or CocoBiotic.

Ocean Vegetables

For many Westerners, ocean vegetables (also called sea vegetables) may be a new food. Don't let the idea of eating seaweed put you off. These vegetables are wonderfully rejuvenating and so high in nutritional value that they are considered a must. You may need to educate yourself a little about them, but soon you will come to love the taste.

Ocean vegetables are really algae colonies or single-cell organisms that grow on rocks or other ocean surfaces. They are red, blue, green, and black; thrive only in clean water; and are harvested like land vegetables. After harvesting, they are dried and packaged. Ocean vegetables contain more protein and amino acids (building blocks of protein) than beans. They are a good source of iodine, carotene, enzymes, and fiber—and high in vitamins A, C, E, B_1, B_2, B_6, and B_{12}. You may be most familiar with the ocean vegetable *nori* from eating sushi, but there are many other varieties, including *kelp, dulse, hijiki, wakame,* and *arame* (see next page for more information on each type).

Ocean vegetables have many benefits, which include:

- Helping prevent aging—in areas of Japan, where ocean vegetables are harvested, women in their 60s often look as if they are in their 30s

- Regulating the thyroid and providing it with a significant source of iodine

- Enhancing and prolonging the color of hair and lips

- Controlling the growth of pathogenic bacteria, fungi, and viruses

- Providing an abundance of easily digested minerals and trace elements lacking in our diets today

- Restoring and maintaining proper acid/alkaline balance in the body

- Strengthening the nervous and immune systems

- Removing radioactive elements, carcinogens, and even environmental pollutants

- Providing calcium and large amounts of chlorophyll

- Keeping the body more alkaline

- Supplying the colon, liver, thyroid, and adrenals with minerals needed to function properly (ocean vegetables are high in mineral salts, and the "toning" effect on the colon can help resolve constipation)

A Selection of Ocean Vegetables

There are many wonderful ways to incorporate ocean vegetables into your diet. They can be added to soups, sauces, and salads, or dried into snacks.

— **Dulse.** High in iron and great for energy and brain food, dulse can be eaten straight from the package. It has a salty taste and used to be served as a snack in taverns in the early 1900s. While tavern owners hoped that the salty taste would increase patrons' desire for alcohol, they didn't know that dulse also balanced alcohol's effect of leaching minerals from the body.

— **Nori.** Typically used to make sushi in Japanese restaurants, nori is a great snack food because of its mild, nutty, salty taste. You can pass a sheet quickly over the stove burner until it changes color from black to green—or buy it already toasted. Eaten alone, enjoyed in sushi, used as a wrap for grains or veggies, or shredded and added to salads . . . there are many ways to experiment with nori. It contains 28 percent protein, and of all the ocean vegetables, it is one of the highest in vitamins. It also provides calcium, manganese, copper, iron, zinc, and fluoride.

— **Kombu.** An excellent medicinal stock for soups or cooking grains, kombu has several benefits and has been known to counteract high blood pressure. It is high in calcium, iodine, potassium, and vitamins A and C. Kombu contains glutamic acid, which can soften food and add flavor. It can also be cooked with beans to improve their digestibility and reduce their flatulence-producing properties. If you dry strips of kombu at a low temperature in your oven, they become crispy like bacon and make a great snack. You can also use kombu as soup stock. Simply simmer a strip or two in springwater for an hour and add vegetables such as cabbage, carrots, and onions to the broth for a quick and refreshing soup.

— **Wakame.** Tender and sweet tasting, wakame has many of the same benefits as kombu. It is high in calcium and vitamins B and C. Wakame is used in Eastern medicine for its benefits to the skin, hair, intestines, blood, and reproductive organs.

— **Agar.** Derived from red seaweed, agar is a natural gelatin that is superior to animal gelatin. It is used to create delicious aspics, puddings, and gelatin desserts. Agar lubricates the digestive tract and has mild laxative properties. It is a source of vitamins, calcium, phosphorus, iron, and iodine.

— **Arame.** A good source of protein, arame has a sweet, nutty flavor and is a good choice for those new to ocean vegetables. It can be tossed into a salad after soaking, with no need for cooking. It can also be added to stir-fries and other cooked meals. A rich source of iodine and iron, it contains calcium and potassium and has beneficial properties to counteract high blood pressure.

— **Hijiki.** With a mild salty or "fishy" flavor, hijiki is the ocean vegetable that is highest in minerals, and it is also known to counteract high blood pressure. A great source of iron, calcium, protein, and trace elements, hijiki makes a wonderful addition to soups and salads.

Just like fermented foods, there are many varieties of ocean vegetables to try, so have fun experimenting! If you seek convenience, consider an ocean-vegetable supplement in order to get the healthy benefits of these superfoods.

Ocean Vegetables and Your Thyroid

With so many people today experiencing thyroid issues, adding ocean vegetables to the diet can be very healing. Thyroid problems can lead to obesity, excessive thinness, hypertension, flatulence, stubborn cases of constipation, fatigue, nervousness, depression, headaches, and neck and shoulder pain.

Ocean vegetables are very medicinal for the thyroid. Within a week or two of eating them every day, you should notice that you feel calmer in both mind and body. Ocean vegetables reduce tension, help you cope with stress, and enable your body to store vitality and energy.

The thyroid also influences the health of the ovaries, prostate gland, and pyloric valve. It's common to have problems with the pylorus, the valve at the end of the stomach, which must open and close at the correct time to allow food into the small intestine. If you suffer from indigestion, it's especially important to eat ocean vegetables.

Fermented Vegetables

One of the many bonuses of eating vegetables that have been fermented is that they enhance our taste buds. The flavors in foods will be stronger and more satisfying.

Fermented vegetables are sour; and when you eat them, you can really taste the natural sweetness in other foods such as carrots, beets, and onions. The sugars found in processed foods will seem unpleasantly and artificially sweet, so you can naturally avoid them. Fermenting vegetables also increases their bioavailability, meaning more of the nutritional benefits are getting through. (See Chapter 15: Fermented Vegetables.)

And if weight is an issue for you and/or you find yourself with constant daily cravings for carbohydrates, alcohol, drugs, and nicotine, it is widely reported that the desire for such destructive substances soon disappears when fermented foods are eaten. At Body Ecology, we are anxious to see more research on this important property of fermented foods and drinks.

Fermented Vegetable Juices

If you already own a juicer, you can put it to good use making *fermented vegetable juices*. Start by juicing cabbage (red and/or green), carrots, ginger, celery, fresh herbs, kale, and dulse; and then ferment the liquid using Body Ecology's Cultured Vegetable Starter (available from **www.bodyecology .com**). These are magnificent digestive aids, immediately boost energy, and put V8 juice to shame. Juices ferment quickly and are ready in 18 to 24 hours.

Go Organic and Buy Local

Organic vegetables are preferred, whenever possible, for their higher mineral content and lack of harmful pesticides. Organic means more than "pesticide free"; it also means that the soil used to grow the vegetables must meet requirements pertaining to mineral richness—much more so than conventional vegetables. Over time, mass-production processes have stripped the land of its minerals.

Some conventional vegetables and fruits, such as avocados and bananas, have such thick skins that the risk of contamination by pesticides is minimal. Others, such as berries and peppers, are particularly risky, so make a special effort to purchase those in organic form. If you must eat conventional vegetables, you can always ferment them to reduce the effects of pesticides.

You may notice that nutrient-dense, organically grown food tastes better; and because it provides you with more nourishment, you may need less of it to feel satisfied—thus effortlessly practicing calorie restriction!

I also recommend that you support your state CSA (community-supported agriculture) program and local farmers' markets, as they promote land stewardship and nonchemical production processes, and also build economically sustainable communities. At a time when one company, Monsanto, owns the entire world's supply of seeds, it is vital that we empower our local farmers and take back control of our food supply from corporate food giants.

No GMO . . . a Call to Baby Boomers

Another benefit of organic foods is that they are not genetically modified. Genetic modification alters the DNA of living organisms intended for human or animal consumption. The goal of gene-altered foods is to make them resistant to herbicides or to improve their nutritional value; however, they have been shown to have adverse effects on health and the environment.

It's important to note that we've been engineering plants for nearly 10,000 years through crossbreeding and cross-pollinating. This type of crop production has been successful because it follows classical breeding practices, which cross close relatives, such as a Yorkshire terrier with a poodle to create a Yorkie-poo . . . *still a dog.*

With new GMO technologies, however, classical breeding is bypassed, so genetic information is crossed from one species to another to create an entirely different species. For example, scientists are experimenting with genes from chicken embryos and insect immune systems to make potatoes resistant to disease. Sounds yummy, doesn't it? When you do this, you disrupt the complex ecosystem in which an organism lives and grows, impacting many forms of life, including bacteria and microbes.

In our immediate-gratification world, we want things bigger, juicier, sweeter, and prettier. If we can create a plant that is resistant to disease, then let's do it, we say, without any care for the long-term consequences. Baby Boomers, in particular, are susceptible to this way of thinking. We are accustomed to getting what we want right away and exactly to our specifications. Our parents never wanted us to struggle or suffer as they did. So we might not have learned that striving, waiting, and moderation are integral to emotional growth and even to our ability to survive.

The fact is, plants are *supposed* to become diseased. They are supposed to be attacked by pests and affected by seasonal and climate changes. This is a natural cycle, with some plants surviving and others not. The death of one organism sustains the life of another. This cycle may not always be pretty, but it is balanced and extremely precious. We really don't know what might occur when we tamper with this process.

We are seeing that genetic modification is not, as scientists have suggested, precise. It can be random and unpredictable, and it can produce significant changes in the natural functioning of a plant's DNA. For example, genetic engineering may cause a plant's genetic makeup to become unstable, resulting in "rogue toxins" that may not show up for many generations after the plant was originally modified.

Seventy to eighty percent of all processed foods contain, or stem from, GMOs. Most Americans are not aware of the potential allergic or toxic reactions they may experience due to these genetically altered organisms. Because of poor labeling and scarcity of data, we may not see the threat of an allergic reaction until it has already hit us. For example, after genetically modified soy was introduced in the U.K., soy allergies skyrocketed 50 percent. Europe no longer allows genetically modified products, and some have suggested that Americans are being used as guinea pigs in a poorly regulated and untested industry.[7]

Jeffrey Smith is an authoritative and outspoken person on this subject. He heads the Institute for Responsible Technology, which investigates and reports the risks of GM foods and crops. On his website he provides a free video on the dangers of genetically modified food. I recommend that you take a look to learn more about this important subject: **www.responsibletechnology.org**.

While it may be difficult to tell whether conventional vegetables are genetically modified, you can watch out for crops that typically are, such as soy, corn, cottonseed, canola, zucchini, Hawaiian papaya, and yellow squash. But there are many more that are being targeted. Go to **truefoodnow.org** for a list of brands of foods that are genetically engineered.

As you move toward whole foods; add some new ones, such as sea vegetables and fermented veggies, to your diet; and reduce your sugar intake, you will be amazed by the youth and vitality you will gain. And you may be surprised to find that after a few weeks of adopting different eating habits, you start to crave vegetables. Your body, as it comes into balance with its newfound energy, will begin to signal you for the foods it needs, and some may be completely foreign to your palate.

The next chapter explores Body Ecology's grain-like seeds, a unique food and a pleasant answer to those universal carb cravings.

Chapter 20

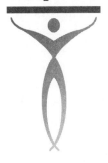

Grain-like Seeds: For Energy, Hydration, and Balance

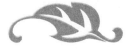

Thousands of years old and venerated by those who grew them, these ancient foods have the power to make us turn back time.

When we were growing up, Wonder Bread was the coolest food around—the bread of choice for sandwiches and eliciting the envy of our classmates. If we cut off the crust, we could roll it up into a gummy white ball. And its white wrapper, dotted with big yellow, blue, and red circles, made it seem even more fun. Little did we know, but we might as well have been eating glue.

Sixty-five percent of Americans eat a diet high in starchy carbs (mostly pasta, bread, and rice); and many of us often start our day with breakfast cereal, a slice of toast, or a doughnut. The recently popular high-protein diets have sought to address the obesity and diabetes issue in America by creating a new mind-set that all carbohydrates are "bad" and must be avoided.

Confused about Carbs?

We now are convinced that carbs are culinary culprits and the cause of all our evils. But just as with fats, this has created a lopsided picture and a heated health controversy. As Chapter 17 pointed out, though, it is the *type* of fats that is important. This is true for carbohydrates as well.

Not all carbohydrates are created equal. Table sugar, fruit, milk, grains, and vegetables are often lumped together into the category called "carbs" because they are made from or contain sugar. At Body Ecology, we disagree with classifying these foods the same, and feel that it adds further confusion concerning what we should and should not eat.

We also make a clear distinction between refined sugars, grains and their flours, and grain-like seeds and *their* flours.

Vegetables should not be classified as carbs, but put into their own unique category. They are simply not "read" by the body in the same way as "carbs." And there is such a wide variety enjoyed by humans—and so many to choose between each day—that this category can be broken down into smaller ones, if desired: *sweet, root, leafy-green, cruciferous,* and *ocean vegetables,* just to name a few. It *is* important to distinguish between starchy and nonstarchy vegetables, because this is a useful guideline when following the Principle of Food Combining. (Refer back to Chapter 19 to brush up on vegetables' countless nutritional benefits.)

Empty, Refined Grains vs.
Ancient, Whole Grain-like Seeds

To simplify the carb issue, bread, pasta, and cereals can be classified together as human-made foods refined from grains—let's call them "empty, refined grains." Because they are empty foods, they should carry the skull-and-crossbones label to indicate they are nonnutritious, poisonous, aging, acid-forming foods. With such a label our mothers would have thought twice about giving us that slice of Wonder Bread!

The category that we would call "grains" would include wheat berries, oat groats, rice (there are many varieties), rye berries, barley, spelt, and so forth. This category may be beneficial for some people *if* the grains are prepared properly. They would be eaten in their whole form, soaked first to remove their enzyme inhibitors, and cooked slowly to make them more digestible. The problem with these grains, even if they are eaten in their whole form, is that they do contain a significant amount of sugar . . . potentially leading to an acid body, infections, inflammation, and earlier aging.

A third category, called "grain-like seeds," would include seeds that have many of the characteristics of grains. They are higher in protein, yet lower in sugar, so they do not feed yeast or create inflammation in the body. Another added benefit is that they do not contain the protein *gluten,* which is present in grains such as wheat, spelt, rye, barley, and oats. Today, many of us are gluten intolerant or are even *allergic* to this protein. These grain-like seeds would still provide us with much-needed fiber and would help us remain calm and centered in the way that whole grains can do. When we eat them for our last meal of the day, they help us sleep better at night.

> *Grain-like seeds provide us with much needed fiber and help us remain calm and centered in the way that whole grains can do. They are also higher in protein, yet lower in sugar, so do not feed yeast or create inflammation in our body.*

Benefits of Body Ecology Grain-like Seeds

Grain-like seeds contain *phytoestrogens,* which help protect against harmful environmental and steroidal estrogens (xenoestrogens) that can get into your body through the food you eat, polluted air or water, or occupational exposure to chemical labs or industrial plants. Once in your body, they can stay in your tissues for years, causing hormone disruptions. Eating grain-like seeds can help balance hormones, support your immune system, and prevent or ease symptoms of osteoporosis and menopause. One important note to keep in mind, however, is that *absorbing phytoestrogens only occurs if you have a healthy gut*—or inner ecosystem—teeming with friendly bacteria.

Gluten Free for Improved Digestion

Gluten is not easy to digest. Most of us have inadequate stomach enzymes, a problem that increases as we age. Without the right digestive enzymes, gluten—like any protein—will not digest properly. And remember what happens when digestion is incomplete or poor—our systems become acidic and attractive to pathogenic bacteria, fungi, and viruses.

High in Fiber and Hydrating

The high fiber content of Body Ecology grain-like seeds is great for your digestive health, feeding friendly bacteria in your colon. These seeds are close enough to grains that they usually stop cravings for the refined carbs and cereals we are accustomed to eating. Grain-like seeds hold moisture in your intestines and help with constipation, which is often created by a dehydrated colon. Bulk fiber encourages peristaltic action in your intestines, moving food through your digestive system. Fiber pushes against the walls of your intestines, and they push back. Think of fiber as a personal trainer for your gut!

Nutrient Dense for Calorie Curbing

Body Ecology grains are very high in nutrients, so you don't need much to help satisfy your body's requirements for proteins, vitamins, and minerals. If you are also eating fermented foods, you obtain even more nutrients from your meal, allowing you to eat less, while being more satisfied.

Now, let's take a closer look at the four grain-like seeds featured in the Baby Boomer Diet—*amaranth, buckwheat, millet,* and *quinoa.*

Ancient Grains

These four superfoods may not be familiar to you yet, but they are delicious and readily available in grocery stores such as Whole Foods and in most health- or organic-food stores. All are high in protein, gluten free, and with the exception of buckwheat, alkaline forming. They are considered some of the most nutritionally complete foods available, and each one has a fascinating story to tell.

Amaranth

Amaranth, also called "Chinese spinach," was nearly exterminated from the planet! Actually a seed from a broad-leaf plant, this ancient yellow grain was a dietary staple among pre-Columbian peoples. The Aztecs, who fermented it into beer and popped its seeds like popcorn, used it prevalently and diversely. It also had a darker history . . . mixed with honey and human blood, it was consumed during religious rituals. For this reason, it was considered evil and was destroyed and banned by early Christian missionaries. It continued to be grown in remote villages in Mexico and Peru, and fortunately for us, it survived.[1]

Amaranth has three times the calcium of milk, so it is an excellent preventive therapy and treatment for osteoporosis. In addition, because it provides all eight essential amino acids (protein) but does not contain fat and cholesterol, it slows down the absorption of glucose into the bloodstream, making it easier to burn fat and lose weight. Unlike other grains, amaranth contains *lysine* and *methionine,* which are both essential amino acids that must be obtained from the diet since they cannot be made by our bodies. Lysine has antiviral properties and is essential in the crosslink formation that stabilizes collagen and elastin—so it helps create younger-looking skin. Methionine helps with the detoxification pathways by supplying the body with sulfur, and it helps the liver process fats.

Uses:

There are 60 species of amaranth in the world. Amaranth has a sweet, peppery taste. Because of its distinctive flavor, many people combine it with other grains. It can be cooked, used as baking flour, added to stews and soups as a thickener, or made into a hot breakfast cereal or pilaf.

How to prepare:

Always wash thoroughly with a strainer under running water for a few minutes. Or soak 1 cup of amaranth in a pan of water overnight. In the morning, drain the old water, and put 3 cups of water in a pan with the amaranth. Simmer for 20 minutes. Drain and pour into a bowl. Add stevia, Lakanto, vanilla flavoring, or cinnamon butter; or eat it plain.

Buckwheat

Buckwheat has been around in America since colonial times, and was particularly common in the northeastern and north-central areas of the country, where it was grown on many farms and used as livestock feed. You might remember the famous 1930s short-film series called *Our Gang* (syndicated as the *Little Rascals* TV show in the 1950s), which featured a character named after the popular and resilient plant. Native to both Northern Europe and Asia, buckwheat was brought to the U.S. in the 17th century by Dutch farmers, who called it *boekweit*, which means "beech wheat." It is a hardy plant that can withstand extremes in temperature and poor soil conditions.

Rich in flavonoids such as rutin (a phytonutrient that acts as an antioxidant) and a good source of B vitamins and magnesium (useful for improving blood flow and relaxing blood vessels), buckwheat contains all eight essential amino acids. Diets that contain buckwheat have been linked to lowered risk of developing cholesterol and high blood pressure. Buckwheat is also a valuable food for diabetics, as it lowers glucose levels.

Uses:

Buckwheat is not a cereal grain, as most people think, but rather a fruit seed, related to rhubarb and sorrel. It is high in oxalates, so it should be avoided if you are on the low-oxalate diet. The hulled buckwheat grains are called "groats," and they make a traditional porridge called kasha. Buckwheat is sold either roasted or unroasted.[2] Unroasted buckwheat has a strong, nutty flavor, which roasting seems to mellow. Buckwheat also makes a great baking flour, is used in crackers and breads, and is a welcome alternative for people with gluten allergies . . . it makes a delicious pancake and fortifying breakfast cereal.

How to prepare:

Soaking buckwheat for at least 8 hours before cooking is recommended. It should be washed and rinsed thoroughly using a strainer. Add 1 part buckwheat to 2 parts boiling (salted) water or vegetable or kombu broth. After the liquid has returned to a boil, turn down the heat, cover, and simmer for about 20 minutes.

Millet

Millet is one of the oldest foods known to humankind, and it is even mentioned in the Bible. First cultivated in China, millet has been used in very hot, dry countries for thousands of years. In India, millet flour is used to make thin, flat cakes

Cancer-Fighting Power of Grains on Par with Vegetables

*R*esearch conducted by Rui Hai Liu, M.D., and his colleagues at Cornell University reveals that whole grains, such as quinoa, contain many powerful cancer-fighting phytonutrients. Until recently, this had gone unrecognized because research methods were flawed.

Researchers have long known the power of phytonutrients, but they've been looking at only the "free" forms of these substances, such as *phenolics*—potent antioxidants—which dissolve quickly and are immediately absorbed into the bloodstream. They have overlooked the "bound" forms of phenolics, which are attached to the walls of plant cells and must be released by intestinal bacteria during digestion before they can be absorbed.

Dr. Liu and his colleagues measured the relative amounts of phenolics, and whether they were present in bound or free form, in common fruits and vegetables such as apples, red grapes, broccoli, and spinach. In free form, the percentage of phenolics was quite high in these foods, while in grains the free form was almost nonexistent. However, these researchers also discovered that 99 percent of the phenolics *were* present in grains, but in "bound" form.

Because previous researchers had been using the same process to measure antioxidants in grains as they did with fruits and vegetables, they have, according to Liu, *vastly underestimated the amount and activity of antioxidants in whole grains.*

These findings, reported at the American Institute for Cancer Research (AICR) International Research Conference on Food, Nutrition and Cancer, underscore the message that a variety of foods should be eaten for optimal health. Says Liu, "Different plant foods have different phytochemicals. These substances go to different organs, tissues and cells, where they perform different functions. What your body needs to ward off disease is this synergistic effect—this teamwork—that is produced by eating a wide variety of plant foods, including whole grains."[i]

---

[i]Rui Hai Liu, M.D., as quoted at the American Institute for Cancer Research (AICR) International Research Conference on Food, Nutrition and Cancer, found at *Hook Up with Health* website, "Amazing Finding: Supplements vs. Whole Food," July 31, 2006, **http:// hookupwithhealth.wordpress.com/2006/07/31/amazing-finding-suppliments-vs-whole-food** (accessed 1/6/10).

called *roti;* and in Africa, it is made into bread, baby food, and a thin breakfast porridge called *uji.*[3] The U.S. has traditionally used millet as livestock feed and birdseed. We are still quite uninformed about this ancient seed's amazing health benefits for humans.

Rich in phytochemicals and one of the least allergenic grains out there, millet is nearly 15 percent protein and contains high amounts of fiber; B-complex vitamins, including niacin, thiamin, and riboflavin; the essential amino acids *methionine* and *lecithin;* and some vitamin E. It is the only grain that won't lose its alkaline state after cooking.

It is particularly high in the minerals iron, magnesium, phosphorus, and potassium, which are beneficial for the heart and can help lower cholesterol. Magnesium can help reduce the effects of migraines. Phosphorus is of particular importance as we age. It is an essential component of lipid-containing structures such as cell membranes, and it is necessary for the metabolism of fats. In addition to its role in forming the mineral matrix of bone, phosphorus is an essential component of numerous other life-critical compounds, including *adenosine triphosphate,* or ATP—the molecule that creates, stores, and transports energy in the body.[4]

Uses:

Millet is related to sorghum, looks a lot like maize, and comes in four varieties, including "pearl," which has the largest seeds and is the kind most often consumed by humans. Millet has a mildly sweet, nutlike flavor. It can be prepared as a cooked cereal; and is used in casseroles, breads, soufflés, and stuffing. It is a grain that mixes well with herbs and other seasonings. It also makes a unique kind of couscous and produces flour that yields a thin, buttery crust.

How to prepare:

Rinse millet off and remove any stones or unhulled pieces. It is recommended that you soak or sprout it for 8 to 24 hours prior to preparing it. Cook millet as you would rice but with more water (3 cups water to 1 cup millet). However, if you soak it, you won't need as much water when you cook it. After soaking, try 1 cup millet to 2 or 2-1/2 cups water. You determine how much water to use depending on how soft you like your grain.

Quinoa

Quinoa (pronounced keen-wah) is native to the Andes of Bolivia, Chile, and Peru. A major staple of the altiplano Indians, and later the Incas, this versatile "mother grain" was believed to have been brought from heaven by a sacred bird called the *kullku*. Grown at 10,000 to 20,000 feet above sea level, quinoa allowed the altiplano peoples to thrive in the harsh living conditions that exist at such altitudes. Because these natives believed their grain was a gift from the gods and contained spiritually enhancing qualities, the ritual first planting of the season was a godlike act performed by the emperor. Considered a god himself, the emperor was responsible for a successful quinoa harvest. He sowed the first seeds of the season with his golden *taquiza,* a planting stick.[5]

During the European conquest of South America, quinoa was scorned by the Spanish colonists as "food for Indians" and even actively suppressed. Because it imparted so much energy and strength, growing it was forbidden, on pain of death. Instead, the Spaniards introduced rice, wheat, and barley. Fortunately, quinoa still grew wild in the higher altitudes, where it could be hidden from the Spaniards, and small amounts were consumed in secret. But its ban had an irrevocable impact on the Incan culture. The grain fell into obscurity for centuries.[6]

Related to the spinach family, quinoa has been called "vegetable caviar" because of its nutrient and mineral density. It is one of the *most complete foods in nature* because it contains amino acids, enzymes, vitamins and minerals, fiber, antioxidants, and phytonutrients. The Food and Agricultural Organization (FAO) has compared its nutritional quality to that of dried whole milk, and the protein quality and quantity in the quinoa seed is superior to those of more common cereal grains. It is higher in calcium, phosphorus, magnesium, potassium, iron, copper, manganese, and zinc than wheat, barley, or corn; and it is rich in calcium and vitamins B and E. It is higher in lysine than wheat or rice, and contains a balanced set of essential amino acids for humans.

Quinoa is also gluten free and considered easy to digest. People living in the Andes consider it an *endurance food*. It is given to pregnant mothers to strengthen them, and is also used for altitude sickness. If you have a milk allergy—or are avoiding dairy, as is recommended in the first stage of The Diet—quinoa is a great alternative.

Quinoa's high mineral content also makes it excellent for bone health. The minerals manganese and copper act as antioxidants in your body to get rid of dangerous cancer- and disease-causing substances, while magnesium helps relax your muscles and blood vessels and positively affects blood pressure. Quinoa may be helpful if you suffer from migraines, diabetes, or atherosclerosis. High in fiber, it is a wonderful way to improve elimination and tone the colon.

Uses:

Quinoa is especially easy to cook and can be enjoyed year-round because it is versatile and light. You can use it in warming winter soups or refreshing summer salads. Quinoa's nutty flavor and rice-like texture make it perfect for stir-fries, but it can also be made into breads and biscuits. When cooked, quinoa is light, fluffy, slightly crunchy, and subtly flavored. Quinoa cooks quickly, which makes it a great breakfast meal; and it can be enjoyed in its whole-grain form, or you can try quinoa flakes made into a hot cereal as a wonderful replacement for oatmeal!

How to prepare:

Make sure you rinse your quinoa, and then soak it for at least 8 hours. Cook 25 minutes . . . and it's ready to mix with a variety of ingredients to create diverse and delicious meals. Adding a little Body Ecology Wholegrain Liquid to the soaking water is recommended. The beneficial microflora help soften the grains before cooking, making them even more digestible.

(*Note:* Some of the nutritional information on these grain-like seeds that is contained in this section was drawn from **www.whfoods.com**.)

For many wonderful recipes using these four grains, please refer to the Body Ecology website or *The Body Ecology Diet* book.

Preparing Grains

It is always recommended that you soak your grain-like seeds for 8 to 24 hours. Grains, beans, seeds, and nuts all have phytic acid, an enzyme inhibtor, in them. It makes these foods difficult to break down in your digestive system. Since most people have weak digestive systems, especially as they age, eating grains without soaking them will mean they will be poorly digested, leading to a toxic, rapidly aging body.

What about Flour Made from Grain-like Seeds?

While the *whole* grain-like seeds are much more nutritious and are better for your digestion, health-food stores often sell *flours* made of buckwheat, millet, quinoa, and amaranth. You can also purchase breads made from these grains. Just like any flour product, the flour from Body Ecology–recommended grain-like seeds is mucus-forming and lacks fiber, which can actually be drying to your colon. If you suffer from constipation, avoid flour products until your inner ecosystem is recolonized with friendly bacteria and your elimination is excellent.

If you feel you must eat flour products, here's a suggestion. To offset the negative side of flour (even that of grain-like seeds), make it a habit to consume these products with fermented foods. Add cultured veggies to a sandwich, for example.

Konjaku—a Noodle Alternative That Won't Pack on the Pounds!

While we at Body Ecology recommend avoiding wheat products, there are wonderful pasta noodles made from quinoa, rice, spelt, and buckwheat (100 percent soba noodles). Another great high-fiber alternative to pasta is *konjaku* noodles, which are made from yam flour from the *konnyaku imo* tuber. A staple in Japan, konjaku noodles (also called *shirataki*) are gluten and calorie free, low carb, and won't feed bad bacteria and yeast in your digestive tract. The fiber in konjaku is called *glucomannan,* and it can control blood sugar and cholesterol and even help with "waist management." This is because konjaku noodles expand to many times their original size, making you feel full on less. They are great with stir-fried vegetables and Body Ecology sauces. Since they absorb other flavors well, season them liberally with herbs and other seasonings.

Putting the Principles into Practice

Grain-like Seeds and the Principle of 80/20

Covered in depth in Chapter 13, this principle shows the value of balancing your meals, with 80 percent vegetables (land and ocean) and 20 percent grains. Following this principle when dining on grain-like seeds or their flour products will go a long way toward creating a healthy digestive system, and it will take the guesswork out of deciding how much of anything you need to include in your diet.

Like any new habit, it takes practice to get used to planning your meals this way. What starts to happen, though, is quite wonderful—you begin to feel comfortable in your own skin again, with less gas and bloating; a healthy weight; and a youthful, glowing appearance.

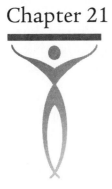

Chapter 21

Hydration Choices: For Rejuvenation and Timeless Beauty

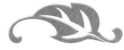

All health—beauty, stamina, strength, and youthfulness—is intimately tied to the body's hydration levels.

Water—the Healing Liquid of Life

In ancient Greek mythology, ambrosia was a substance that granted immortality to anyone who consumed it. Although it was never quite clear what this liquid "nectar" might actually be, it was very cleansing and purifying to all those who drank it or bathed in it. Hera (Juno in Roman mythology) used ambrosia to "cleanse all dirt from her fair body,"[1] and it was believed to undo the cumulative toll of years. Its restorative attributes could turn back the hands of time.

There is really only one liquid on the planet that has the purifying reverse-the-clock qualities of ambrosia . . . and it's water—literally, the elixir of the gods.

Approximately 60 to 70 percent of the body and 85 percent of the brain is composed of water, H_2O—a universal solvent and the most abundant substance inside of us. Since the beginning of life within Earth's primordial ocean, we have essentially been water-based life-forms. And virtually all of our chemical and physical processes; nerve transmissions; and circulatory, motor, and immune functions occur in or depend on this water-based terrain.

But this is just the tip of the iceberg, so to speak . . . the work of Masaru Emoto has demonstrated water's unique trans-spiritual qualities as well, and its startling ability to be transformed by positive or negative energy.

A doctor of alternative medicine, Emoto gathered water samples from around the world, slowly froze them, and then photographed them with a dark-field microscope to capture their aesthetic and structural differences. Emoto discovered that there were radical discrepancies in the crystalline structures of water depending on its source and the surrounding environment. For example, water from a pure mountain spring might reveal a beautiful geometric design, while water taken from a polluted or heavily industrial area might show structures that were random and distorted.

Noting how water changed in different environments and under different conditions, Emoto began to wonder if music, words, and even thoughts might also affect the crystal structures. He then conducted a number of experiments where he exposed water in glasses to different words, pictures, or music. He photographed these as well.[2]

The resulting images are truly astounding, and you can easily find some examples of them on YouTube. Once you've seen the shimmering jewel of *peace* versus the jagged-edged cavity of *anger*, you can't help but be convinced of the transformative impact that we have on water and that water has on us. If so much of who we are is made up of water, consider how important our own thoughts and intentions can be to our health and well-being.

Dehydration—What It Means and What It Does

We often hear of nutrients that are "good for" radiant skin and hair, or are "essential" to a strong heart or proper digestion. But most of us don't realize how much of our physical and mental well-being depends on being well hydrated.

You may be excited to learn that water can be a therapy, a healing substance for your body.

What does it actually mean to be *dehydrated?* Most people think of dehydration as simply the body lacking in water. But a more accurate discussion of dehydration would include looking at *where that water is located.*

Like fish in an aquarium, all of our cells are surrounded by a complex *modified* water called the extracellular fluid. When we become dehydrated, 66 percent of the water loss is from the *interior* of our cells (the intracellular fluid) and 26 percent is lost from the extracellular volume.[3] Dehydration causes the blood to become concentrated.

The mineral-rich extracellular fluid creates a kind of buffer zone against toxins. Some physiologists refer to this fluid *and* the complex network of fibrous connective proteins as the extracellular *matrix*—a distinct system within the body, even larger than your skin surface. According to the matrix theory, you are only as healthy as your matrix. It provides nutrition to your cells,

Dehydration causes the blood to become concentrated, a biological nightmare both inside and outside the cells.

removes waste, regulates your internal environment, "reads" your external environment, defends your cells against free radicals, and more.[4]

But when the *interiors* of cells become dehydrated, it is nothing short of a cellular nightmare. Acid builds up inside, the cells become poisoned, and DNA damage occurs. Enzymes and amino acids lose their effectiveness. Brain cells, lacking useful amino acids, cannot manufacture brain chemicals, such as serotonin. The electrical and magnetic energy inside each cell is lost, weakening its vitality. The list goes on and on.

The initial impact of *mild* dehydration in adults appears when the body has lost about 2 percent of its total fluid. Some of these mild dehydration effects[5] include:

- Thirst
- Loss of appetite
- Dry skin
- Flushing
- Dark-colored urine
- Dry mouth/cotton mouth

- Fatigue/weakness
- Chills
- Head rushes

If dehydration is allowed to continue to a fluid loss of 5 percent, the following more severe effects can be experienced:

- Fatigue
- Headaches
- Nausea
- Increased heart rate
- Increased respiration
- Decreased sweating
- Decreased urination
- Increased body temperature
- Muscle cramps
- Tingling of the limbs

When 10 percent fluid loss occurs, conditions have become quite dire, and this level of fluid loss is often fatal. The effects of severe dehydration include:

- Muscle spasms
- Vomiting
- Racing pulse
- Shriveled skin
- Dim vision
- Painful urination
- Confusion
- Difficulty breathing
- Seizures
- Chest and abdominal pain
- Unconsciousness

However, when dehydration is long-term or "chronic," even if low-grade, the symptoms take on the additional characteristics of chronic degenerative diseases:

- Fatigue/energy loss
- Constipation
- Digestive disorders
- Feeling irritable
- Feeling depressed
- Not sleeping well
- Increased cravings
- Fear of crowds or of leaving the house
- Poor circulation and congestion of lymph glands
- High or low blood pressure
- Gastritis and stomach ulcers
- Respiratory troubles
- Acid/alkaline imbalance
- Excess weight/obesity
- Eczema
- Elevated cholesterol
- Cystitis and urinary infections
- Rheumatism
- Premature aging
- Skin aging, including wrinkles and loss of elasticity

In short, the health effects of chronic dehydration are profound.

F. Batmanghelidj was a renowned medical doctor who wrote extensively about water's healing properties for more than 22 years. His research revealed that the issue of dehydration is sorely misunderstood—even by medical doctors and by the alternative-health community.

Drinking enough water to stay well hydrated is one of those issues that we understand *intellectually:* "Yes, I know I should be drinking more water, but . . ."

This can be a difficult habit to learn, as most of us didn't grow up watching our parents or grandparents drink water. The trend of carrying around bottled water is a very recent one, and many of us still do not understand water's profound importance.

Dr. B (as he was affectionately called) was not saying that you could heal diseases with water alone, but that if you want to stay young, and even reverse many of the signs and symptoms of aging and disease, you must address and correct your lifelong problem of not being well hydrated.

Young bodies are blessed with optimal hydration. A baby's body is 80 percent water, while that of an adult is only 60 to 70 percent. As we age, this percentage continues to drop. To regain our youthfulness, we must be mindful to keep water nearby and make a conscious effort to achieve optimal hydration at all times.

The Amazing Benefits of Water

Batmanghelidj's first book, *Your Body's Many Cries for Water*, is a testament to the extensive health benefits that can be accomplished solely by restoring sufficient hydration levels. In this book he documented the many diseases he was able to reverse with just ordinary water, minerals, and sea salt.

Most hydration cures are related to the fact that water is the primary transport system in our bodies. It carries nutrients and oxygen into the cells and waste products out. When hydration is not at an optimal level, blood turns acidic, so it thickens and becomes more condensed. As it does so, circulation decreases, there is poor oxygenation of tissue, and inefficient removal of CO_2 and toxins. All this creates a low-grade state of metabolic acidosis. Remember, when we're too acidic, our bodies become *dis*-eased.

When toxins and waste products accumulate in our cells, the cells then deteriorate or even die. As these tissue cells die, aging results. Skin sags, hair falls out, energy drops, memory fails, hormone levels plummet, libido wanes, and heart attacks and aneurysms can occur. Further, dehydration prevents accumulations from being washed out of the cells and tissues. These accumulations, such as cholesterol, lactic-acid wastes, pyruvic crystals, or calcium, muck up the cell membranes, clog the efficient pathways of arteries, and inhibit the smooth motion of the joint capsules; and thus contribute to such chronic degenerative diseases as arteriosclerosis, arthritis, gout, kidney stones, and gallstones, to name a few.

Water is the substance that takes the toxins and carbon dioxide out and carries vital nutrients in. That is why it can and should be considered an anti-aging remedy!

Its benefits[6] are numerous:

- Water makes the skin smoother.

- Water helps reduce fatigue.

- Water makes the immune system function more efficiently.

- Water helps with weight management.

- Water helps prevent the loss of memory as we age; and reduces the risk of Alzheimer's, Parkinson's, and Lou Gehrig's disease.

- Water can help offset the progression and symptoms of hormone-related health issues such as hot flashes and osteoporosis.

- Water is the main lubricant in the joint spaces and helps prevent arthritis.

- Water rids the body of toxins.

Dehydration = Pain

Batmanghelidj also showed that dehydration causes your body to produce excessive amounts of cholesterol. Why would this be so?

Batmanghelidj called cholesterol a "waterproof bandage." When blood becomes dehydrated and therefore too concentrated and imbalanced, it rushes through our arteries and capillaries, creating abrasions and tears. Cholesterol is produced to cover them up. If this "bandage" were not there, then blood would get under the arterial membrane and peel it off, soon killing us.[7]

How Do We Get Dehydrated in the First Place?

Through activities of daily living, the average person loses about three to four liters (about 10 to 15 cups) of fluid a day in sweat, urine, exhaled air, and bowel movement. We lose approximately one to two liters of water just from breathing. The most common cause of increased water loss is exercise and sweating. The evaporation of sweat from the skin accounts for 90 percent of our cooling ability.

Pain is a sign of water shortage. Wherever there is pain, there is dehydration.

Exercise, sweating, diarrhea, temperature, or altitude can significantly increase the amount of water we lose each day. Even though we are all at risk of dehydration, the people most vulnerable are infants, elderly adults, and athletes. They are either not able to adequately express their thirst sensation or to detect it and do something in time.

What we lose must be replaced by the fluids we drink and the food we eat.

Tips for Staying Hydrated

Staying properly hydrated is one of the best—and easiest-to-implement—anti-aging strategies around, but it is one we must be vigilant about.

- It's important to drink regularly, not just when you "feel" thirsty. Most likely, as you grow older, your thirst sensation will completely disappear, and you will not be able to recognize that your body is dehydrated. In other words, don't depend on the symptom of a "dry mouth" to alert you to the need to drink water again. Keep a glass or bottle beside you at all times.

- To keep your body well hydrated, drink at least half your body weight in ounces. If you weigh 200 pounds, drink ten or more 12-ounce glasses of water per day. If you weigh 100 pounds, you need at least four or more 12-ounce glasses per day. If you are physically active or live in a warm climate, drink even more.

- A hydrated body produces clear, colorless urine every three to four hours. If your urine is yellow, you are dehydrated—but only moderately so. If your urine is orange or dark colored, you are severely dehydrated.

- If your water-drinking habits are poor, try this tip: Set a timer for 60 minutes. Every time it goes off, drink one cup of water. Set the timer again. If you don't like the idea of using a timer, another suggestion is to keep a running list of what you drink each day on a notepad at your work desk or perhaps on your refrigerator at home. That way you can see when you are falling behind. If necessary, place sticky notes everywhere that remind you to pour a delicious, life-lengthening glass of water.

- When you wake up in the morning, *immediately* drink two glasses of water to rehydrate after loss of fluids during the night. You wake up dehydrated, toxic, and in need of energy to start the day. It's best to then wait at least 30 minutes before consuming other foods. Water early in the morning gets your circulation going and herds those toxins out of the body.

- To keep your body and brain functioning at peak performance, consider having at least half your daily water intake before noon . . . it really revitalizes a dehydrated body.

- Drink two glasses of water 30 minutes before lunch and again before dinner. This will help your digestive tract (and liver) do a better job of processing the food you eat.

- Do not drink water with meals. Large amounts taken with a meal will dilute stomach acid. Instead, try chewing each mouthful of food at least 30 to 40 times before swallowing.

- Wait about one hour after each meal and drink another glass of water.

- Sipping on a warm cup of tea with meals has a positive effect on digestion. While warm liquids (including soup) with a meal can aid digestion, ice-cold drinks halt it and, in general, are a shock to your system. You can also sip on three to four ounces of one of Body Ecology's probiotic liquids, such as CocoBiotic. Served in a pretty champagne glass, it is a superior substitute for wine.

- Dr. B taught that water combined with other ingredients has an "agenda" and cannot be counted as part of your daily water intake. However, minerals and sea salt can be added. The more water you drink, the more salt you need. The ocean and your blood are nearly identical in the proportion of mineral electrolytes.

- Forget the coffee break. Take water breaks instead. Water is the source of true energy, and coffee is dehydrating.

- If you find it difficult to up your daily amount of water, it is strongly suggested that you read Dr. F. Batmanghelidj's book *Water for Health, for Healing, for Life: You're Not Sick, You're Thirsty!* This is an update to *Your Body's Many Cries for Water.* It will definitely convince you to drink more water.

The Search for Pure Water

The best water in the world—the ambrosia of those early Greeks—is found very deep in the earth, about two miles down. It is called "primal water," and it is water that has been untouched by the atmosphere. It surfaces through fissures in rocks. Unfortunately, this water is largely unavailable to us and quite costly. Scientists also fear that even it may contain some undesirable constituents such as metals, radioactivity, and even hydrocarbons.

Sadly, healthy water is not available anymore from our city water systems. Water-treatment chemicals and additives (for example, chlorine, chloramines, aluminum, and fluoride); microorganisms; pollution; heavy metals; and even medicinal drugs such as antidepressants and antibiotics that cannot be filtered out (from human and animal urine) have compromised our drinking and bathing water, perhaps forever.

These contaminants have caused people from developed countries—including half of all Americans—to turn to bottled water as their primary source of drinking water. The bottled-water craze, which began in the 1990s, has grown steadily to a $100-billion-a-year industry. The results are predictably negative:

- It's expensive. At up to $2.50 per liter ($10 per gallon), bottled water costs more than gasoline in the United States.

- A lot more energy and raw materials are required to produce and transport bottled water compared to tap water. Worldwide, some 2.7 million tons of plastic are used to bottle water each year.

- Most plastic bottles are not recycled, and end up in the ocean or in a landfill.

- Even though the very *best* bottled waters may start out chemically and biologically pure, plastic bottles may pose some risks, as they can leach chemicals into the water itself, especially if they have been sitting in the hot sun.

What You Can Do

Make your first priority the installation of a water-filtration system in your home. You should be aware that roughly 40 percent of bottled water starts as tap water, so simply switching from tap to bottles is not the best answer.

Why not go green, especially if you are traveling away from home? Carry a *refillable, protected* glass water bottle or an HDPE (#2 high-density polyethylene) plastic bottle, preferably made by a trusted supplier (such as Nalgene). Never choose a plastic bottle (#7 Lexan or polycarbonate), which can leach BPA, a toxin, into the water. *Note:* At Body Ecology we do not recommend stainless-steel bottles because most are manufactured in China and can leach metals (including troublesome nickel) into the pure water.

At home, the very best way to keep water pure is in a refillable glass bottle.

Differences among Waters

Bottled Waters

Distilled water has long been popular among people who embark upon a fast or detoxification regimen, although the benefits and risks have been the subject of debate for many decades. The problem, some opponents argue, is that distilled water is so "pure" and chemically "hungry" that it will dissolve minerals out of the body. Proponents of distilled water argue that the amount of minerals supplied by water is insignificant compared to dietary minerals, so this is a moot point. They claim that the benefit of extracting toxins from the body's tissues outweighs any negative aspects. Yet another perspective is that as soon as distilled water mixes with the stomach fluids, it quickly loses much of its chemical "hunger" and is no different from other low-mineral sources.

Distilled water is water that has been boiled and evaporated. The vapor (or steam) leaves the impurities behind, then cools and condenses back to pure water. This is the process nature uses to recycle water on planet Earth. Water evaporates from the oceans, and the wind currents carry it over cooler mountainous areas, where it condenses into rain and snow. This process eradicates virtually all microbiological impurities—including protozoa, bacteria, and viruses—and heavy metals. It contains no minerals, so it is able to actively absorb toxic substances and eliminate them from the body quickly.

You should be cautious about using distilled water (or any low-mineral-content water) during fasting, especially if you are deficient in minerals already, as you might experience heart irregularities and a rise in blood pressure. If you are eating a healthy diet or supplementing the distilled water with a mineral mixture, this should balance the potential removal of minerals.

Those toxic soft drinks and colas that so many uninformed Americans consume are made with low-mineral-content water. Added to this are acidic ingredients such as phosphoric acid and high-fructose corn syrup. This combination results in the loss of significant amounts of calcium, magnesium, and other trace minerals. The more mineral loss, the greater the risk for osteoporosis, osteoarthritis, hypothyroidism, coronary artery disease, high blood pressure, and a long list of degenerative diseases associated with premature aging.

Generally, the consumption of distilled water as a means of hydration should be limited unless an adequate diet and complete mineral supplementation are in place.

A Water Process You Can Live With:
Reverse Osmosis + Coconut-Shell Activated Carbon

At Body Ecology, we recommend a water filter that uses both reverse osmosis and coconut-shell activated carbon. This tank-less system is the most effective, practical, and economical for making the highest-quality, contaminant-free water for drinking and cooking. If you use ice, make sure you are using this pure, high-quality water . . . and, of course, you'll want to also give it to your pets. Information on this water filter can be obtained at: **www.bodyecology.com**.

Sparkling Water vs. Still Water—
Some "Fizzy" Misconceptions

Although sparkling waters are consumed all over the world, most people aren't aware that they vary widely in taste, quality, purity, and origin. It is important when choosing "fizzy" over "flat" that you select only those that are naturally carbonated. What does "naturally carbonated" mean? Certain geological conditions can produce naturally carbonated water, such as volcanic activity. When water comes in contact with certain geological formations, it takes on a strong and healthy mineral composition, which the carbon dioxide in the water helps absorb. Some waters may have been formed only 30 days before bottling, whereas others are more than 20,000 years old. It's the mineral content that really makes these waters uniquely curative.

Ideal for the human body is alkaline water, which contains minerals such as calcium, silica, and magnesium. This is why sparkling water may be a better option than still, and is certainly better than distilled, which has no "life force" energy.

There is a long-standing belief that sparkling water is not as healthy as springwater, but new research indicates otherwise.

A study published in *The Journal of Nutrition* was designed to assess the difference in health benefits between women who drank sparkling mineral water and women who drank still mineral water. Study participants were asked to drink one liter of either the sparkling or still water each day for two months, followed by two months on the other water. During the study, the participants underwent a number of tests, including blood pressure and cholesterol levels.

Compared to the still mineral water, the drinking of sparkling water brought about significant reductions in the level of LDL cholesterol (generally regarded as a risk factor for heart disease), as well as a significant increase in levels of HDL cholesterol (generally taken to reduce heart-disease risk). These and other biochemical changes induced by drinking sparkling water were estimated to reduce the women's risk of developing heart disease over the next decade by about one-third.[8]

Researchers aren't completely sure why sparkling water is good for so many of us, but they suspect it has something to do with the high mineral content in naturally carbonated water and its ability to stimulate bicarbonate (HCO_3) secretion in both the stomach and the duodenum. (Remember, though, this is not necessarily true for all carbonated waters such as those with little mineral content or the wrong kind.) Although such waters are often high in sodium—a mineral that has often been maligned and erroneously linked to high blood pressure and heart problems—it is believed that the bicarbonate alkalinity and the other minerals in sparkling water help balance any negative effects sodium may have in the body.

Minerals also determine differences in taste. As with wine, subtle flavor distinctions can be caused by the soil, climate, and geography of where the water is "harvested." The amount of mineral elements in water is commonly referred to as "total dissolved solids" (TDS) and is expressed in milligrams per liter (mg/l) or parts per million (ppm). TDS is made up of positively charged cations (sodium, calcium, magnesium, potassium, phosphorus, iron, manganese, copper, and strontium) and negatively charged anions (chloride, bicarbonate, carbonate, sulfate, fluoride, and silicate)—and many trace elements. Altogether, there are about 80 mineral-element building blocks. The higher the mineral content, the more distinctive the taste. You might think of low TDS as comparable to white wine, with more of a neutral taste that's less weighty. Waters with high TDS feel heavier and have more of an aftertaste, rather like a robust red wine. In the U.S., bottled water must contain at least 250 mg/l TDS in order to qualify as "mineral" water.[9]

Other studies have suggested that the magnesium and bicarbonate content of natural mineral water can result in favorable changes in urinary pH and magnesium and citrate excretion, and may inhibit kidney-stone formation (from oxalates).[10]

But not all sparkling waters are what they seem (or what they're promoted to be). For example, many people consider Perrier the "aristocracy" of carbonated waters, but the truth is that Perrier (475 mg/l TDS) is a still water that has been aggressively infused with CO_2 bubbles, creating unusual acidity (pH of 5.5).

Instead of Perrier, drink Apollinaris (1,600 mg/l TDS) or a water from Germany called Gerolsteiner (2,527 mg/l TDS). Gerolsteiner is almost like taking a mineral supplement. Classified as naturally carbonated, with a low pH, this water has been a famous health tonic since 1888. (It is interesting to note that the TDS of these waters is so high that they exceed the maximum allowed for drinking water in the U.S.)

For more information on where to purchase the finest waters and to find out which ones are the healthiest, go to: **www.aquamaestro.com/step1.asp**.

For additional information on fine waters, go to: **www .finewaters.com**. Or read the book *Fine Waters: A Connoisseur's Guide to the World's Most Distinctive Bottled Waters,* by Michael Mascha, which can be purchased at: **www.finewaters.com/ Bottled_Water_Guide_Book.asp**.

The Important Role of Salt and Minerals in the Water You Drink

As you increase the amount of water you drink, you should also increase your intake of mineral-rich sea salt and other minerals.

Body Ecology's **Ancient Earth Minerals** is an excellent choice for minerals from a *land* source, while **Celtic sea salt** is the recommended way to obtain minerals from the *ocean*. Ideally, you want both. Selina Naturally (**www.selinanaturally .com**) has delicious-tasting sea salt from France, Hawaii, and the Polynesian islands.

Don't be afraid of salt . . . not if it is high-quality, mineral-rich sea salt. Salt is not bad for you. It does not raise blood pressure if you also have adequate amounts of other minerals, especially potassium, calcium, magnesium, and zinc, in your diet. These key minerals work with sodium to keep the right balance of water inside and outside the cells (osmotic balance). You'll be reading more about the importance of real sea salt in the next chapter.

If you want to begin reversing the signs and symptoms of aging, balance your sodium intake with your water consumption—drink more water, yes, but also consume sea salt and minerals. Dr. Batmanghelidj's many years of research clearly showed this. His recommendation is to take a quarter teaspoon of sea salt per *quart* of water—that's every four to five glasses of water.

Ancient Earth Minerals can be taken in the morning with your first two glasses of water. Put approximately one-eighth teaspoon of sea salt on your tongue just after drinking the water.

Take this same amount of both minerals once again at bedtime. Doing so will help you sleep more deeply at night.

Other Hydration Choices

A dangerous misconception has many of us thinking that other fluids such as coffee, tea, soda, wine, alcoholic beverages, juices, and milk count toward our daily water requirements. Dr. Batmanghelidj made it very clear that these other fluids have their own "agenda." This means they contain chemicals that alter the body's chemistry at its central-nervous-system control centers. Even milk differs from water—it should be considered a food, not a substitute for water.[11]

Your body was designed to drink pure water that has no agenda. Although other healthy hydration choices appear in the pages to follow, please remember that none should take the place of the right amount of pure water your unique body needs each day. *Nothing is a substitute for water!*

Super Green Drinks

You may be familiar with a variety of supernutrient green drinks sold in powder form that are widely available in health-food stores today. These drinks are quite popular, and rightly so. Typically, a blend of powerful, energizing, whole foods and herbs, in a base of cereal grasses and microalgae, is stirred into water or juice. Green drinks are easy to digest and provide an excellent all-alkaline option first thing in the morning. This will help bring your body, which becomes more acidic at night, back into balance. Green drinks are a great way to help correct nutritional deficiencies—you get so many amazing nutrients in one drink—and they are much easier than taking supplements.

Look for a green drink that has healing benefits of aiding digestion; creating energy; and providing protein, enzymes, vitamins, minerals, and probiotics. Many green drinks have spirulina, collards, and kale, which in raw form can suppress the thyroid. But this is not so when they are fermented! A well-blended formula can be such an excellent energizer in the morning that you might find that it replaces your need for caffeine. A whole-food green drink also works well if you are having a midafternoon slump and need a pick-me-up.

Body Ecology's green drink, **Vitality SuperGreen,** does all of the above. Potent Proteins is another excellent protein powder. One hundred percent of its ingredients are fermented. Over 50 percent of this is predigested, fermented spirulina.

Tea

Tea has many healing qualities, including polyphenols and tannins. Polyphenols in tea provide antioxidants, increase white blood cells, and may have anticancer properties. They also absorb cholesterol in the digestive tract and bloodstream. Tannins and oils in tea can aid digestion and fat emulsification.

Green teas vary in taste because of differences in soils, harvesting, and processing. Green tea is not processed as heavily as other teas because the freshly picked leaves are dried and then heat-treated to prevent oxidation. With the finer varieties, traditional handmade methods are often used; and the resulting tastes can range from sweet, buttery, nutty, and smoky . . . to grassy and floral.

More and more research substantiates the health benefits stemming from regular consumption of green tea. Specifically, it contains a group of antioxidants known as *catechins,* which protect our cells from free radicals. They can actually prevent tumor-generating conditions that can lead to cancer. Catechins may also prove beneficial for the treatment of existing cancer and the prevention of heart disease.[12]

Research has also shown that green tea increases your metabolism, acts as an antiviral, inhibits oral bacterial plaque, is a rich source of vitamins, and has anti-aging properties. It, as well as ginger tea, is an excellent digestive aid. There are several other teas with medicinal properties, too. Cat's claw, echinacea, and pau d'arco (also known as Brazilian bark or taheebo) are especially healing and antifungal. Burdock-root teas, dandelion-root teas, and Yogi Stomach Ease are also quite healing. Fruit teas and teas with citric acid are best avoided, as they often have mold growing on them. Teas such as tulsi (also known as holy basil) and chamomile are calming and can help to manage stress and regulate sleep.

Consider using teas as a means of warmth and comfort, consumed in addition to your daily water requirements, but not in place of water. As mentioned previously, having a cup of warm tea or a bowl of soup adds liquid to your meals, and helps facilitate the digestive process. Tea can also be your between-meal snack, providing warming, healthy liquid—and even a touch of sweetness—to satisfy a craving. If you like your teas a little sweet, be sure to use stevia instead of processed sugar or artificial sweeteners.

You can find many green teas in grocery stores today, but there is often a big difference in quality, purity, and taste. If you fancy yourself a tea connoisseur, then you will certainly enjoy the rare and unusual varieties offered by artisan tea maker Silk Road Teas (**www.silkroadteas.com**).

Unlike most tea companies, Silk Road buys its teas direct, and is always searching for new regions that produce unique-tasting varieties. They sell only 100 percent unadulterated leaf. Their teas are certified organic, too, which means they are grown without the use of chemicals and pesticides, with no added flavorings, colorings, perfumes, oils, or preservatives. With a mission to support the artisan or traditional tea farms in China, Silk Road delivers teas that have a nuanced, healthful taste; and that are now widely recognized for their unparalleled quality and purity.

Wine

Many readers will be very disappointed to learn that wine is not the anti-aging beverage that the media has led us to believe. It's true that red wine has *resveratrol,* the anti-aging substance that mimics calorie restriction. But wine is also, like all alcohol, very dehydrating.

Dr. Batmanghelidj's research clearly showed that alcohol stops the emergency water-supply system to important cells, such as the ones in your brain.

Wine is fermented, yes, but it is fermented from fruit and is not good for anyone with candidiasis. It is not as healing as the other fermented foods and liquids mentioned throughout the book. If you are really serious about reversing the signs of

CocoBiotic:
A Naturally Fermented, Refreshing Probiotic Drink Made from Young Coconuts

*A*ll probiotics are not the same! Many probiotic products are synthesized in a laboratory . . . even worse, many of them are genetically modified.

Not CocoBiotic.

A naturally fermented drink created from wild-crafted young Thai coconut, CocoBiotic utilizes Grainfield's proprietary *FermFlora* organic fermentation process. The gut-friendly bacteria and yeasts in this delicious beverage are derived entirely from nature . . . from organically certified plant sources.

With a light, refreshing, and slightly fizzy taste, this beverage has long been a favorite of Body Ecology customers. While CocoBiotic is *not* exactly the same thing as young coconut kefir, and not made in the same way, it *does* similarly embrace Body Ecology's emphasis on fermentation, and provides you with an amazing range of health benefits. Fermented young coconut juice was included *by design* . . . because of the many benefits coconut-kefir users have reported over the years, such as:

- Improved digestion

- Reduced sugar cravings

- Greatly increased energy

- Improved cleansing of the liver

aging in your body, avoid wine. If you feel you must drink it, limit it to special occasions and celebrations, and be sure to take in even more water as soon as possible, especially water with minerals. A meal with a glass of wine *and* a serving of cultured vegetables will help balance the negative side effects of the alcohol.

Make Your Celebrations Healthy— Now That's *Really* Something to Toast!

Instead of wine or bubbly, pour InnergyBiotic or CocoBiotic into that pretty champagne glass. It lends a little elegance to your meals and aids in digestion. It is also a great way to celebrate a special occasion because you can drink it knowing you are going to live a long and healthy life.

Become a Tea Aficionado

While many of us are accustomed to learning about and enjoying different types of wines—finding out about the regions they come from and discovering the subtleties of taste and how well they pair with certain foods, we can also bring the same enthusiasm to tea. There are so many varieties, each with its own unique properties that benefit the body in some specialized way. Consider experimenting with tea with the same zest you bring to your wine tasting!

Juices from the Sour-Fruit Family

There are many *unsweetened* fruit-juice concentrates that can be used to make excellent energy-boosting juices in the morning. Look for cranberry, black-currant, pomegranate, açaí, noni, mangosteen, and blueberry *concentrates.*

Read the labels carefully and purchase them only if they are unsweetened.

Unfortunately, many manufacturers and marketers of these juices add water, additional fruit juices and concentrates, sweeteners, chemical preservatives, and other unwanted and unnecessary ingredients. This is done to lower costs, improve flavor, increase sweetness, and speed production runs.

The sour juices mentioned in the following pages are gaining in popularity and are often called "super fruits." Consider adding them to water, young coconut kefir, or milk kefir for a delicious, hydrating drink first thing in the morning.

- **Noni:** Traditionally an important fermented food for those living in the Polynesian islands, noni is high in minerals; contains trace minerals; and has numerous health benefits, including helping increase production of serotonin, strengthening immunity, increasing microbial population in the intestines, and regulating blood sugar and energy levels. Unfortunately, noni has to be pasteurized or it would continue to ferment during shipping, and the glass bottles would explode. **Genesis Today**'s noni juice is a recommended brand.

- **Mangosteen:** From Thailand and Myanmar, this fruit's rind has been shown to have medicinal qualities. In Southeast Asia, it has been used to treat dysentery and skin disorders, such as eczema. Mangosteen is a free-radical scavenger. It supports healthy inflammatory processes, strengthens the immune system, and promotes youthful cell regeneration and thus, healthy aging. Genesis Today's mangosteen juice is 100 percent pure, wild-harvested, and is made the traditional way, just like it was 1,000 years ago. Mangosteen is pasteurized, also.

- **Açaí:** A purple berry from Brazil, açaí falls into the category of "super fruit." It is thought to have anti-aging and anticancer benefits, along with promoting improved digestion, mental focus, and energy. More studies are being done to better understand the health benefits of açaí. Genesis Today also has premium-quality unsweetened açaí juice. Açaí is pasteurized. (The frozen pulp may not be pasteurized.)

- **Pomegranate:** A fruit that grows wild in many parts of the world, pomegranates are rich in phytochemicals, and have been shown to inhibit hormone-dependent breast-cancer-cell growth. A report published in a recent issue of *The American Association for Cancer Research* reveals that compounds found in pomegranate have a suppressive effect on the proliferation of breast-cancer cells.[13] Pomegranate has also been shown to lower bad cholesterol and to reverse plaque buildup in the arteries.

- **Black currant:** This fruit is revered in Europe as an adrenal tonic to provide energy. It also helps

soothe an upset stomach and stimulates appetite.
It is great for anemia, is high in vitamin C and rich
in antioxidants, and strengthens the bladder while
helping to alleviate urinary tract infections. It also
stimulates peristaltic action in your colon. Try a glass
of water with unsweetened black currant juice (and
stevia to taste) first thing in the morning. Austria's
Finest, Naturally imports an excellent black-currant
juice (**www.austrianpumpkinoil.com**).

- **Cranberry:** This berry strengthens the bladder and
alleviates urinary tract infections. Research shows
compounds in cranberry juice prevent pathogenic
bacteria from adhering to bladder walls.

- **Blueberry:** This unassuming little berry packs
a wallop—with possibly the highest antioxidant
capacity of any fruit or vegetable because of its large
concentration of anthocyanin (the pigment that gives
it its free-radical-fighting powers and which is also an
anti-inflammatory). Blueberries have also been shown
to slow down vision loss, improve brain functioning,
and be anti-hypoglycemic. And recent studies point to
this berry's benefits to diabetics due to its ability to
improve fasting glucose and insulin sensitivity.

Body Ecology's Use of Fruit

Although the USDA food pyramid has long given almost
equal priority to fruits and vegetables, Body Ecology recommends that you *favor land and ocean vegetables in your diet*, and
give fruit less emphasis.

Certain fruits are healthy and provide a natural sweet taste
that our bodies love. This is especially useful if we want to move
from being too contracted—as we are when we first awake in
the morning—into a more balanced state. Fruits are expansive
and help balance this dehydrated/contractive condition.

But fruit, if it is too sweet, weakens the adrenals—not good
when you need energy to start your day. In fact, your adrenals
need a boost of energy in the morning to get you up and
going. The very sour juices listed previously are wonderfully
energizing morning beverages. To make a really great,
youthening "energy tonic," simply combine one ounce of juice

concentrate (using one of the sour super fruits) with one of Body Ecology's probiotic liquids such as InnergyBiotic, Dong Quai, or CocoBiotic.

Fruits have an alkalizing effect on the body when metabolized and are usually very good for us, but if your diet is high in sugar or if you feel as if your health, immunity, or energy levels are less than ideal, sweet fruit is harmful. While the sugar is "natural," it feeds opportunistic yeast and parasites, and, as mentioned previously, it can be especially weakening to your adrenals, particularly in the morning. For this reason, there is a protocol for how to incorporate fruit into your diet. (See the chart at the end of the chapter.)

If your health, immunity, and energy levels are strong, eating fruit following the rules for food combining in Chapter 13 is recommended. This will ensure that you can enjoy it and digest it well without setting your body up for an inner-ecosystem imbalance. Fruits are cooling and hydrating, so as you follow the protocol, consider adding more during the summer when they are naturally in season.

The chart to follow shows the suggested protocol for including fruit in your diet. You'll notice that a distinction is made between sour, acid, and sweet fruits. Remember, the sour varieties have many health benefits and do not feed opportunistic yeast and parasites. If you are experiencing low energy levels or immune-related illness, only eat sour fruits.

Pay attention to the signals your body is giving you as you experiment with fruit in your meals. As with anything you add to your diet, start with one food at a time and see if you notice an increase in cravings or ups and downs. Whenever you do eat fruit, always eat or drink something fermented.

Lemons and Limes

Lemons and limes contain unique flavonoid compounds that have antioxidant and anticancer properties. They also are an excellent source of vitamin C, which is a powerful antioxidant that has been shown to be helpful in reducing some of the symptoms of arthritis. Vitamin C supports the immune system, and a little extra can be a great preventive first step when you feel a cold coming on. There are also compounds in citrus fruits—called *limonoids*—that have been shown to help fight cancers of the mouth, skin, lung, breast, stomach, and colon.

Additionally, lemon juice can help alleviate symptoms of indigestion—such as heartburn and bloating—and, in general, it helps your body to eliminate waste more efficiently, mitigating problems with constipation and diarrhea. Better yet, it stimulates the liver, helps dissolve uric acid and other poisons, and liquefies bile.

Sour fruits are wonderful, hydrating, nutritious, antioxidant-rich, and refreshing foods that can be part of your anti-aging arsenal. But be careful to follow your body's signals as you learn to develop a sense of when and if you need the expansive, cooling properties of fruits. Keep in mind the principles that allow your body to best assimilate them.

Dehydration plays a big role in the aging process, turning our juicy, plumlike cells into dried-up, wrinkly prunes. Chapter 24 addresses some of the other ways to restore proper hydration levels in your body again, including colon therapy, which helps cleanse your cells of toxins.

The next chapter will look at condiments—those embellishments we tend to ignore—and some of their remarkable healing properties.

Protocol for Including Fruit in Your Diet

If Health, Immunity, and/or Energy Levels Are Low	
Sour, Acidic Fruits	Uses and Benefits
Lemons	Stimulates peristaltic action in your colon—try a glass of water with fresh-squeezed lemon and stevia (BED lemonade) to start your morning. Aids in digestion of protein. Has antiseptic properties and cleanses your digestive tract.
Limes	Same benefits as lemons.
Unsweetened black-currant juice	Soothes upset stomach and stimulates appetite. Great for anemia, high in vitamin C, and rich in antioxidants. Stimulates peristaltic action in your colon (try mixed with a glass of CocoBiotic with unsweetened black-currant juice and stevia to taste first thing in the morning). Strengthens the bladder and alleviates urinary tract infections. Excellent for the adrenals, the organs that provide energy.
Unsweetened cranberry juice	Strengthens the bladder and alleviates urinary tract infections (try 1 ounce of unsweetened cranberry-juice concentrate in 4 ounces of InnergyBiotic). Compounds in cranberry juice prevent pathogenic bacteria from adhering to the walls of your bladder.

Protocol for Including Fruit in Your Diet (cont'd.)

As Health, Immunity, and Energy Levels Improve, Add These Fruits in the Order Listed Here	
Fruit	Uses and Benefits
Grapefruit	Low in sugar and has enough acidic qualities that it doesn't feed opportunistic yeast and parasites. The juice made from sour grapefruit is also beneficial.
Kiwi	Low in sugar and doesn't feed opportunistic yeast and parasites.
Berries— blueberries, raspberries, strawberries, bing cherries, and black-berries	Contain vitamins, minerals, and phytochemicals that may prevent disease. Dark-colored berries are high in antioxidants, which can help slow the aging process.
Sour green apples— Granny Smith	As you listen to the signals of your body and you are eating grapefruit, kiwi, and some berries with no symptoms, add Granny Smith apples. Fermenting green apples with your cultured veggies is a great idea because the microflora will use the natural sugars in the apple for food. Also, when you make a green smoothie, a sour green apple adds a touch of sweetness but not too much. It's a much better choice than carrots, beets, or fennel.

Chapter 22

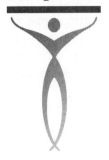

Healing Condiments:
Delicious and Age Defying

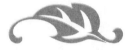

*Healthful, high-quality condiments can mean the
difference between an average meal and
an inspiring one. From starter herbs and spices
to delicious finishing oils, these culinary niceties
should never be left to chance!*

We don't typically think of condiments as anything more
than flavor-enhancing substances that we add to foods to make
them taste better. But many are healthy and life giving! This
chapter reviews some of the little-known health secrets of a
few of our favorite condiments.

Apple-Cider Vinegar

Apple-cider vinegar is rich in potassium and helps reestablish a healthy inner ecosystem with friendly bacteria. Thanks
to apple-cider vinegar's mineral content (especially potassium), it has the ability to normalize your body's acid/alkaline

291

balance. Its antiseptic qualities cleanse the digestive tract. The acidity aids in the removal of calcium deposits from joints and blood vessels, but has no effect on normal calcium levels in the bones or teeth. Pectin in unfiltered apple-cider vinegar promotes elimination and healthy bowels. The potassium in the vinegar regulates growth, hydrates cells, balances sodium, and enables proper performance of the nervous system.

Sipping on a glass of apple-cider vinegar and water during a meal will help increase stomach acid.

Vinegar is also linked to satiety—the feeling of being full. Researchers at the Department of Food Technology, Engineering and Nutrition at Sweden's Lund University recently reported on a study in which 12 healthy subjects ate four "meals" of white wheat bread. One of the meals consisted of bread alone (a control meal), while the others were supplemented with different amounts of vinegar: 18, 23, and 28 grams. Each meal was separated by a week, and each was eaten in the morning after an overnight fast. For two hours, at specific intervals after each meal, subjects rated their feelings of satiety, and researchers took several blood samples from each subject.

The results: compared with the control meal, the highest level of vinegar intake (between two and three tablespoons) was associated with significantly lower blood sugar and insulin responses and an increased satiety score.[1]

While you may have seen apple-cider vinegar in the grocery store, it may not be the raw, fermented kind that has so many medicinal benefits. Several different companies manufacture apple-cider vinegar. Some bottles are labeled "filtered," but the recommended kind is labeled "unfiltered." Select unpasteurized apple-cider vinegar, which contains the "mother" of the vinegar (a natural sediment with pectin, trace minerals, beneficial bacteria, and enzymes) that you can see floating at the bottom of the bottle.

Adding one tablespoon of apple-cider vinegar to water (you can add stevia to soften the sharp taste) can help alleviate arthritis, aid digestion, combat a sweet tooth, and balance your body at the first sign of cleansing (when it is overly acidic). In fact, sipping apple-cider vinegar in water can be used as an antidote if you've overindulged in sugar or salt. If you feel as if you're coming down with the flu or have signs that a fever blister is about to break out anywhere on your body, immediately sit down to rest and sip on a glass of water with apple-cider vinegar.

One note of caution: Brush your teeth after drinking water with vinegar, as the acid can slowly eat away at the enamel on your teeth if you don't. Another option is to use a straw to protect your teeth.

Apple-cider vinegar is good for your liver and can help with insulin sensitivity (too much blood sugar). You can use it drizzled on your vegetables and as a dressing. It is just one more way to add the sour taste, and it supplies more of those important beneficial microflora that the body needs and loves.

Sea Salt

High-quality, mineral-rich sea salt is essential for life and has medicinal value. It is grounding, contractive, and stimulates digestion.

The conventional wisdom calling for avoidance of salt because it raises blood pressure is a grave misunderstanding that surfaced when medical research showed that the "salt" Americans were consuming (in large amounts) did indeed increase blood pressure. But here is where we were duped. We were not actually eating salt. The salt in processed foods and in those dark blue cylindrical containers is so refined that none of the beneficial minerals remain; and it is loaded with additives, including sugar, chemicals, bicarbonate of soda, and preservatives. Perhaps the cute little girl on the package should be replaced with a warning sign such as the skull and crossbones.

High-quality, mineral-rich sea salt is essential for life and has medicinal value. It is grounding, contractive, and stimulates digestion.

Salt does not raise blood pressure. If yours is high, ask yourself these questions: "Am I drinking enough water for maximum hydration? Do I drink alcohol and wine, causing further dehydration?" These are usually the true underlying causes of elevated blood pressure.

Because salt has an alkalizing effect, we naturally have an innate desire to sprinkle it on acid-forming foods such as animal protein. In fact, salt is the most alkalizing of all foods and can help correct an over-acid condition in the body.

If I could prepare an evening meal for you, I'd serve an appetizing entrée using a grain-like seed (such as quinoa); a dark green, leafy vegetable (such as kale); and a tasty (naturally salty) ocean-veggie dish (such as arame). Of course, a serving of cultured veggies and a champagne glass of one of Body Ecology's probiotic liquids (such as InnergyBiotic) would accompany your meal. Everything would taste wonderful, I promise. Spices and herbs and a high-quality sea salt (Celtic) would be added during cooking to give the dishes more delicious flavor and medicinal value. There would be a nice "finishing salt" (such as Selina Naturally's Hawaiian Sea Salt) on the table to use as you wish. Your body naturally knows how much salt it needs, and when the salt you sprinkle on your food is of excellent quality, you will flourish upon it.

When using sea salt, listen to your intuition and add just enough of this true salt to make your food taste delicious. This means that the flavors will be enhanced, but your food won't taste "salty."

Naturally occurring sodium is an important mineral for the adrenals—remember those two little organs that are responsible for much of your energy? They naturally crave the minerals that sea salt provides. While this alone won't resolve your mineral deficiency, your craving for salt is a "sign" that you need to add many more minerals to your diet and focus on nourishing your adrenals in other ways as well.

But don't forget the Principle of Balance. If you eat too much salt, you may find that you start to crave expansive sweets, as salt is contracting, and your body will always seek balance. Do you remember going to the movies when you were a kid and eating a greasy bag of *salty* popcorn, then rushing back to the concession stand for a *sweet* soda to wash it down? If so, then you are already familiar with the body's built-in urge for balance.

So how do you know how much salt is the right amount for you?

That question is impossible for me to answer because according to the Principle of Uniqueness, your need for salt will be unique for you and will fluctuate. We all require differing amounts of sea salt, so there is no "one size fits all" approach. In the summer you will find you desire less salt, and in the winter

The Truth about Iodine

*T*here are many misconceptions today concerning salt and iodine. As Selina DeLangre puts it, "It is my intention to sprinkle the truth about salt out of our shakers."

Because of salt's unfortunate link with hypertension, many people have gone to great lengths to reduce their sodium intake. This has resulted in an iodine-deficient diet. One of the most-often-asked questions about Celtic sea salt and Selina Naturally Hawaiian and Portuguese salts is, "Do they have iodine?"

Selina, who has researched this subject for many years, has been kind enough to share her thoughts:

"Iodine is *not* salt, and all salt does *not* have adequate levels of iodine. In other words, you cannot meet your body's needs for iodine with sea salt alone. You must obtain it from other sources as well. Nor can all salts be measured equally.

"There exists in the public eye (and ear), a huge discrepancy and a confusing conspiracy regarding the facts, probably because of the FDA, American Heart Association, and the Surgeon General's office are all proclaiming to the public that one must reduce sodium/salt intake. This stigma has had a detrimental effect—people assume this also means reducing or completely eliminating all salt from their daily diets.

"The confusion resulting from the various claims is understandable—one source states: 'Get your iodine from salt,' while the other states: 'Reduce your sodium intake.' Thus, through the elimination of both substances, we've neglected to accept the importance of each of these sacred substances and how they define our well-being.

"According to Dr. David Brownstein, author of the book *Iodine: Why You Need It, Why You Can't Live Without It*, iodine is a very important nutrient, essential for proper thyroid function and brain development. In addition, he maintains that all glandular tissue, including prostate, breasts, ovaries, and all white blood cells, needs sufficient iodine for optimal health.

"Did you know that only 20 percent of all the salts Americans consume contain this important micronutrient? Did you know that most of the popular 'designer salts' usually do not have iodine in them? The type of commercial table salt to which iodine is added is in itself highly toxic!

"Due to the toxicities we are exposed to on a daily basis, such as bromide, fluoride, pesticides, and chlorine derivatives, we require iodine to assist in purging these from our systems. Many 'iodine-fortified table salts' fall short of the nutritional-recommended levels required (and found) in the diet—particularly if you tend to follow a diet without ocean fish or sea vegetables, low-sodium diets, strict vegan diets, or if you just generally consume a diet high in bakery products (such as breads/pastas) that contain bromide.

"In order to reduce the sludge of toxic buildup, you must increase your body's iodine levels. This daily process involves drinking plenty of water to maintain balanced hydration, taking 3,000 to 6,000 milligrams of vitamin C, and consuming unrefined (unbleached) sea salt supplemented with iodine. One of the simplest things we can do in curing our iodine deficiency is to examine what we are pouring into our saltshakers! We must make sure that it is unbleached, unrefined pure sea salt."[i]

[i]Information on iodine provided by Selina DeLangre in conversation with Donna Gates, March 1, 2010.

you'll be using more, especially if you live in a cold climate. Our need for salt becomes more and more intuitive as we create a healthier body.

Men need more salt than women, and children need the least of all. Babies don't require any additional dietary salt during the first two years of life and can obtain their minerals from the foods they're eating. In fact, too much salt can stunt a baby's growth. This can be seen in Japan, where high-salt diets before the Second World War contributed to shorter, stockier adults. After the war, milk (a more expansive food because of the fat) was introduced into the diet of Japanese children, and the next generation grew much taller.

When a woman's body becomes too contracted from a lot of sea salt, she will have extreme cravings for sugary, sweet foods as it attempts to balance itself. This can even affect her temperament and cause mood swings . . . making her feel uptight and cranky.

A woman should be especially mindful of her salt consumption during her monthly cycle. She should cut way back on the amount of sea salt she eats from the moment she begins to ovulate until the beginning of her period (monthly cleansing). This way her body will relax and easily "open up," expanding ever so slightly to release the uterine lining. When a woman eats too much sea salt during her monthly cleansing, she can become too contracted, perhaps bringing to a halt this important opportunity to shed the lining and even eliminate toxins. After the lining is shed and her period is over, she can increase her use of sea salt and contracting foods a bit. Doing so helps the ovary contract and release the tiny egg smoothly at ovulation.

What's in *Your* Shaker?

Buy the best-quality sea salt available—one that retains the high percentage of minerals, trace elements (including iodine), and nutrients that are inadequately represented in our diets today. Minerals, in particular, balance the sodium and chloride in our bodies, and they can't be found in traditional refined salt. A plethora of sea salts are available on the market today, but not all are equal. The ones used in Body Ecology recipes are from *Selina Naturally* (**www.selinanaturally.com**).

Selina DeLangre, who has followed in the footsteps of her father-in-law, Jacques DeLangre, owns Selina Naturally. More than 30 years ago, Jacques founded the Celtic Sea Salt

---

Garlic—Give It a Place of Honor in Your Pantry

*G*arlic has been around, well, forever! It is noted in 4,000-year-old Sumerian cuneiform records and is depicted on the walls of ancient Egyptian tombs. It is mentioned in the Bible as a staple of the wandering tribes of Israel. In America, the early colonists became interested in garlic after they noticed how Native Americans used it to treat everything from intestinal worms to scurvy to snakebite.[i]

Chock-full of minerals and nutrients, garlic has powerful antibiotic, antifungal, anticancer, antiparasitic, antioxidant, and antiviral properties. Nearly all cultures attest to its amazing healing potential, and it has been used to treat a wide range of ailments, from athlete's foot to typhoid. New clinical trials are showing that garlic is effective in preventing cancers of the digestive system, including esophagus, stomach, colon, and rectum.[ii]

In fact, some people believe garlic should be classified as a drug. If you know someone who eats garlic regularly and rarely gets sick, it may be because of its special ability to heal wounds both inside and outside the body.

Culinary garlic originated in central Asia, but it was transferred to many other cultures. It does not grow wild today, but was one of our first cultivated plants. As far back as the 1st century A.D., Dioscorides, the Greek physician to Emperor Nero's army, stated that garlic "clears the arteries and opens the mouth of the veins." Two thousand years later, science confirms that garlic is, indeed, a blood thinner or anticoagulant, and protects against heart disease by lowering blood pressure.[iii]

Chewing, chopping, or crushing garlic causes a natural ingredient in the plant called *alliin* to change into the antibiotic substance *allicin*. When garlic cells are ruptured by cutting, they release an enzyme called *allinaise,* which chemically changes the inherent *alliin* into *allicin,* and also results in the pungent garlicky scent we know so well. Today, garlic is once again being prescribed by doctors as a treatment for colds and bronchitis. Like chili peppers and other hot foods, garlic works by turning on the body's natural "fire-fighting faucets" to cool the heat. This prompts the lungs and bronchial tubes to produce more fluids, which in turn thins the mucus and helps flush it out of the body.[iv]

In Ayurvedic medicine, garlic is one of the few foods thought to embody five of the six tastes. The only one it lacks is sour . . . perhaps we should try fermenting it!

---

[i]"Glorious Garlic," from *Optimal Diet* website, **http://homodiet .netfirms.com/otherssay/letters/garlic.htm**, October 4, 2003, adapted from *Healing Foods from the Bible,* by Bernard Ward (accessed 3/4/10).

[ii]Lisa Fayed, "Garlic and Cancer: Can Garlic Prevent Cancer?" from **About.com** website, **http://cancer.about.com/od/prevention/a/ preventgarlic.htm**, updated May 25, 2006 (accessed 3/4/10).

[iii]Christopher Hobbs, "Garlic: The Pungent Panacea," 1998, from **http://www.christopherhobbs.com/website/library/articles/ article_files/garlic_01.html** (accessed 3/4/10).

[iv]Vitamins & Health Supplements Guide website, **http://www .vitamins-supplements.org/herbal-supplements/garlic.php** (accessed 3/4/10).

Company and introduced the original brand of Celtic sea salt to Americans. From his own study of the human biological terrain, Jacques realized that we were consuming the wrong type of salt, not only for flavor but also for optimal health. The premium *sel de mer* from Brittany, France, was made famous through his efforts, and he established the standards that all other sea salts with that name attempt to duplicate.

Selina Naturally Celtic Sea Salt® is unprocessed whole salt from one of the most pristine coastal regions of France, harvested by salt farmers using the same method employed by the ancient Celts more than 2,000 years ago. This farming method preserves the purity and balance of ocean minerals. It also contains no anticaking agents, bleaching agents, or other additives.

With the same dedication and passion as Jacques, Selina has developed an exciting selection of salts from natural sources around the world. They can be purchased in health-food stores or from **www.selinanaturally.com**. Look for Celtic, Portuguese (a very light and delicious "finishing" salt), and Hawaiian salt; and Organic Herb Blends made with Celtic sea salt. Today, more than 600 medical professionals use and recommend the Selina Naturally brand.

Herbs and Spices

Herbs and spices are a great way to add flavor and medicinal properties to your meals. Organic varieties are widely available now. Body Ecology has always promoted their use as medicinal healing foods; and now research is showing that the phytochemicals in some spices can actually help with inflammatory diseases such as cancer, diabetes, Crohn's, multiple sclerosis, asthma, arthritis, allergies, Alzheimer's, psoriasis, and AIDS. Spices mentioned in the studies are ginger, basil, rosemary, garlic, red pepper, cloves, anise, fennel, tumeric, and pomegranate.[2]

Other great options are bay leaves, chives, coriander, dill, Italian and Mexican seasonings, mustard powder, marjoram, oregano, black pepper, poppy seeds, sage, tarragon, thyme, nutmeg, and cinnamon.

Here are some recommended brand-name herbs:

- Sea Seasonings Dulse, Dulse with Garlic, Nori with Ginger, and Kelp with Cayenne

- Herbamare (blend of herbs and sea salt)

- Trocomare (blend of herbs, sea salt and cayenne pepper)

Experiment with your favorite herbs and spices as you try the various recipes on The Diet. You can have a new taste experience just about every day as you vary what you cook and how you flavor it.

Fiber

As you've learned from reading thus far, healthy digestion is essential to feeling your best—and fiber goes a long way toward facilitating this process. Fiber feeds healthy microflora and provides bulk so that as food moves through your digestive tract, cleansing is greatly enhanced. Fiber is also very important because it helps the colon to hold water long enough for maximum hydration.

There are two kinds of fiber—*soluble* and *insoluble*. Most vegetables are about two-thirds soluble, while fruits are about one-third, so they contain a nice balance of both.

Soluble fiber is fiber that dissolves in water. It can have an almost gelatinous quality, and that's why it makes you feel full and satiated after consuming it. Soluble fiber slows down the absorption of nutrients in the small intestine and also functions as a food for short-chain fatty acids, such as *butyrate,* which your cells use as a fuel for keeping the colonocytes (colonic epithelial cells) functioning optimally. These colon cells need to be healthy and strong because they're being exposed to large amounts of free radicals, as well as microbial by-products and toxins found in semisoft and solid bowel movements that are in close and constant contact with the colonic lining.

Insoluble fiber has great value for digestion. It actually pushes against the muscular receptors of the colon and allows for normal peristalsis. Without enough insoluble fiber, your bowel movement becomes small and hard. The colon has to contract harder to move it. Over time this will predispose people to *diverticulosis*—small pouches in the lining of the colon or large intestine that bulge outward through weak spots. When these pouches become inflamed, it can result in a condition called *diverticulitis,* which can lead to bleeding, infections, and small perforations or blockages in the colon.

The other great value of insoluble fiber is that it binds up everything—from fungal toxins to bacteria to heavy metals—that we ingest all the time. The extra bulk in insoluble fiber helps transport these pathogens out in large and healthy bowel movements.

If you're on a plant-based, high-fiber diet and you're well hydrated, you should enjoy healthy eliminations all the time. The Body Ecology program is 80 percent plant based, so it offers many good sources of fiber.

Chia Seeds

Long used by Native Americans in the Southwest for their medicinal and nutritional benefits, chia seeds are rich in omega-3s and omega-6s, calcium, and antioxidants. The soluble fiber in chia seeds is an excellent source of energy and provides a steady release of glucose into the bloodstream. In fact, just one ounce of chia seeds contains 43 percent of your daily fiber! This is great for stamina and strength.

Psyllium and Flax

You may be familiar with psyllium or bentonite as a bulking agent for colon cleansing. These substances virtually pull impacted waste material off the colon walls. When using psyllium, it's crucial to drink a lot of water. Actually, at Body Ecology we try to steer people away from psyllium because it can cause constipation unless you wash it through with at least eight glasses of water per day. We prefer gentler products such as ground flax fiber and EcoBloom (both found in Vitality SuperGreen), along with chia seeds. Plant foods provide the kind of fiber that your body loves best.

Research on flax fiber shows that it protects your colon from cancer and is antiviral, antibacterial, and antifungal. The Body Ecology grains, soaked and cooked for a long time, porridge-style, also provide excellent stimulation to the intestines, helping to create a really healthy stool.

EcoBloom Made from Chicory Inulin (FOS)

Chicory inulin (FOS) is another great form of fiber that also acts as a "prebiotic" food for the healthy bacteria in your system. Chicory inulin helps your body remain hydrated, and you may see it listed as an ingredient in several products in health-food stores. FOS also supports your immune system and helps maintain a healthy cholesterol level. Inulin is a good companion with dairy foods and other products that are high in calcium because it assists calcium absorption.

Fiber has been removed from fruit and vegetable juices, flour products, and most processed foods on the market today. Keep this in mind as you plan how you will eat. Choosing foods that are in their natural form, with fiber intact, goes a long way toward achieving and maintaining optimal health.

Finishing Oils

On the Baby Boomer Diet, oils pressed from olives, nuts, and seeds are used as flavorful toppings to add taste, subtlety, and variety when sprinkled on dishes.

— **Olive oil:** Extra-virgin olive oil can be drizzled onto everything on your plate. Meat, fish, eggs, vegetables, and grain-like seeds all complement this almost sacred oil. Use it generously and watch your skin grow moist with each passing day. It's an anti-aging miracle.

— **Flaxseed oil:** Use flaxseed oil in salad dressings and mixed into smoothies or as a dip for veggies and bread. Always buy flaxseed oil from a refrigerator case at your health-food store.

— **Pumpkin-seed oil:** This delicious oil adds a nutty flavor when drizzled over salads and veggies or stirred into milk kefir.

— **Macadamia-nut oil:** This is another flavorful alternative to olive oil and has been linked to appetite suppression. Use it as you would any other condiment.

Note: Ideally, avoid cooking with these seed and nut oils, as they are unstable at high heats, become toxic, and their nutritional value is destroyed. As with all oils, store in a cool, dry place (away from the stove!). Flaxseed oil should always be refrigerated (or frozen) to extend its shelf life.

A Healthy Twist on Two Favorites

— **Mustard:** Mustard made with apple-cider vinegar makes a sweet and tangy condiment that is a great topping to turkey burgers. Add it as a salad dressing. A quick recipe appears at the bottom of the page.

— **Mayonnaise, with grapeseed oil:** If you're not into making your own, the only recommended store-bought mayonnaise is from Follow Your Heart. Read the label carefully and choose the one that contains grape-seed oil. (The company has other varieties of mayonnaise.) This egg-free mayo is great for vegans and uses minimally refined grape-seed oil (known for its cholesterol-lowering and antioxidant effects). Mayonnaise, diluted with a little water, makes an excellent salad dressing when combined with roasted pumpkin-seed oil, mustard, dulse flakes, sea salt, and a pinch of cayenne.

So, we are ending our discussion of foods appropriately with a culinary "flourish"! I hope you will enjoy experimenting with the wide variety of foods available on the Baby Boomer Diet program. The final section of this book offers some innovative anti-aging strategies—a few may already be a part of your health routine, but others will be exciting new discoveries for you as you continue on your journey toward growing younger.

Mustard Sauce

1 Tbsp. Dijon-style mustard
1 tsp. dry mustard
8–10 drops stevia liquid concentrate
2 Tbsp. apple-cider vinegar
1/2 cup olive oil (or 1/4 cup olive and 1/4 cup flaxseed oil)
1/2 cup chopped fresh dill, or 1 tsp. dried

Whisk the Dijon, dry mustard, stevia, and vinegar together in a medium-size bowl. Slowly add the oil, continuing to whisk the mixture until it is thick and well blended. Stir in the dill. Cover and refrigerate at least 1 hour.

Chapter 23

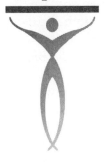

Where to Begin: A Day in the Life of the Body Ecology Program

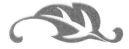

A very important aspect of digestion is eating the right foods at the right times. In this chapter you'll find some simple guidelines for how to get started on Body Ecology's Baby Boomer Diet, and the kinds of foods that work best at different points in the day.

Morning

When we wake up in the morning, our bodies are dehydrated, contracted, and naturally acidic. We also need energy to start our day. With the Principle of Balance to guide us, it will be best to drink liquids that hydrate us while giving us energy, relax us a little, and also help us become more alkaline. Our bodies are still waking up and need time to get into full gear, so nutritionally dense, easy-to-digest, liquidy foods and drinks are a must.

What would the perfect beginning to the day look like?

First, drink several glasses of water. Nothing hydrates like water, and water with minerals added to help alkalize is best.

Then, drink a "probiotic juice" that acts as an adrenal tonic and also provides the "sweet taste" you need when you are too contracted. Choose a sour juice such as cranberry, pomegranate, açaí, noni, mangosteen, or black currant; and put this into a probiotic liquid, like young coconut kefir or InnergyBiotic. Add stevia to sweeten.

A cup of an energizing green tea sweetened with stevia, and a grapefruit sprinkled with sugar-free Lakanto, is comforting on a cold winter day. Kiwi or a handful of berries provides more energy and antioxidants as you begin your day.

Stir Body Ecology's Vitality SuperGreen into some young coconut kefir, and add some chia seeds. Let this thicken for several minutes and you have a great drink that will nurture your intestines.

I always find time to mix a half teaspoon or more of Body Ecology's Potent Proteins (fermented protein powder) into InnergyBiotic. In minutes my energy increases even more.

You can whip up a nutritious anti-aging "Green Morning Smoothie" with water, two stalks of celery, two leaves of romaine lettuce, a small zucchini, a small cucumber, some soaked chia seeds, a handful of mint, a large squirt of Barlean's 3-6-9 Swirl Essential Oil, and a few drops of stevia. It's an amazing, alkalizing, high-fiber drink, too.

If your body likes casein (the main protein in dairy foods), pour some homemade milk kefir over a bowl of your favorite berries. Milk kefir is a European favorite in the hot summer months because it is cooling. This cooling quality is great to combat inflammation (internal heat) all year round and is another reason why it is an anti-aging food. Or take the berries and your freshly made milk kefir and add stevia to create a delicious berry smoothie. Milk kefir, a splash of roasted pumpkin-seed oil, some vanilla flavoring, and Lakanto and/or stevia is another tasty smoothie combination.

This light yet extremely nourishing start to your day is a perfect example of practicing calorie restriction with optimal nutrition. These are all good options that hydrate, give you energy, are filling, and are properly combined. An acidic meal is inappropriate, so bacon, eggs, toast, oatmeal, and cereal with milk (a food-combining nightmare) are not on the Baby Boomer Diet.

While all the suggestions above are easy to digest, you may want to take digestive enzymes if you feel you need them. For example, even though fermenting helps with digestion of the casein in the milk kefir, it may still be difficult for those with weak digestion. If you have this problem, try taking a digestive enzyme with HCl and pepsin to promote digestion of casein in your stomach and a second enzyme with pancreatin that breaks it down when it reaches your small intestine.

Midday Meals

The best time of the day to eat heavier proteins (such as animal proteins and nut and seed pâtés) is between 11 A.M. and 2 P.M. Your liver is ready to accept proteins at this time, and you are more active and need the extra concentrated energy. Many of us would benefit from eating two smaller protein meals. For example, around 11 A.M., eggs, cultured vegetables, and a small leafy-green salad makes an energizing brunch. Eggs are great for your thyroid and your brain and help create energy. At 1 P.M., have a tasty protein-and-veggie lunch served with a small champagne glass of CocoBiotic.

Afternoon Snack

If you need or want to gain weight, have an energizing, alkaline snack such as Vitality SuperGreen mixed into young coconut kefir around 3 or 4 P.M. This will give you a midafternoon boost of energy to get you through that period when you feel a bit sleepy or unfocused. Satisfying those afternoon cravings with something healthy will give you more motivation to prepare an evening meal that is balanced and unrushed.

Final Meal of the Day

Your last meal of the day should be vegetarian. Your digestive tract starts to slow down around sunset, so difficult-to-digest, complex meals are not wise. Eat early, and have a light vegetarian meal. You've had a busy day, and it won't be long before you will want to prepare for a great, rejuvenating night of deep sleep. You'll sleep better and awaken refreshed if your last meal is 80 percent vegetables, with a gluten-free, grain-like seed such as quinoa, millet, buckwheat, or amaranth.

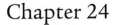

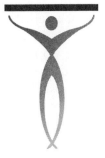

Chapter 24

Anti-Aging Basics: Gifts Granted to Us at Birth

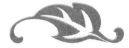

The simplest things give us nourishment—sunlight; oxygen; deep sleep; and pure, clean water. But we often take these everyday elements for granted, ignoring their power to heal and replenish our bodies and minds!

Therapies that recognize and honor such life-essential basics as breathing, rest, and basking in the sun are what you should consider first when you begin your journey toward restoring youthfulness and vitality.

Sunlight and Vitamin D

Sunshine is as vital to our health as food, oxygen, and water. Certain ultraviolet rays (UVBs) help us make vitamin D, a potent anti-aging hormone and powerful nutrient that offers us countless health benefits. Anthropologists now believe that the pigmentation in our skin actually became lighter as an evolutionary mechanism to acquire more vitamin D when our ancestors migrated away from the equator.

The health benefits of vitamin D fill volumes of scientific journals, and its current widespread deficiency has been identified as a serious epidemic in the U.S., showing up in 80 percent of people of all ages—even newborns. This deficiency will cause us to age quickly . . . very ironic when most of us have been told to avoid the sun because of those ugly brown sun spots and wrinkles. This is why it is so important today to use sunlight wisely, which means obtaining moderate amounts *directly on the skin* and also taking vitamin D supplements.

Your body begins making vitamin D when the UVB rays of the sun react with the 7-dehydrocholesterol in your skin. However, vitamin D does not become a useful hormone until it travels via your bloodstream into the liver to become 25-vitamin D. (A 25-OH vitamin D test is what doctors often use to measure the vitamin D in your blood.) It then travels on to enter your kidneys and become the active form of vitamin D called 1,25-dihydroxyvitamin D_3, also known as calcitriol or 1,25-DHCC. Presence of vitamin D signals your intestines to absorb calcium from your diet to build strong bones and teeth. (Please note that the health of your liver and kidneys is important for making vitamin D.)

Researchers at first believed that the kidneys made all the active vitamin D needed by the body, but by the mid-1990s studies began to show that cells in other organs create active vitamin D as well. In other words, the cells in your brain, lungs, colon, and breasts or prostate make it, too. Your brain cells, for example, take up 25-OH vitamin D, convert it into 1,25 vitamin D (the active form), and then consume it.

Vitamin D's importance to our overall health is indisputable. It has now become one of the most intensely studied hormones. A deficiency is serious and well worth your immediate attention.

Why Are We Afraid of the Sun?

As with many of today's health fads, sunlight phobia is a fairly recent phenomenon. We evolved in the sun, and our ancestors embraced and honored it for its life-giving qualities— some even worshipped the sun as God.

It is probably no coincidence that as people grow older, they

The Big D—It's Not Just for Bone Health

*W*e have known for a long time that vitamin D plays an important role in bone health, but it does so much more. In fact, it can be called a natural "gene therapy" because it positively influences the functions of at least 2,000 genes. Every tissue and cell recognizes and has a vitamin D receptor (VDR) for active vitamin D, even the white blood cells in the immune system. When 1,25-DHCC links to its VDR and then moves into the nucleus of the cell, then the correct programming of these vitamin D–related genes begins. Like a piano player who touches certain keys, it is the selective activation of these genes that determines the overall status of the immune system and its control of inflammation.

This helps explain why vitamin D is a potent weapon against osteoporosis, diabetes, rheumatoid arthritis, multiple sclerosis (MS), high blood pressure, inflammation, Sjögren's syndrome, and thyroid infection. There is also an unmistakable connection between vitamin D deficiency and breast, prostate, and colorectal cancers. You'll notice that all these diseases typically occur later in life.

Immunity

By strengthening our natural immunity and protecting us from viruses, bacteria, and fungal infections that cause inflammation, vitamin D prevents and helps heal inflammatory skin autoimmune conditions, like psoriasis and dermatitis. This is true for types of intestinal inflammation such as IBS, Crohn's disease, and ulcerative colitis as well. Vitamin D also inhibits dangerous autoimmune reactions, where the body turns on itself, as in the case of Hashimoto's disease, a disease of the thyroid gland.[i]

Muscle Mass

Essential for maintaining muscle mass throughout life, vitamin D helps preserve the Type II muscle fibers that are prone to atrophy in older people. In addition, recent research reveals an association between higher vitamin D levels and improved physical functioning as we age.[ii]

Heart Disease

Researchers from the University of Warwick, England, evaluated 28 studies involving almost 100,000 men and women across different ethnic groups. The data revealed a strong association between high levels of vitamin D and significantly lower risk of both cardiac and metabolic disorders. Compared to those with low levels, men and women who had high levels of vitamin D had a reduced risk of developing cardiovascular disease by about 33 percent, elevated blood sugar by 55 percent, and metabolic syndrome by more than 50 percent.[iii] Vitamin D also regulates insulin secretion by the pancreas and may increase insulin sensitivity better than some diabetic drugs such as Metformin.[iv]

Weight Loss

Vitamin D and sunlight should be included in any successful weight-loss program. Believe it or not, even your fat cells have receptor sites for vitamin D. Give them adequate amounts and they become more active and burn up calories more efficiently. Also, your fat cells secrete a hormone called leptin that tells the brain when you are full. A deficiency of vitamin D prevents this hormone from working well so that you are less able to control your appetite.

---

[i]M. D. Griffin, N. Xing, and R. Kumar, "Vitamin D and its analogs as regulators of immune activation and antigen presentation," *Annual Review of Nutrition,* 23 (2003): 117–145. (First published online as a Review in Advance on March 19, 2003.)

[ii]"Vitamin D Status Associated with Physical Function in Older Men and Women," *Life Extension,* April 30, 2010, **http://www.lef .org/newsletter/2010/0430_Vitamin-D-Associated-with-Physical-Function-in-Older-Men-Women.htm?source=eNewsLetter2010Wk18-2&key=Archive** (accessed 10/6/10).

[iii]J Parker, O. Hashmi, D. Dutton, A. Mavrodaris, S. Stranges, N. B. Kandala, A. Clarke, and O. H. Franco, "Levels of vitamin D and cardiometabolic disorders: Systematic review and meta-analysis," *Maturitas,* 65(3) (March 2010): 225–236, as found in article by Allen S. Josephs, M.D., "Vitamin D Continues to Dominate," **Vitacost.com** website, February 24, 2010, **http://www.vitacost.com/Vitamin-D-Continues-to-Dominate-printable?csrc=EM-FYH20100225:print** (accessed 10/6/10).

[iv]K. C. Chiu, A. Chu, V. Liang W. Go, and M. F. Saad, "Hypovitaminosis D is associated with insulin resistance and ß cell dysfunction," *American Journal of Clinical Nutrition,* 79 (May 2004): 820–825.

tend to gravitate to warmer, sunnier climates such as Florida, California, and Arizona. Perhaps intuitively we know that to stay young and healthy, we need even more of this anti-aging hormone. Yet the American Academy of Dermatology, well funded by the sunscreen industry, has created so much fear of the sun that many of us never go outside, or only go out with chemical-laden, potentially cancer-causing sunscreens.[1]

Only the negative effect of UV rays is presented to the public. Yes, *chronic* or *excessive* exposure does, indeed, increase the risk of nonmelanoma (basal- or squamous-cell) cancers, but these types of skin cancer rarely spread, are rarely lethal, and can be easily removed by surgery.

There is very little evidence that the potentially deadly form of skin cancer, melanoma, is caused by *sensible* amounts of sun exposure. In fact, new research indicates that sensible amounts *decrease* the risk of cancers, including melanoma, by controlling cell growth and inducing cells that are malignant to become normal or to die of apoptosis (programmed death). While skin-cancer cases total about one million per year in the U.S., they are lethal in only about 2,000 cases, which is only .5 percent of all cancer deaths.[2]

Vitamin D regulates up to 200 genes that control cell growth and cellular differentiation, so it is not surprising that it prevents up to 16 other types of deadly cancer that *do* spread and *do* kill. So the benefits of the sun may far outweigh the small risk of skin cancer.

To harness the power of the sun safely, it's important to understand the difference between UVA and UVB rays. UVA rays penetrate deeply, and when you are out in the sun too long, they have a negative effect on the elasticity of the skin. They cause wrinkles and brown or white pigmentation, sometimes called sun spots. UVA rays are the major cause of the potentially lethal melanomas. UVB rays, on the other hand, redden and can potentially burn the skin, but are the only rays that make vitamin D. Over time, without proper protection from sunburn, UVB rays can cause skin cancer. Once again, it's a matter of prudent sun exposure.

Sun Sensitivity . . .
Could Our Poor Diets Be a Clue?

What explains our hypersensitivity to the sun these days? After all, skin cancers were at one time fairly uncommon.

Remember, the first step in making vitamin D begins when the sun reacts with a type of cholesterol in your skin. Dietary fats and oils affect the quality of cholesterol in your body.

Our supersensitivity to the sun seems to coincide with the dietary changes that occurred at the beginning of the 20th century when we began eating fats and oils that were heated, refined, bleached, and deodorized. Instead of having small amounts of healthy, vitamin D–rich raw butter and ghee, we've been consuming margarine and trans fats for generations. The liver, which plays a key role in producing vitamin D, is also damaged by toxic fats and oils.

Even as you begin eating the recommended healthy fats and oils, poor *absorption* of dietary fats becomes another concern. Your liver and gallbladder may be in need of special care and attention, and your digestion of fats (which occurs in your small intestine) may be inadequate and will contribute to low levels of vitamin D.

The good news is that a probiotic diet, with lots of fermented foods, will improve the health of your liver and gallbladder and greatly assist in your digestion of fats. As the beneficial microflora work to keep your intestines optimally functioning, your liver benefits as well.

How Much Vitamin D Is the Right Amount?

This is an area of much controversy, and there is a lot of negative information floating around on the Internet. With so much confusion, it is smart to turn to the experts out there who are doing the cutting-edge research, people like Dr. Michael Holick and Dr. John Cannell.

Dr. Holick's excellent book, *The Vitamin D Solution: A 3-Step Strategy to Cure Our Most Common Health Problem* (Penguin/ Hudson Street Press, 2010), is an excellent place to turn for credible information and a list of charts that tell you how long to expose yourself to the sun depending on where you live and the color of your skin. Dr. Holick is the scientist who discovered the active form of vitamin D and has worked closely with other experts in his field uncovering the truth about this essential anti-aging hormone. See his website: **www.vitamindhealth.org**.

Also, it would be wise and commendable to join (and financially support) Dr. Cannell's nonprofit organization, called the Vitamin D Council (**www.vitamindcouncil.org**). This way you can stay updated on the fascinating and extensive research being done around the world. If you spend time on his website, you will be thoroughly convinced that vitamin D is for you. Dr. Cannell sends out an informative, educational newsletter that is free.

Both Cannell and Holick are comfortable recommending at least 5,000 IUs per day of a vitamin D supplement (for an adult). After testing, you may want to increase the amount to 10,000 IUs per day. However, evidence is mounting that even higher levels may be needed by many of us. The larger amounts are important if you have not been out in the sun or have signs of osteopenia, osteoporosis, or cancer.

If you are overweight, you will need to take more (perhaps twice as much) because vitamin D gets locked into fat cells and cannot be released. Anyone with intestinal disorders, like Crohn's disease, inflammation problems, or diarrhea, requires larger amounts, and supplements may not be useful at all. (See the "Tanning Beds?" section later in this chapter.)

Can you take too much vitamin D in supplement form? This is a hotly debated subject among researchers today, and many currently believe that you can. (You can never overdose on vitamin D made from sunlight or food.) Symptoms of vitamin D toxicity (from taking too much from a supplement) include nausea, loss of appetite, vomiting, and elevated blood pressure. If you experience these problems and excessive supplementation continues, you could suffer kidney failure.

Currently, however, your doctor will want you to reach blood levels of 54–90 nanograms per milliliter (ng/ml) of blood (or 135–225 nmoles/L). These numbers are ones to watch, however, as newer research suggests that levels of 80–90 ng/ml (or 225 nmoles/L) are even better. (Lifeguards often have levels as high as 100–200 ng/ml.) If you want to rejuvenate and experience greater vitality, then levels in the low 30s will be grossly inadequate.

As extensive, worldwide research continues to unfold, it's still not clear what the precise "ceiling" vitamin D levels might be. However, levels higher than were originally thought safe are now proving to be quite harmless and even beneficial (even up to 200 ng/ml) as long as simple blood tests show that your parathyroid hormone levels and your calcium-to-phosphorus ratio remain normal.

You can obtain your own levels of vitamin D by visiting your doctor or by ordering an inexpensive blood-test kit from the Vitamin D Council website, or from **www.zrtlab.com**. (You should retest three or four times per year.) Blood levels do change. If your levels are high at the end of the summer, they may be quite low in the winter, so retest. As new information on the benefits of vitamin D, as well as the recommended blood level and supplement dosage, is being compiled monthly, choose a doctor who is up-to-date on the latest research. Also, joining Dr. Cannell's nonprofit will keep you current. As new guidelines become available, you'll be one of the first to know.

A Supplement Isn't Enough . . . Embrace the Sun

A supplement alone isn't sufficient if you are truly serious about rejuvenation. Vitamin D from sunlight remains in the body at least twice as long as that derived from diet. What's more, there are unique substances in sunlight, called "photoproducts," that you cannot obtain from food or a supplement. Scientists, including Dr. Holick's group, are now looking carefully at these photoproducts, feeling certain that if they are there, it must be for a biological reason.

You'll definitely feel happier from sunlight. Research shows that when you go into the sun, keratinocytes in your skin cells actually create endorphins, which improve feelings of well-being.

Exposure to the sun helps regulate our circadian rhythms. We sleep better and are far less likely to suffer from depression and seasonal affective disorder (SAD). (Supplements do not improve circadian rhythm.)

What Is "Prudent" Sun Exposure?

You should never go into the sun and get burned. Start sunbathing for short periods at first, and slowly and carefully build up a base tan. Prior to the Industrial Revolution, working outdoors probably helped build a resistance to sunburn. It appears that those who have developed higher vitamin D levels (like roofers and lifeguards) do not burn as easily. Therefore, correcting your vitamin D deficiency with supplements before spending time in the sun might be wise, especially if you are fair-skinned and tend to burn easily.

Midday is the best time to sunbathe because the rays reach us directly. In the morning or afternoon, they are coming in at angle and are not as effective.

Most people can go into the sun starting with 10 minutes at first and then building up to as much as 60 minutes at midday (depending on how intense the sun is in your area). If you must remain outside longer, you

You'll definitely feel happier from sunlight. Research shows that when you go into the sun, keratinocytes in your skin cells actually create endorphins, which improve feelings of well-being.

should then apply a chemical-free, broad-spectrum sunscreen that shields you from UVA and UVB rays. Badger sunscreen, which is zinc oxide and herbs (no chemicals), was rated the safest sunscreen of more than 600 tested by the Environmental Work Group (**www.ewg.org**). See **www.badgerbalm.com** for more information.

You'll want to protect your face and hands by wearing sunscreen and/or a hat. The less clothing you wear, the more vitamin D your body will make. If you are fortunate enough to live in a sunny region of the country, only 20 minutes in the sun a day will give you what you need. If you are an African American with darker skin, Dr. Holick suggests that you may need as much as three to ten times that amount of exposure.

Tanning Beds?

Tanning beds have been shown to dramatically increase vitamin D levels in the blood. If used properly, they can safely produce vitamin D in the winter months when it is impossible to get enough sun to prevent disease. However, they must be used in moderation and responsibly. Dr. Holick tells his readers to find a facility that has been certified by the International Smart Tan Network. He recommends that you make sure they use low- or medium-pressure fluorescent lamps. He also warns that you must be just as cautious as you would with regular sunlight and protect your face and lips with sunscreen and your eyes with goggles.

If you have an intestinal-absorption problem (due to surgery, Crohn's disease, celiac disease, or diarrhea from infections), you may not respond well to vitamin D supplementation. Tanning beds could be a good alternative for you.

Simple Dietary Secrets That Will Unleash the Power of Vitamin D

Certain nutrients are "cofactors" that are essential for the assimilation of vitamin D. The most important cofactor is magnesium, but your diet and supplements should also include sources of vitamin K$_2$, zinc, boron, and a small amount of vitamin A. For example, all the enzymes that metabolize vitamin D require magnesium. Basically, vitamin D won't work in the body without it. If you try to elevate your vitamin D levels and are deficient in magnesium, you will only intensify your magnesium deficiency. If, after taking vitamin D, tests show that your levels are not rising, look elsewhere for the problem.

Simply taking your vitamin D supplements with your largest meal of the day may quickly improve your blood levels of D. Researchers at the Cleveland Clinic examined 17 patients who were not getting better under treatment. By taking vitamin D *with* their biggest meal, they boosted the level of vitamin D in their blood by an average of 56 percent.[3]

Sun-dried mushrooms such as dried shiitake (often exposed to extra sunlight during the growing process to create even more vitamin D) are your richest dietary source of this wonder nutrient. Fresh mushrooms don't supply nearly as much, but are still quite good.

Wild or wild-caught salmon and albacore tuna are excellent sources of vitamin D. Farmed salmon never has the vitamin D content of wild or wild-caught salmon. The term *wild-caught* means the salmon are born in hatcheries and released into the wild. Every year in Washington State, elementary-school classes vie for the privilege of performing this task—really! All hatcheries mark these fry (the fish, not the kids!) by clipping their fins so they can't be confused with the truly wild salmon.

Sockeye salmon cannot be farmed, so it's your best choice. Atlantic salmon from your local supermarket is always farmed. Canned salmon contains vitamin D but is overcooked and difficult to digest.

Canned sardines, mackerel, and tuna can also provide you with vitamin D. Depending on the brand, cod-liver oil (**www .greenpasture.org**) is right up there with wild salmon as a good source of D. However, upping your intake of cod-liver oil above two tablespoons a day could cause an overdose of vitamin A. Fermented milk kefir, butter, ghee, and egg yolks provide only small amounts of D, so you can't correct a deficiency relying on these alone. Ocean's Alive Marine Phytoplankton (**www .sunfoods.com**) is a high-quality, vegan source of vitamin D.

Please don't think you can get vitamin D from fish-oil capsules. While a potentially excellent source of omega-3 fatty acids (depending on the company and quality), fish oil does not contain vitamin D.

Remember that vitamin D tells your intestines to absorb more calcium and is essential to the uptake of this mineral in your diet. So increase your dietary calcium by eating plenty of dark green, leafy vegetables such as kale, collards, escarole, bok choy, and Brussels sprouts. Sea vegetables are another excellent source of calcium. Avoid calcium-depleting nutrients, especially sugar, and too much fruit, alcohol, and caffeine. Drugs like prednisone and diuretics also deplete calcium.

By increasing your intake of vitamin D and calcium, doing resistance exercises that work against gravity (yoga, Pilates, walking, weight training, climbing stairs, or dancing), and making sure you digest your food well (with enzymes and fermented foods and drinks), you are well on your way to creating superhealthy bones that will be resistant to breaks and deterioration as you age.

Breathwork

Most of us use only a fraction of our full breathing capacity and, particularly when we're stressed, breathe from the chest in short, gaspy intakes. Proper breathing should originate from the diaphragm—full, deep, and rhythmic.

Right now, take a long, slow, deep breath. Did your abdomen expand?

Deep abdominal breathing has many benefits for anti-aging. For example, did you know that breathing directly affects your body's pH balance? Poor breathing also results in chronic fatigue, muscle cramps, cold hands and feet, heartburn, PMS, impaired concentration, and more.[4] Proper breathing can help you metabolize your food better and improve your ability to concentrate and remember.

If breathing is so basic to life, why do we breathe so poorly? Some people believe that as infants we breathed perfectly. But over time we developed "muscle armoring," beginning with the diaphragm and continuing to the pelvis, chest, back, legs, and throat.[5] These muscular tensions, along with poor posture and self-consciousness about keeping our stomachs flat, compromise the easy, effortless breathing we enjoyed as babies.

There are a number of breathing techniques you might try to dismantle this muscle armoring, including bioenergetics, the Alexander Technique, and various styles of yoga and yoga meditations. Holistic retailers such as Gaiam offer CDs that guide listeners through simple breathing exercises.

With regular practice, breathing correctly will begin to become second nature. You will feel new levels of stamina, as well as improved digestion and elimination. Many people who have practiced deep breathing regularly report that it generates a profound feeling of contentment and alleviates anxiety and nervous tension.

Hyperbaric Oxygen Therapy

Hyperbaric Oxygen Therapy (HBOT) is a treatment dating back to the 17th century, although it has only been recognized in conventional medicine since the 1940s. It involves breathing 100 percent oxygen while under increased atmospheric pressure. In this way, the oxygen concentration in the body increases up to 20 times its normal amount at the cellular level. Basically, the increased pressure deposits a lot of oxygen into the blood plasma in all bodily cells, tissues, and fluids.

The treatment, which is painless, consists of lying down on a bed inside a pressure chamber. Patients can sleep or even read while in the chamber—there is no need to wear a hood or a mask. Some people can experience a popping in their ears due to the increase in pressure, similar to what is experienced when changing altitude in airplanes. Chewing gum or swallowing hard can alleviate this.

My friend Raymond Crallé introduced me to HBOT in 2008. Raymond, who has been a practicing physical therapist in Delray Beach, Florida, for 35 years, believes that when HBOT is delivered on a long-term basis, it can slow down the aging process. He uses it in his practice to treat a variety of brain and sports injuries. Ray himself is testament to the anti-aging benefits of oxygen therapy. He is the proud father of two amazingly calm yet alert and intelligent little girls. His oldest daughter received oxygen from birth. His youngest began doing so while she was in the womb.

In their book, *The Oxygen Revolution,* authors Paul G. Harch and Virginia McCullough argue that hyperbaric oxygen actually acts at the DNA level to stimulate growth and repair hormones. Although HBOT has long been an effective treatment for burn victims and those suffering from decompression sickness, many healers are beginning to see that it has a much more far-reaching impact in promoting natural healing and can be used to treat a wide range of conditions, including Alzheimer's, fibromylagia, viruses, and immune-system disorders. Others, like Harch and McCullough, believe that HBOT can literally rejuvenate our "tired brains," which have suffered chemical and toxic insults over the course of a lifetime that have contributed to premature aging.[6]

As you know by now, according to the Principle of Balance, everything has two sides. We must always look for the negative one so we can balance or fix it. For example, antibiotics have saved millions of lives. But had we known 60 years ago to look for their downside, we might have prevented hundreds of millions of yeast or fungal infections.

What is the drawback of HBOT? Oxygen, while it does much good, also creates more free radicals. Hyperbaric oxygen therapy also puts a burden on and stresses the liver.

So what can be done to undo the negative side effects of HBOT yet still reap its many benefits? How would you create balance? There are three recommended actions:

1. Significantly increase the amount of antioxidants you consume during your weeks of therapy. Your diet should include even more of the enzyme-rich fruits and vegetables recommended on the Baby Boomer Diet. Fermented foods

Activated Air

"*B*iophysically altered" air is another way to counter free radicals or oxidative stress. The Active Air device, manufactured by Eng3, can be used at home. A valuable healing and anti-aging tool, it can help strengthen your immune system and accelerate recovery from illness. It is also a great way to create energy.

The Active Air device creates higher levels of oxygen in the body, but it does so in a different way than HBOT. Unlike HBOT, which delivers concentrated air, this technology delivers an oxygen level that is the same as regular air. Because of the free-radical damage done by pressing oxygen into the system, hyperbaric treatments should be considered a short-term solution, while an activated-air machine actually repairs and protects against free-radical damage.

Go to **www.eng3corp.com** to learn more.

and liquids are the ultimate antioxidants, so consume large amounts.

Increase your levels of glutathione, a master antioxidant. A green shake made of Vitality SuperGreen combined with un-denatured whey-protein concentrate helps increase glutathione. Up the amount of minerals you take in via food and supplements to keep your body more alkaline.

2. Cleanse more actively. Cleansing your colon at this time with home enemas or with a visit to your professional colon therapist is key.

While undergoing HBOT, the mitochondria in your cells receive significantly more oxygen. This increases energy in your body (the positive). But what happens when your energy goes up? Your cells immediately start to cleanse and push *out* toxins. These toxins put a greater burden on your liver (the negative).

Yes, you may be having a healthy elimination each day . . . but this is a time when your body will need to eliminate even more than usual. Colon therapy is wonderful way to create balance.

3. Take extra special care of your liver. Body Ecology's protocol encouraging a mostly raw diet is especially appropriate during HBOT because a raw diet is best for the liver. Take care to eat few or no fats or oils at this time, avoiding cooked saturated fats in particular. Take a liver-cleansing supplement such as Body Ecology's LivAmend, which works by increasing bile flow. Bile is produced in your liver, and toxins are dumped into the bile and then sent to your gallbladder. When you eat, this stored bile is deposited into the colon, where it stimulates peristaltic movement so that the toxins can be eliminated with the bowel movement. Because the daily bowel movement is usually not sufficient to remove toxins fast enough, colon cleansing at this time is highly recommended. If you're having a daily HBOT session, then a daily enema or at least four colon-therapy sessions per week is best.

Sleep

Insufficient sleep plagues 50 million to 70 million Americans today, especially women. Yet, sleeping deeply like a newborn baby is crucial for restoring your prenatal jing. It is absolutely fundamental for staying young, healthy, and vibrant. And . . . it's free!

As the years pass, sleep often becomes more elusive. If you are not falling asleep, staying asleep, and waking up on time feeling refreshed, you'll want to change this as soon as possible. The Principle of Step by Step tells you to first and foremost create more energy to heal or to reclaim the vitality you had in your mother's womb.

It *must* be important to sleep; there is not an animal on the planet that doesn't do it. A really great night's rest is an investment in your anti-aging bank account. Insufficient sleep is associated with increased risk for diabetes, heart disease, depression, and obesity.

Your brain is very much affected by the *quality* of your sleep. Research clearly confirms what you've probably already observed—your mood, cognition, and memory are negatively affected by sleep deprivation. Notice the vast difference in what you are willing to do for yourself and for others when you've gotten a great night's rest.

In fact, a recent study with university students found that sleep can help you remember something you need to do in the future. After giving a series of tests to 24 students who slept after processing and storing the idea of a planned task, researchers found that these students were more likely to follow through on their intentions than those who tried to tackle their plan before going to sleep. Researchers believe that this process, called *prospective memory,* occurs during slow-wave sleep (an early pattern in the sleep cycle) and involves communication between the brain's hippocampus (memory formation) and its cortical regions (memory storage).[7]

But it's not only your mood and memory that are impacted by sleep. Your very life depends upon it! The North Carolina DMV's *Driver's Handbook* offers up this little cautionary statistic: "Anyone who has had less than five hours of sleep the night before is four to five times more likely to crash than someone who got eight hours of sleep."[8]

And a team of British and Italian researchers determined that if you regularly sleep less than six hours a night, you are 12 percent more likely to die prematurely. *Chronic insomnia* (the inability to fall asleep or remain asleep for an adequate amount of time) also elevates one's risk of an earlier death. Interestingly, these researchers—after analyzing 16 sleep studies that included more than 1.3 million people—also found that sleeping *too much* (more than nine hours a night) might be an important sign of a serious or potentially fatal illness.[9]

So the solution is to sleep within an optimal range of seven to nine hours every night. But bear in mind, this applies to adults only. Babies and toddlers spend many more hours in sleep a day, around 10 to 14. Children require between 10 and 12, and teenagers need at least 9 hours. By contrast, older adults tend to sleep a little less, more lightly, and to take more catnaps.[10]

The Mechanics of Sleep

Early in the night, there is a greater amount of slow-wave deep sleep, which is the most restorative sleep. Growth hormone is produced during the initial onset of nightly sleep. Go to bed early and you'll not only become "healthy, wealthy, and wise," you'll also look and feel younger. Smaller pulses of growth hormone are also released later in your sleep cycle, so if

Boomers on the Cutting Edge

Ceragem Massage Beds

One of my most recent discoveries for combatting aging is the Ceragem Jade Massager, an at-home thermal massage bed that stimulates the body to heal itself. Ceragem utilizes far-infrared light, the warm, penetrating rays naturally produced by the sun. This far-infrared light is combined with the gemstone jade to provide deep and healing heat to the body. It is an excellent way to detoxify, increase circulation, reduce inflammation, and alleviate stress.

As the heated jade slowly rolls over your back, the spine is stretched, and knots of tension are released. Decompression takes place, giving more space for the disks and the nerves, thus improving the communication that takes place between the brain and the various organs via the nervous system. This spinal alignment not only positively affects the health of every organ in the body, it can relieve chronic backaches and sciatica pain as well.

Ceragem is at its best as a detoxifier: The polished jade safely heats deep into the body, increasing circulation, while mobilizing toxins from fat cells, thus aiding in the elimination of heavy metals, chemicals, cholesterol, and lactic acid, as well as hundreds of other toxins. Removal of such toxic residue from the body improves cellular function, enhancing overall health and slowing down the aging process.

Deep relaxation is another of the many benefits of the 40-minute treatment. In fact, it's so relaxing that within just a few weeks of use, disturbed sleep patterns are usually normalized; and sleeping through the night, one of nature's greatest healers, is once again possible. The abdominal program is not only excellent for removing extra inches, it also brings the healing far-infrared heat to all the digestive organs while stimulating the peristaltic action of the colon, helping to restore regular bowel movements—a necessary component to turning back the clock.

For more information or to order a Ceragem Jade Massager, contact Oasis Wellness Center at: **www.oasis-wellness.com**.

you only sleep for five hours, you won't obtain enough of this rejuvenating hormone.

Rapid eye movement (REM) or "dream" sleep is active sleep—important for the development and health of your brain. REM increases later in the sleep cycle and just before you naturally awaken.

Melatonin, often called the most potent antioxidant in the human body, is critical to restorative sleep. A natural hormone secreted by the pineal gland in your brain, melatonin increases with darkness, causing drowsiness. It then decreases with the morning light, and you begin to wake up. Because the production of this important hormone is suppressed by light, working late into the night, especially on the computer, or watching late-night television might be cutting off years from your life.

Tips for Sleeping Long and Well

Most of us look for shortcuts when it comes to sleep. As with weekend-warrior exercise, we think we can "make up" weekday deficits by sleeping in on the weekend. But that's not how it works. Here are a few suggestions for restorative sleep:

— Reset your circadian rhythm. Get up early and start to move. Try stretching with the ancient yoga posture called the Sun Salutation. A walk in the morning light will help you sleep better that night. In the spring, summer, and fall, sunbathe midday for 20 to 30 minutes.

— Start to unwind as the evening begins. Take a Chinese herbal formula called Peaceful Spirit (available from **www .jingherbs.com**). The herbs open your heart, calm your spirit, and relax your nervous system to prepare for the evening ahead. The main ingredient, *reishi,* is often called the "mushroom of immortality" and is also an excellent source of vitamin D. Called their "happy formula" by Jing Herbs, Peaceful Spirit is used as a treatment for sadness and anxiety because another ingredient, the *polygala root,* strengthens the connection between your heart (shen) and your adrenals (jing). The Chinese asparagus "puts a wing on your heart."

— As bedtime approaches, begin to celebrate the ritual of sleep. Take a hot bath and create a "sleep sanctuary," with soft organic bedding, candles, soothing incense or aromatherapy, gentle music, and the like.

— You may need to take something to help you sleep. Noncaffeinated teas such as chamomile, tulsi, skullcap, and valerian have a mildly sedating effect. In Chinese medicine, the "shen herbs" are calming.

- If you have issues with an overactive mind that won't shut off and let you sleep, Bupleurum & Dragon Bone (also from Jing Herbs) can help. This classic formula has been used for more than 2,000 years with great success. It differs from Peaceful Spirit because it addresses an overactive liver energy that causes inner "chatter." It also moves the energy out of your head and into your heart, where your "spirit resides during sleep," giving you a sense of well-being and of feeling like you are at home in your own skin. Because of the calming and grounding qualities, Bupleurum & Dragon Bone formula is used for insomnia; however, other modern-day applications are: anxiety; angina pectoris; and addictive behaviors such as smoking, drinking, drug use, and overeating.

- If you can't sleep because of hot flashes, night sweats, dryness, and irritability, then Jing Herb's Winter Yin Formula is a modified classic formula for clearing "heat" and for those who have depleted their reserves of energy.

- Melatonin supplements can be purchased at your local health-food store and can help regulate sleep. When taken short-term, melatonin is safe and is especially useful when you travel and change time zones. Side effects may include morning grogginess, vivid dreams, and a lower body temperature. Melatonin also suppresses your desire for sex. Supplements can be purchased in one- to five-milligram capsules. You will have to experiment to find the best dosage for you. Start with the lowest amount and increase if necessary. Taken 45 minutes before bedtime, and time-released versions may be a better choice if you awaken often during the night.

— Aim for eight hours of sleep a night. Some of us will require a little more, while others will function just fine on seven hours if it is quality sleep. Napping works for many, and you may feel the need to take rejuvenating catnaps during the day. (See "Power Napping" below.) What's most important is that your sleep be restful and restorative, with three to five complete sleep cycles that take you from drowsiness, into light sleep, followed by deep and then deeper sleep, and ending in REM.

— Your last meal of the day should have been a calming grain-like seed (quinoa, millet, buckwheat, or amaranth) that helps create more serotonin (which then turns into melatonin).

— Try to go to bed and wake up around the same time. This also helps set your biological clock. A good rule of thumb is to avoid anything that is too "stimulating" before bedtime. That includes alcohol, caffeine, and sugar, which disturb circadian rhythms.

— Light also interferes with production of melatonin, so get rid of the night light in your bathroom or bedroom. Several hours before bed, withdraw from visually stimulating activities like television, the Internet, take-home work, and so on. Vigorous exercise can also be a bit too exciting to the body, leaving you energized rather than calm. Try more soothing kinds of exercise, like yoga or stretching or a leisurely walk, if you need to relieve tension.

Power Napping

Not only is regular and restorative sleep important, research reveals that taking naps can also improve cognitive performance and your ability to absorb new information.

A study at the University of California–Berkeley recruited 39 healthy adults and assessed their ability to learn and memorize with or without naps. The participants who napped between learning sessions (for 90 minutes) improved their scores by 10 percent, while their non-napping counterparts saw scores dropping by 10 percent.[11] Napping can also be beneficial for those who have insomnia issues or problems with sleep apnea.

Many cultures, especially those in hotter climates, have long known the value of napping . . . think of Spain and their famous afternoon *siestas*. However, in America's corporate culture, it can be a bit more challenging to find time for napping,

Boomers on the Cutting Edge

The Earthing Pad

*R*emember free radicals . . . those oxidizing villains that result from chronic stress and environmental toxins? Sixty years ago, we Baby Boomers began to wear shoes with synthetic soles and unknowingly lost our connection with the greatest free-radical neutralizer, Mother Earth.

Throughout most of human history, we walked barefoot or slept on the ground. When in contact with the earth, its tranquil energy naturally transfers to any conductive object— whether it is a metal rod, a wire, a tree or plant, an animal, or a barefoot human—and it becomes "grounded." The known effect of grounding is to discharge and prevent the buildup of electrical stress.

Our bodies are mostly water, and minerals are excellent conductors of electricity (electrons). The free electrons on the surface of the planet are easily transferred to the human body as long as there is direct contact. Unfortunately, synthetically soled shoes act as insulators so that even when we are outside, we do not connect with the earth's electric field. When we are in homes and office buildings, we are also insulated and unable to receive the earth's balancing energies.

Having your bare feet touch the ground connects you with an infinite supply of *free* electrons. The Earthing Pad is a unique tool for neutralizing the painful and chronic inflammation that causes autoimmune and degenerative diseases, including aging.

In fact, the patented Earthing technology is the only way, without standing directly on the ground, to connect with Earth's electrons. It allows you to connect to the earth during sleep or while you work. As it neutralizes free radicals in your body, it supports your immune system; reduces stress and anxiety; and is fundamental to sound, restorative sleep. There is no question that maintaining a functionally "young" immune system is an excellent strategy for preserving the quality of life and slowing senescence. As Earthing greatly reduces oxidative stress, it is expected to increase life expectancy and improve health.

To learn much more about this simple but essential healing tool, read *Earthing: The Most Important Health Discovery*

Ever? by Clint Ober, Stephen T. Sinatra, M.D., and Martin Zucker.

To purchase an Earthing Pad for your desk or bed, go to **www.longevitywarehouse.com**. The products offered on this website allow you to conveniently ground yourself when indoors. They are "barefoot substitutes."

Everyone in your family should be working and sleeping on an Earthing Pad. An affordable anti-aging tool, it should be under your feet while you work on your computer and on your bed at night.

especially if you work at an office and follow a typical 9-to-5 schedule. You might consider taking a 30-minute nap during your lunch break after you've eaten. Some companies even provide "meditation" rooms for employees who need to "recharge their batteries" for a little while.

The famous Sunday-afternoon nap, in a favorite armchair or hammock, was once practically an American institution . . . and for many of us who want to stay youthful and young looking, it certainly should become one again!

A Few Things about Napping

- You are an experiment of one, so try taking a few afternoon naps and observe how you feel afterward. If you complain of waking from naps groggy and disoriented, it may be that you have gone into deep sleep (stages 3 and 4), which means you won't wake as easily. But if your nap only takes you through the first two stages of sleep, you will most likely wake up feeling energized and more alert. As the first two stages of sleep take about 10 minutes each, the best napping time is around 20 minutes.[12]

- Don't nap late in the day, as this can interfere with your regular sleep schedule. The prime napping time is between 1 and 3 in the afternoon.

- Try not to nap for more than about 30 minutes. Longer than that may actually have the opposite effect of what you intend, and you may wake feeling tired and listless. You might want to set your watch or phone alarm to make sure you don't "over-nap."

- Try to find a darkened room or use eye pillows or a mask to create daytime darkness. Quiet is essential.

How Do You Know If You Need a Nap?

One method is to sit in a comfortable chair with your feet flat on the floor, back upright but supported by the chair. Then simply breathe into and out of your belly slowly for about five to ten minutes. If you are tired when you do this, you will usually fall asleep. If that happens, lie down or just take a nap in the chair. Even if you don't feel sleepy, you will benefit from the quiet contemplation and deep-breathing exercises. Even taking a mental siesta for ten minutes here and there during the day will improve your outlook and attitude.

Now that we've covered the basics, it's time to move on to some truly innovative, cutting-edge approaches to anti-aging. These recommended therapies and products are the latest and greatest in the life-extension field of medicine. Let's start with detoxification therapies.

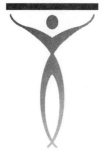

Chapter 25

Anti-Aging Therapies #1: Detoxification

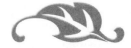

Pure, clean, well-nourished cells are the secret to longevity. End of story!

Chapter 3 taught that one of the principal causes of aging is the buildup and storage of toxins in the body. Unfortunately, many of us begin life on this planet with toxins in our cells. Some we inherited from our parents and grandparents, and even more toxins entered our cells at birth. In fact, in those days general anesthesia for women in the delivery room was standard practice!

As infants, we received vaccinations, many of which contained mercury. Later, we probably took antibiotics that destroyed the beneficial bacteria we needed for healthy digestion. And as the years passed, we Boomers continued to be assaulted by a "chemical soup" of pollutants—from processed foods in aluminum foil (TV dinners) to household pesticides. I actually remember one summer my brother and I entertained ourselves by taking the mercury from a thermometer, rolling it into a ball, and playing with it—our own version of toxic Play-Doh.

No one knew. . . .

Toxins from the Inside and Out

Many of the toxins that harm us are *exogenous*. They are found in the external environment—our food, water, and air. They are in the pots and pans we cook with, the fillings in our teeth, and the cosmetics we put on our faces. Many of us are experiencing symptoms of heavy-metal toxicity that our overstressed organs of elimination are simply not able to handle.

Other toxins are *endogenous*. They are internal, and can be created by viruses or parasites or too much stress. These, too, have an energy-draining effect on our bodies. By the time we reach our 40s, many of us have already begun to feel the symptoms of a poisoned system, ranging from chronic fatigue to constipation to sore joints. When this toxicity remains unchecked, far more serious health problems occur as we age.

As the focus of this book is on physical health, this chapter will emphasize toxins that affect our bodies, and offer suggestions to eliminate them. However, it is worth mentioning that one can be *emotionally* and *spiritually* toxic as well. Holding on to anger and resentment can wreak havoc on the body just as surely as a high-sugar diet or nicotine does. With today's economic and social pressures, many of us will find ourselves in jobs and relationships that sap our strength. The disconnection we experience between our bodies and the earth, or between our passions and our heavy responsibilities, can express itself in a kind of listlessness and depression from sources we may not even recognize.

Toxins are a virtually inescapable part of life today, and unfortunately, they are not going away anytime soon. The good news is that we have built-in mechanisms for cleansing, and they are as natural and predictable as the changing seasons. Our bodies will joyfully and capably push out toxins if we have the energy to cleanse and are able to do so regularly.

Before some of the various therapeutic options for cleansing are described, it might help to note a few of the common symptoms of toxicity that you may already be recognizing in yourself.

The Signs of a Toxic Body

Toxins exit our bodies along detoxification pathways. If these pathways are blocked—when our bodies have more toxins trapped inside than can come out—certain symptoms of toxicity will emerge. Here are just a few of them:

- Chronic fatigue
- Headaches
- Arthritis/joint issues
- Hormonal imbalances
- Constipation or diarrhea
- Insomnia
- Breathing issues
- Congestion/runny nose
- Teary eyes
- Vomiting

When we remove toxins from our systems, everything begins to work and move around more smoothly.

A good analogy might be when you drain and change the oil in your car. Afterward, your car performs more efficiently and will be less susceptible to breakdowns. This is true of your body as well. With a pure, clean body, all the parts work better. They have greater resiliency and longevity. You manage stress better, you're much happier, and your quality of life greatly improves.

Detoxification Times and Seasons

There are three "seasons" when the body naturally cleanses—spring, summer, and "Indian summer." In the spring, we may notice that we feel achy and that our joints are sore. This is a sign that the liver has gone into a cleansing mode. Summer is also an excellent time for our cells to get rid of impurities, as we tend to be more physically active. The hot weather allows us to eliminate toxins through our sweat glands. We also consume more watery foods that naturally help cool and detoxify. Fresh vegetables and fruits, readily available in this season, aid in the cleansing process.

As fall approaches, the weather turns cold and then, more often than not, suddenly turns warm again for a few more delightfully beautiful days. This is Indian summer; and it can frequently trigger a runny nose, a chest cold, or perhaps even a fever. We often mistake this for disease, but it is nature's way of allowing us one more opportunity to cleanse before we begin to consume fats and salty foods so that we can be warm and comfortable during the colder winter months ahead. Fats, animal proteins, and mineral-rich salts are warming.

When we remove toxins from our systems, everything begins to work and move around more smoothly. It is one of the most important ways to stay young.

Although your body can push out toxins at any time, it is usually not a good idea to choose to go on an intense detoxification program in the winter. Winter is a time for rest and stillness—a time to accumulate energy, not to cleanse.

With plenty of accumulated energy and with the coming of another spring, new life begins. Spring is a season for renewal, and you can't renew without cleansing. So the cycle begins again.

This cycle of the seasons and the chance to purify is an extraordinary arrangement that we haven't really valued or understood. Honoring nature's laws of cleansing is vital because cleansing is one of our most important tools for staying young.

The body is always cleansing. But when you do decide to aid it in eliminating some of its toxins with a more aggressive cleansing program, it's best to start your cleanse on the days when you're not particularly busy or highly stressed. Many people make Saturday or Sunday their cleansing days, as the weekend tends to be less harried, and there is more time to focus on self-care.

Who Shouldn't Cleanse

Because energy is necessary before we cleanse, there are certain individuals who should not cleanse, either because they need to conserve their energy or because they don't have enough of it to make cleansing viable:

- People who are very weak or recovering from an illness
- People whose immune systems have been compromised or who are critically ill
- People with low blood sugar or diabetes
- People over 70, who must restore energy before they can cleanse
- Pregnant or nursing mothers—it's better to cleanse *before* conception (lower-bowel enemas are fine if constipated)

Cleansing Therapies

Toxicity and detoxification is the number one health concern on many people's minds today. But because we are very busy, we often look for quick fixes—reaching for harsh herbal supplements and laxatives, instead of changing our lifestyles and the way we eat. These quick fixes are often stressful and even harmful to the body. For example, many colon-cleansing products contain strong herbs that deplete the body of important minerals and also drain the adrenals. Many liver-cleansing products have maple syrup, molasses, and honey in them that feed yeast. And the suppositories and chelation therapies (for removing heavy metals) that are available at local health-food stores are a bit like putting the cart before the horse. Most people do not have detoxification pathways that are open enough for these therapies to be effective. These pathways (via organs of elimination) must be strengthened and opened before they will work efficiently.

The Body Ecology program prepares and strengthens the body so that detoxification can occur. The most important way it does this is by promoting foods that create energy and restore digestion. Other therapies help as well.

Foods as Cleansers

By now you have learned quite a lot about the wonderful healing and cleansing properties of food. Below are just a few reminders of why the Baby Boomer Diet is an extremely effective detoxification program.

— **High-fiber vegetables and grain-like seeds.** Fiber grabs up the toxins and binds them for removal, and it helps reduce constipation. When a stool remains in your colon for too long, the toxins are simply reabsorbed over and over again instead of being eliminated.

Fiber ensures that your food moves through the digestive tract more efficiently, forms a healthier stool, and then leaves your body with ease. It also gives you a feeling of fullness that prevents you from overeating, so it helps with weight loss. In addition, fiber helps regulate your blood sugar by slowing down its absorption rate. When blood sugar is too high or too low, your body becomes acidic (toxic).

Apart from fermented foods, fresh fruits and vegetables are the most cleansing, but fermented foods have the added benefit of assisting with digestion, while raw ones can actually be more difficult to break down (unless pureed, as in a green smoothie). A nice balance of fermented, cooked, and raw vegetables, including sea vegetables, is always best.

— **Probiotic foods (fermented foods).** Body Ecology has been the leader in promoting fermented foods. Over the years we've received wonderful testimonials about the effectiveness of these foods in helping our bodies become cleaner. The microflora are powerful scavengers of toxins, including heavy metals.

The good bacteria also kill and suppress the growth of harmful pathogens that produce inflammation and endogenous toxins in your gut. Both pathogens and beneficial microflora can "translocate," but with beneficial microflora as watchdogs, your intestines will contain fewer toxins, and that means that every cell in your body will be healthier. Clean cells live longer, and *you* live longer.

While fermenting young coconut kefir is something new, coconut water has always had a wonderful reputation for helping to cleanse the heart, kidneys, and liver.

Adding a half cup or more of cultured vegetables to your meals gives you another powerful tool for purging toxins. Cultured vegetables, a good fiber source, are usually made with cabbage and may include kale and collards. These veggies are members of the cruciferous family and contain potent, natural antioxidants called *indoles* and *isothiocyanates*. These compounds ramp up your immunity and help protect against cancers of the colon, breast, and respiratory system. Indole-3-carbinol, specifically, protects your cells from damage and hunts down and destroys free radicals; while isothiocyanates are sulfur compounds that have been shown to disrupt the growth and division of cancer cells.

The Principles and Cleansing

The Body Ecology Diet is the ultimate cleansing diet because it quickly strengthens your body and creates more energy. One of its 7 Principles is cleansing. But let's review the other six, as they can be of great help to you as you put this principle into practice.

— **The Principle of Uniqueness.** The phenomenon of cleansing is embedded in the very essence of your physical being. Just as you have no control over the rising and setting of the sun, you can't stop your body from pushing out toxins. Some of us are born with a lot more toxins; others have accumulated less. Some of us have more power to cleanse than others. Toxins come out when *they* want to—the best you can do is to help them out. Don't suppress them if you want to grow younger.

— **The Principle of Balance.** Toxins keep us in a constant state of imbalance. Throughout our youth, our bodies make a valiant attempt to stay balanced. At some point they can no longer do so, and those early signs of aging start to show. Actively eliminate toxins and assist your body to achieve balance. Always striving for balance is another phenomenon that was embedded in your body's very creation, but it is always wise to help your own cause.

— **The Principle of Acid/Alkaline.** Toxins keep the body in a constant state of acidity. You already know what that means. Toxic bodily fluids are the perfect environment for fungi, viruses, and even cancer cells to thrive. You want to strive for clean cells that are never too acidic.

— **The Principle of Food Combining.** Undigested food is toxic. Following the food-combining rules creates more efficient digestion and fewer toxins.

— **The Principle of Step by Step.** Incremental steps are particularly important for detoxification, as cleansing should be slow, steady, and deliberate. Cleansing too rapidly can weaken us or even make us ill. Go slowly, but be persistent, never stopping. Cleansing is a lifelong process. The myth that going on a 10-day (or 30-day) cleanse will rid the body of toxins has been circulating around the natural-health community for decades. The assumption is that doing this occasionally is enough. It's just not so.

This principle also helps us better understand the cleansing process. You'll remember from reading Chapter 3 that cleansing is also related to creating more energy, correcting nutritional deficiencies, and conquering infections.

- **Creating energy:** Because The Diet quickly strengthens your body and creates more energy, the first thing your cells want to do is push out toxins. They must do so to live. As you create more energy, you can expect to have moments of joy and occasional moments of discomfort. These ups and downs are all a part of the process of becoming healthy and strong.

- **Correcting nutrient deficiencies:** When you correct deficiencies, your cells come alive again as the missing nutrients work their magic. This creates more energy, giving you even more power to cleanse and create even healthier cells.

- **Conquering infections:** Viruses, fungi, bacteria, and other parasites cause serious endogenous toxins. As your cells and bodily fluids become cleaner, these pathogens won't find you a desirable host.

The Two 80/20 Rules

Follow these two simple rules when you eat:

- **Rule #1:** Do not fill up your stomach completely when you eat a meal. This puts too much food in the digestive tract at one time. Digestion of food is much more efficient when you leave about 20 percent of your stomach empty. When any food takes too long to break down (or does not do so thoroughly), it becomes another toxin.

- **Rule #2:** At least 80 percent of your meal should be alkaline forming (mostly plant foods), and 20 percent can be acid forming (animal proteins). Too many acid-forming foods are, as their name implies, acidic and create a toxic environment in your cells.

Colon Cleansing (Colon Hydrotherapy)

Colon cleansing has been around for centuries, and is mentioned in Egyptian historical documents as early as 1500 B.C. Russians have long included colon-therapy tools in their spas, recognizing the radiant effect these cleansings have on the skin.

A 4-Day Starter Cleanse

Foods to avoid:
- Animal proteins
- Fats and oils
- Dairy products
- Grains and grain-like seeds

Alkalizing foods to include:
- **Sour fruits** and their **juices**
- **Vegetables**—80% raw, 20% cooked*
- **Ocean vegetables**—rich in minerals
- **Cultured vegetables** and **probiotic liquids**—extremely important
- **Cleansing herbs**—LivAmend helps increase flow of bile from the liver
- **Adaptogenic herbs**—build more energy during your cleanse
- **Water**—add minerals, and drink a gallon per day to flush out toxins
- **Lemon juice in water**—also helps flush out toxins; drink as desired

*Cruciferous vegetables, such as kale and cabbage, should not be eaten raw. Prepare your vegetables in an easy-to-digest format, such as puréed soups and smoothies. These give your detoxification organs a much-needed rest.

In the U.S., colonics were used quite extensively in the 1920s and '30s, and were considered a common health practice. For the next 70 years or so, their use dramatically declined, along with interest in bowel health in general, and only in recent years has there been a comeback.

Many of the actors and actresses gracing the covers of today's popular magazines don't want us to know that colon-cleansing sessions are their secret tool for remaining young, well hydrated, and healthy. Yes, from beautiful lingerie models to famous opera singers, people find that regular colon-cleansing sessions help with performance and offer wonderful cosmetic benefits. Colon therapy not only keeps our skin glowing and healthy, but it also helps us to maintain an ideal body weight. It is now commonly known that the ability to keep off those excess pounds and inches is directly linked to good colon health.

Finally many doctors "in the know" are recommending colonics before a patient undergoes a colonoscopy, in lieu of the highly potent magnesium treatments that can be traumatic to some people.

Safe, painless, and convenient enough to do at home, colon cleansing definitely helps reverse the signs and symptoms of aging. No, you won't find many research studies on colon therapy, but isn't it just common sense? Removing toxic buildup (accumulating inside our intestines for decades) can help revive us and even reverse some of the most serious reasons why we age—inflammation, free radicals, nutrient deficiencies, and cellular debris.

Colon therapy helps correct these issues and also promises improved energy. You will also feel more calm and focused; sleep better; become more creative; and have a happier, more positive outlook on life. While it helps reduce the risk of gastrointestinal problems and colon cancer, another important yet little-appreciated benefit of colon therapy is that it is an excellent way to hydrate every cell in your body. And as you know from reading Chapter 21, we also age very quickly when we become dehydrated.

Because of its ability to hydrate and then draw out toxins and remove them as they accumulate in your stool, colon hydrotherapy, especially in repeated sessions, actually eliminates toxins from cells everywhere in your body, not just your colon.

Fortunately, colon therapy has become a respected health profession and practice that is undeniably essential due to the increasingly toxic world in which we live. Colonics, enemas, and colema boards offer highly therapeutic interventions.

Not Just for Colon Health— Colon Therapy Is Deep-Cell Cleaning

Colon hydrotherapy is a simple procedure that allows purified, temperature-controlled water to flow slowly into the large intestine, where it gently stimulates the colon's natural peristaltic action to release softened waste. This process is repeated several times in a session and results in better colonic function and elimination. A clean colon is a happier colon.

Clean cells have less inflammation—they live longer, and so will you. Because both disease and health begin in your intestines, you can understand how every cell in every organ and structure in your body—from your brain, lungs, liver, and heart; to your eyes, skin, muscles, and even your bones—benefits from removal of toxic waste from your intestines.

One of the first systems to improve with colonics is your lymph system, which defends your body against infections and the spread of tumors. Lymph nodes (an organized collection of lymph tissue) are numerous in the blood vessels of your intestines and can easily become cancerous when toxic.

Hydrotherapy is an excellent way to remove waste from the small intestine as well. Because the colon and small intestine are connected, when the colon eliminates its material, it signals the small intestine to start eliminating, too.

Labeling such an effective anti-aging tool "colon" therapy downplays its value, because this process also has a profound effect on the emotions. Indeed, your abdominal region houses a very sophisticated nervous system, affectionately termed a "gut brain." This mass of cells in your abdomen is connected to the mass of cells in your skull and to the rest of your central nervous system. It influences the production of neurochemicals, including serotonin and dopamine. When you release toxic material from your gut, toxic emotions (like sadness and anger) leave as well. These emotions are extremely aging, so eliminating them helps you feel more cheerful and serene.

Imagine what will happen if we Baby Boomers choose *not* to do colon therapy. We'll soon have a country with 79 million grumpy old men and women who won't be very effective at fulfilling our greatest mission—to restore peace and harmony to our planet before we leave here.

There are basically two types of colon therapy: colonics performed by a professional therapist; and those you do at home with an enema bucket or a colema board (see below).

Working with a Professional

If you are new to colon cleansing, you may feel more comfortable with a professional—at least at first. There are two methods available today: the open system and the closed system.

The *open system* delivers a constant, low-pressure stream of water through a small, pencil-sized speculum. You control both the filling and the release of water from your colon with the open system. This method is ideal for those who prefer

---

Boomers on the Cutting Edge

Gently Eliminate with the Luis Rojas Method

While each colon therapist has his or her own unique style, our preferred method at Body Ecology is the Luis Rojas method. Usually, colon therapists are trained to fill the colon with water and then release all the water and the waste that flows out with it. With the Rojas Method, the colon is filled with water not only at the start, but throughout the entire session. Water is slowly and gently infused into the colon until it is well hydrated. When the client feels the need to release, the hydrotherapist turns a knob on the instrument and the softened waste material is eliminated. While releases do flush out plenty of waste material, not all of the water is eliminated from the colon before the therapist initiates another slow fill. At the end of the session, all the water is eliminated in a final release.

In this way, the water remaining inside the colon through the entire session continues to soak and hydrate the older waste material. This gentle method keeps the colon well hydrated and softens material that will be released in the next session.

being left alone in the colonic room, but with a certified therapist nearby to assist as needed. This method offers an ultraviolet filtration system; an odorless vent system; and a sterile, disposable rectal tube. Waste material is flushed away with consistently flowing water but can be seen through a clear view tube.

In a *closed system,* the speculum nozzle is closer to the size of the actual rectum, and waste material goes directly into the speculum and from there into a viewing tube. In the closed-system procedure, a certified colon therapist remains in the room with you, controls the instrument, and gives you the colonic. The closed system involves a very thorough release, and the waste material can be viewed and assessed by the therapist.

What should you look for in each session? Thanks to the view tube, you can see some of what you are eliminating. Certainly you'll release recently eaten food and older waste material, but much of what you are removing cannot be seen. *Invisible toxins*, including pathogenic bacteria (even those in biofilms), and *toxic chemicals* (from heavy metals, pesticides, preservatives, and air pollution) are also being removed during each session.

An effective colon-therapy session may involve much more than just the release of waste matter. To help facilitate the process, many therapists offer reflexology, acupressure, massage, and emotional-cleansing techniques that help relax you or prepare you emotionally and physically for the session.

You can find a certified colon therapist in your area on the website of the International Association for Colon Hydrotherapy: **www.i-act.org**.

How Often Should You Cleanse?

A frequently asked question is: "How many colon cleansing sessions will I need?" Unfortunately, there is no simple answer, as according to the Principle of Uniqueness, each of us is different.

As you begin your cleansing sessions, you will soon be able to judge how many you need. However, cleansing all the cells in your body by working through your colon is not something you do once or twice. Clearing away decades of toxic accumulation is, indeed, a process—one that should continue for as long as you live.

Fortunately, when done properly, colon hydrotherapy is safe, gentle, and effective and will not lead to dependency. In fact, the expansion and contraction of the colon as the water fills and releases will help to tone and strengthen the muscle over time. The hydration is priceless.

When you first begin, you will need to schedule your colon-cleansing sessions more closely together. If done correctly, water from each previous session will also be softening the more stubborn material that may not be released until the next visit.

It can take time to soften this material, but it will eventually be released in the future sessions. Most colon therapists, naturopaths, and doctors who now recommend colonics suggest you start by having at least four sessions close together.

In future visits, give your colon a chance to rest—at least one day between each session is best. A professional colonic has more "fills" and "releases" than an enema and can cause your colon to become fatigued if continued for too long on one day. That is why sessions are scheduled for 45 minutes each. With a home enema, you can continue until the water is clear and, if needed, repeat the enema the next day. Questions to ask yourself at the end of the session are: "Did I eliminate well in this session? Should I come back for another right away?"

After Your Colonic

After your colonic, you should go home and take it easy for the rest of the day. Eat a light meal. A liquid or pureed soup is best. Eating or drinking probiotics is also wise.

You will always benefit from a colon-cleansing session either with a professional or at home when you are experiencing signs of toxicity, such as pain, fatigue, depression, bloating, dry skin and lips, or swelling and puffiness anywhere in your body. If you feel flu-like or if you have the flu, cleansing your colon is a must. You will soon learn to recognize your body's unique way of saying, "I need to eliminate toxins quickly."

Does Colon Cleansing Wash Away Good Bacteria?

Many physicians (who in all truth have usually never experienced colon therapy) have stated that flushing the colon with water depletes it of healthy microflora. But remember, most microflora are in the stool anyway and would leave naturally with daily eliminations (if these eliminations are even occurring). Trillions do remain and are not disturbed by the colonic water because they have colonized or settled into healthy mucus.

The fact is, most people are so toxic that when they begin The Diet, they don't have healthy microflora anyway. This is why it's so important to eat the foods on the Body Ecology Diet, especially probiotics such as young coconut kefir and cultured vegetables, as well as probiotic liquids. Nutritious and geared toward intestinal health, these powerful foods constantly replenish your colon with healthy microflora.

Anyone on a high-fiber, sugar-free, probiotic diet like the Body Ecology Diet will have excellent colonics. Beneficial microflora in the fermented foods act like microscopic Roto-Rooters. They are quite masterful at softening the material that has accumulated for years in both your small and large intestines. Imagine millions of microscopic "Pac-Men" working away inside you, helping you to eliminate years of improper eating. This is why colon therapists tell us that their clients on The Diet have the best eliminations during their sessions. Over time, with continual colonics (as needed), years of accumulation in the small intestine will also be cleansed. Your ability to absorb nutrients will increase tremendously, also helping you rejuvenate and live a longer, happier life.

Cleansing at Home

The Home Enema

Only two generations ago, it was common for homes to always have an enema bag. Doctors were even trained in medical school to prescribe an enema when someone fell ill.

An enema flushes out approximately five to ten inches of the lower portion of the colon with water or a special solution. Afterward the person uses the toilet for elimination.

You can find a great deal of information, instructions, and even videos on how to do an enema on the Internet. Enemas have been an important part of our BEDROK (Body Ecology Diet Recovering Our Kids) program for years. Parents of children recovering from autism have found that enemas are very effective at removing toxins, heavy metals, and pathogens quickly—speeding up recovery time.

Enemas are an excellent healing tool for anyone of any age. They are also safe throughout most of a pregnancy. (Stop once the mucus plug is released, usually a week or two before the birth.) Breast-feeding mothers will find that their milk is less toxic and even more nutritious when they practice proper colon cleansing with nutritive implants. Find a holistic ob-gyn or naturopath who understands their value if you prefer to discuss home enemas with a professional.

One of the benefits of cleansing your colon at home is that you can follow your cleansing enema with a "nutritive implant." Wonderful medicinal herbs and nutrients are combined in a cup or two of liquid (tea or water) and are retained in your colon. This idea is not a new one, as practitioners of Ayurvedic medicine call these implants *bastis*. And they are not new to Western medicine either. In fact, Taber's medical dictionary mentions the use of nutritive implants.

The Colema Board

Cleansing your colon with a colema board is very much like the professional open-system colonic, but can be done at home, where it is private and you can add your own mineral supplements.

To do a colema, you fill a five-gallon bucket with filtered water at body temperature. A strong folding chair is placed facing the toilet. The colema board is placed on the toilet and chair so that you can rest on your back. A pillow and folded towel will make the board comfortable during your colema. The bucket should be placed on a sturdy surface no more than four feet above your colema board. You will then siphon water through the surgical tubing so that it is flowing freely through the rectal tip. Stop the flow of water, lubricate the tip with organic extra-virgin olive oil, and position your body so that you can insert the tip no more than three inches into your rectum. Once it's inserted, you can open up the flow of water for your colema session.

Setting up and storing of the colema board can be an issue if you live in a small space and only have one bathroom.

As many of us are now committed to recovering the energy of our youth, I foresee that housing for Baby Boomers will need to change dramatically in the near future. To reflect our passion for rejuvenation, we need smaller homes that require less care but will have wellness amenities that include colonic equipment, a soaking tub, a steam shower and/or infrared

Boomers on the Cutting Edge

A Professional Unit for Home Use—*The Traveler*

A portable yet professional-grade home-colonic machine called The Traveler is available from Clearwater Colon Hydrotherapy. A three-day training at their facility in Ocala, Florida, is required in order to qualify for purchase so that you learn to use and care for the equipment correctly. The Traveler is not inexpensive, as it is of the same quality as what your colon therapist would use in his or her office or spa. However, the price also includes three days of instruction. Given that colonics are a lifelong anti-aging tool, and many families have more than one member in need of colonics, the price then appears much more reasonable.

The disposable specula and waste tubes to use for each colonic can also be purchased from Clearwater (**www.colonhydrotherapy.com**).

sauna, and a massage table (for in-home visits). We'll also seek homes with plenty of sunlight, a great kitchen for preparation of healing meals, a serene bedroom, lots of thoughtful storage, and definitely a home office. Of course, while we're planning away here, let's not forget that separate suite for our children and grandchildren, who may often visit for their own spa needs as well!

A Note on Colon-Cleansing Herbs and Laxatives

Unfortunately, when people experience constipation or digestive trouble, they often turn to harsh laxatives for relief. Most (senna, aloe, cascara sagrada, and rhubarb) work by irritating the colon wall so that it will eliminate unnaturally. These should be used sparingly, if at all. Over time, these laxatives can become habit forming, and the colon will no longer move without their stimulation. They do weaken the adrenals and will continue to deplete your prenatal jing.

For thousands of years, Chinese herbalists created customized formulas for their patients and used a combination of the gentler herbs to stimulate the colon to eliminate. Ayurvedic medicine, which also takes a much more gentle approach, uses an ancient herb called *triphala,* which can be taken every day and is not habit forming.

For better elimination, you can also encourage your liver to produce more bile, which in turn stimulates peristaltic movement in both intestines. (Body Ecology offers an herbal formula with Jerusalem artichoke, sarsaparilla, wasabi, and milk thistle, called LivAmend, which is very effective for this.)

Consistent use of digestive enzymes, especially ones with hydrochloric acid (HCl), pepsin, and pancreatin, also helps improve elimination and stubborn constipation. Of course, eating plenty of fiber in your diet and drinking water so that you are maximally hydrated is a must. (The 80/20 Principle, where 80 percent of your meal is from land, ocean, and cultured vegetables, guarantees an abundance of fiber.)

Herbs and herbal products that stimulate bile or even gentle laxatives like triphala are best taken *with* meals. They then travel down with the food you eat and help it to move along more effectively. Over time this can help retrain a sluggish colon. But again, chose a gentle herbal colon-cleansing formula and use it short term.

Even if it seems strange to you, gently infusing water into your colon to hydrate and cleanse the cells throughout your entire body to purify your lymph system, liver, and small intestine should become one of your most valued anti-aging tools. Whether in the hands of a skilled therapist or at home with enemas or a colema board, you will soon learn to recognize how often to use this wonderful tool to help your body become cleaner and turn back the clock.

Exercise

The ability to move with strength, confidence, and grace is a wonderful gift—and one we become more appreciative of as we grow older. Many of us already know how great exercise makes us feel, flooding the body with endorphins and raising serotonin, dopamine, and norepinephrine levels. But more and more research is showing how exercise combats and even reverses many of the degenerative conditions of aging.

An article in *Newsweek* magazine noted the many ways exercise improves brain functioning. Scientists have found that vigorous exercise can cause older nerve cells "to form dense, interconnected webs that make the brain run faster and more efficiently." Aerobic exercise also helps pump more blood to the brain, which means more oxygen to nourish brain cells. Scanning technology reveals that exercise actually causes the frontal lobes to increase in size, challenging the old belief that loss of brain cells as we age is permanent. It has been shown that physically active adults have less inflammation in the brain, so they also have fewer small (and often-unnoticed) strokes that can impair cognition.[1]

But exercise doesn't just affect the brain. Vigorous physical activity has been shown to reduce blood pressure, increase healthy HDL cholesterol, and strengthen cardiovascular capacity. It also increases bone density and size, which helps prevent osteoporosis and sarcopenia (loss of lean muscle mass), two common conditions of aging.[2] Exercise allows your body to modulate blood-sugar levels because it helps create skeletal muscles. Along with your liver, your skeletal muscles help absorb blood sugar, saving your insulin receptors from overload. Without lean muscle mass, blood sugar that is not used by your body is absorbed as fat, which then sends out inflammatory signals, further disrupting insulin receptors. Regular exercise is also a highly effective mental-health therapy, and has been shown to improve sleep, decrease anxiety, and elevate mood.

Using Exercise to Detoxify

Some kinds of exercise are especially effective at helping you cleanse. For example, it's important to exercise the lymph system when you are detoxifying. It has no pump like your heart, so you must activate it through movement. Daily bouncing on a mini trampoline is the best way to stimulate and move the lymph system. At Body Ecology, we recommend the Bellicon, an excellent-quality rebounder from Germany (**www .QiBounding.com**), but any exercise that results in movement followed by ample hydration and healthy elimination through your intestines (through a normal daily bowel movement or colon therapy) can facilitate cleansing of your lymph system.

Getting Started—Exercise Tips

1. **Try to get at least 30 minutes of moderately intense exercise (an activity you can do while breathing harder than normal) a day.** It doesn't work to follow the "weekend warrior" method of cramming an entire week's exercise into Saturday and Sunday. Overzealous weekend exercise often results in injury and undue stress.

2. **Choose forms of fitness that make you happy.** Many Baby Boomers have mixed feelings about exercise because of how we were introduced to it as children. You may have felt humiliated rather than encouraged, or you might have been alienated by the intense competitiveness of team sports. And the "no pain, no gain" philosophy of many fitness programs makes exercise sound more like an ordeal than a pleasure. If you are coming to exercise later in life and don't know where to begin, you may feel self-conscious about trying something new. Don't despair! Everyone can enjoy some kind of exercise, whether it's walking, biking, Pilates, or ballroom and belly dancing. Experiment and then select those activities that you most enjoy and can excel at.

3. **Set step-by-step, small goals and gradually challenge yourself more.** It can be elating to achieve a health or fitness goal, whether shedding a few pounds or completing a marathon. Listen to your body and follow your own unique pace.

4. **Mix it up.** It's important to give all of your muscles a workout, with a good blend of cardio, strength, and flexibility exercises. This can be accomplished through cross-training. We Boomers who are die-hard runners might find ourselves struggling with tendonitis and knee issues as we get older. If you're a runner, consider complementing your runs with some core exercises or by taking a Pilates or stretching class for flexibility. If you're an avid golfer, you might consider rounding out your routine with a more cardiovascular-oriented activity such as swimming or biking. As you get in touch with what your mind and body need, you may find that you choose different types of exercise at different

periods of your life. Walking, yoga, and t'ai chi are three types of exercise that are excellent for longevity and can be pursued no matter what your age.

5. **Stretch and warm up.** As we age, our muscles get sore faster and stay sore longer. Heating cold and stiff muscles with 15 minutes of warm-up exercises or stretching not only prevents soreness, it also protects us from injury, and allows our muscles to repair themselves more quickly.

Other Sweating Therapies

Saunas

In the earlier chapter on cleansing, I spoke of the body's natural ability to rid itself of waste. One of the principal ways it does so is through the skin, our largest eliminative organ. According to Mikkel Aaland, who wrote a book on bathing customs, sweating is essential not only for detoxification, but as a way to regulate body temperature and to keep the skin pliant.[3]

Interestingly, the appeal of the sauna surged in the 19th

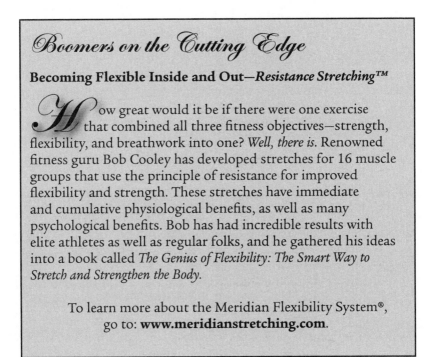

Boomers on the Cutting Edge

Becoming Flexible Inside and Out—*Resistance Stretching*™

How great would it be if there were one exercise that combined all three fitness objectives—strength, flexibility, and breathwork into one? *Well, there is.* Renowned fitness guru Bob Cooley has developed stretches for 16 muscle groups that use the principle of resistance for improved flexibility and strength. These stretches have immediate and cumulative physiological benefits, as well as many psychological benefits. Bob has had incredible results with elite athletes as well as regular folks, and he gathered his ideas into a book called *The Genius of Flexibility: The Smart Way to Stretch and Strengthen the Body.*

To learn more about the Meridian Flexibility System®, go to: **www.meridianstretching.com**.

century after Louis Pasteur's work encouraged more hygienic conditions during surgery and in hospitals. The country that really took the idea and ran with it was Finland, and the Finns have mastered the art of the therapeutic sauna. Other cultures have used some form of the sauna as well, such as the ceremonial sweat lodge of a number of Native American tribes.

Saunas are a very effective detox therapy. Most environmental toxins are fat soluble, and so they have an affinity for body lipids or fatty tissue. Metabolic organs such as the liver convert fat-soluble substances into water-soluble chemicals to facilitate excretion. Sauna therapy can enhance this process by moving these poisons from storage sites like the liver and putting them "back into circulation," where they can then leave the body through our perspiration.[4] (Colon therapy also helps remove them quickly.)

There are other benefits from saunas! They can restore energy levels, lower blood pressure, improve mental clarity, and enhance liver and immune function.

Nasal Cleansing—the Value of the Neti Pot for Eliminating Airborne Toxins

Once viewed as "one of those weird Eastern things," neti pots have entered the mainstream now. They are simply little water pitchers, usually metal or ceramic, used to cleanse the nose, nasal passages, and sinus cavities using salted water. For thousands of years, neti pots have been a basic tool in Ayurvedic medicine, used to wash away dust, pollen, and other kinds of airborne pollution. From the yogis of India to the common man, woman, or child, when we all wake up in the morning, there is an excess of mucus in the upper part of our bodies that needs to be cleansed away.

This type of water cleansing is easy to do and involves tipping your head to the left and pouring water directly into the right nostril so that it flows back out of the left, then switching sides. Use one heaping teaspoon of sea salt to two cups (half liter) of purified water.

Performed daily, just like teeth brushing, cleansing with a neti pot will also improve the health of your eyes, ears, throat, and even your immune system. It is a must if you have allergies, chronic respiratory infections, asthma, or sinus headaches. It reduces sinus congestion and helps prevent colds and flu.

To fight a pathogen or even to prevent exposure to one,

Boomers on the Cutting Edge

Infrared Saunas

*I*nfrared saunas are a little different from conventional saunas. Rather than turning red-hot, they produce an invisible, gently radiating infrared heat through a ceramic heater. In infrared saunas only 20 percent of the energy is used to heat the air; the rest is used to heat the body. The temperature is adjustable and allows a person to sweat more quickly but also to tolerate longer periods of time inside the sauna.

Infrared saunas are excellent at ridding the body of a wide range of toxins, from heavy metals to other fat-soluble chemicals. They can be an effective treatment for many toxicity-related disorders, such as chronic fatigue; and offer many additional health benefits, such as weight loss, improved circulation, pain relief, more vibrant skin, elevation of energy, and reduction of stress.

You can also obtain the benefits of infrared-heat therapy in a mat form. The "Biomat" is an FDA-approved medical device that combines therapeutic infrared light, negative ions, and amethyst quartz as a way to reduce inflammation, eliminate toxins, and improve immune-system function. Learn more about it at: **www.biomat.com**.

---

you can also add a few drops of antimicrobial essential oil (eucalyptus, tea tree, oregano, or thyme) to the salted water. The water should be close to body temperature—lukewarm-ish. Most health-food stores now carry neti pots that come with instructions for use. Worth owning and using, they're an inexpensive but valuable longevity tool.

Emotional Cleansing

Toxic buildup can occur in our hearts and spirits, just as it does in our physical bodies. We Boomers have stockpiled decades of negative memories, traumas, and unresolved conflicts and resentments. The mind and body are not isolated from one another, but are inextricably linked, and we can see the psychological and emotional origins of many illnesses today. Many of us, particularly those who struggle with chronic anxi-

Boomers on the Cutting Edge

The LifeLine Technique™

The LifeLine Technique is an advanced holistic system developed by Dr. Darren Weissman that discovers, interprets, and releases the root cause of physical symptoms and stress. It is a compilation of more than 14 natural-healing modalities—ranging from Applied Kinesiology, acupuncture, and the Five Element Theory of traditional Chinese medicine, to Ayurvedic medicine and the chakras, shamanism, chiropractic, homeopathy, and Neuro-Linguistic Programming—into one seamless system.

The LifeLine Technique facilitates your awakening to the root cause of the painful, scary, or stressful experiences that are manifesting as symptoms, such as physical pain, stress, or anxiety. Until the subconscious is made conscious, we are unable to make a choice or take action based on what we are truly experiencing in any given moment. Coupled with the Five Basics of Optimal Health—the proper quantity, quality, and frequency of water, food, rest, exercise, and owning your power—this technique allows you to create the best possible conditions for the body to heal itself.

Find out more about The LifeLine Technique at:
www.drdarrenweissman.com.

ety and depression, may benefit from traditional talk therapy with a licensed mental-health-care professional. For others, who may have had limited results in therapy or who are looking for something less time-consuming and costly, there are other helpful methodologies for releasing pent-up emotions and tensions. Many are benefiting from therapies such as Emotional Freedom Technique (EFT), and The LifeLine Technique developed by Dr. Darren Weissman (see sidebar).

Empowering vs. Toxic Relationships

Have you ever spent an afternoon with a friend or relative and returned home feeling worn-out and depressed? It could be that your "friend" *is toxic*. A toxic person is someone who isn't happy until his problems become yours. Are there people in your life who spend a lot of time complaining or blaming others for their troubles? Are you involved with someone who spends all of your time together talking about herself? What about that co-worker who gossips incessantly every time you meet for lunch?

We've all known people who want us to take care of them rather than learn how to take care of themselves. They can sap our energy, and their negativity leaves us feeling helpless and on edge.

We can never entirely avoid toxic people—they are every-where!—but we can limit the time we spend with them and establish boundaries so that their impact on our emotional lives is slight. Cheryl Richardson, who wrote *Take Time for Your Life*,[5] suggests some questions you might ask yourself about someone you think might be toxic:

1. "Am I able to be myself with this person? Do I feel accepted by them?"

2. "Are they critical or judgmental of me?"

3. "Does the relationship provide an even give-and-take exchange of energy?"

4. "Do I feel upbeat and energized when I'm around this person, or depleted and drained?"

5. "Does this person share my values? My level of integrity?"

6. "Is this person committed to our relationship?"

7. "Can this person celebrate my success?"

8. "Do I feel good about myself when I'm with this person?"

In short, it is important to connect with people who support us, who celebrate our successes, and who want to give to us as much as to receive. Find these people, and hang on to them! (And encourage them to take better care of themselves, too, so they'll be around for a long time.) They make living joyful and rich.

So the main take-away from this chapter is this: *you will* cleanse on The Diet, and *you must* do so to regain the energy of your youth. Wise Boomers will spend the rest of their lives honoring this important principle.

Next, in the second chapter on anti-aging therapies, you will get an in-depth look at ways to restore and increase your energy—methods to bring back your precious prenatal jing.

Chapter 26

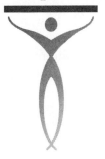

Anti-Aging Therapies #2:
Energy Restoration

*Today, the wisdom of the ancients has merged
with ingenious, constantly evolving energy
therapies. Along with pure water, sun, and air,
these age-defying techniques make it easy and fun
to restore our precious jing.*

By the time we reach our 40s many of us have strongly ingrained habits that are often harmful. For example, women often get stuck in the "caretaker" mode and feel guilty when they spend money or time on themselves. Many of us, both men and women, have become true workaholics and can't simply just "be here now." And of course, we Baby Boomers were far more fortunate than our parents and grandparents; and we still have an almost programmed, unquenchable desire to experience and have it all. This has cost us dearly in terms of our precious prenatal jing energy.

Now you've arrived at the time in your life when you *must* start to find therapies to restore that gift given to you at birth.

When you begin to search for rejuvenation treatments to increase your life-force energy, you'll quickly discover that there are an overwhelming number of therapies available now, and many more will be emerging in the future. When the choices become confusing, always remember that your time and money are best spent on those who will replenish your prenatal jing. This chapter features a few favorite options.

So, how does one choose the therapies that are best for your unique brain, body, and spirit?

The *Principle of Step by Step* is your road map. It teaches that before you can restore your prenatal jing, heal from anything, or even look and feel younger, you must first and foremost create energy. With it, your body will have the vitality to consistently eliminate physical and emotional toxins. With more energy you will digest your foods better and your cells will no longer be craving vital nutrients. More energy provides the immune system with the power it needs to overcome fungal, viral, and bacterial infections. And, as each of these causes of aging is overcome, you'll find you once again have more energy. You will be creating a "benevolent" cycle . . . quite the opposite of a vicious cycle that spirals downward, causing you to grow old far sooner than you should.

The *Principle of Balance* is also about energy. As you practice this Universal Principle, your goal will be to increase your core energy by creating balance in your body, in the foods you eat, in your relationships, and in the way you structure your time. All of these should be carefully nurtured. Are they making you feel more alive? Or are they draining your inner essence? So it is time right now to begin seeking out those therapies that add more energy, and carefully evaluating those things around you that take away from your constitutional life force.

The Great Healers of Chinese Medicine

No other practitioners of health and healing have focused on creating energy in quite the same way as the great sages of Chinese medicine. For thousands of years, these brilliant healers, who used acupuncture, acupressure, and herbs as natural daily routines, understood that if you "tonify the chi" or create a sufficient amount of energy on a day-to-day basis, your body will take any surplus energy and replenish your prenatal jing while you sleep.

Those of us with more of a Western mind-set might find the concept a little easier to understand if we think in terms of money instead of energy.

Remember your rich "Uncle Freddie" in Chapter 3? He gifted you with $5 million when you were born. Well, let's say that your parents, who were very wise, added to this great inheritance. As you grew up, they taught you to replace any money debited from your account with new deposits as quickly as possible. For example, perhaps you did odd jobs (babysitting or cutting grass or lifeguarding) to make the spending money you needed each week so you didn't have to tap into your inheritance. Even better, you might have often added a little extra to your account knowing that you might need it in the future—to go to college, perhaps, or to buy a house or have a baby. Nevertheless, you didn't touch your precious inheritance unless it was prudent and farsighted to do so.

Now reread the above paragraph and replace money with energy. Your ancestors gifted you with energy. By creating at least enough to use each day, you were careful to never deplete it. At night your body stored what it didn't need. You were mindful to create a way of life where you could often *increase* your energy. At times when you needed to expend extra (to create a baby or if you were traveling, changing jobs, or moving), you always had enough in your energy account to never deplete your original inherited energy.

Many Baby Boomers are focused on creating, conserving, and saving money these days. That's great and very necessary. However, because of the number of years we've spent literally depleting our constitutional energy, we must now also start accumulating more energy than we spend each day to create a reserve.

It's never too late to start saving and restoring your jing. Whatever you do to replenish your original prenatal energy will enhance the quality of your life. It is also the secret to longevity.

The sun on your skin; the air you breathe; restful sleep; stress-management techniques; the quality of the water you drink; a probiotic-rich, sugar-free diet; the right supplements; and doing exercise that you enjoy will all become important tools to replenish that life-force energy. But can there be anything more? Absolutely yes! Stem cells; restoring youthful hormone levels; and even an active, loving sex life can also be powerful tools. So keep reading.

Chinese Herbs for Energy and Longevity

Chinese herbs have always had a prominent place in Asian cultures. They are associated with long life, slowing the aging process, radiant health, physical energy and vitality, mental acuity, and sexual vigor. Entirely natural, these herbs provide special nutrients for physical and mental health, and can be used to treat a variety of conditions, from anxiety to weight problems.

In a conversation with my friend the herbal master George Lamoureux (**www.jingherbs.com**), he gave this advice on restoring prenatal jing:

"In Chinese medicine, there are two organ systems that must be 'tonified' or strengthened as you restore your prenatal jing—your digestive system and your lungs.

"Healthy digestion is crucial for obtaining the nutrients we need from our food, while healthy lungs are crucial for acquiring 'nutrition' from the air. These two energies together create our daily chi—our bodies live and move on them. Create more than enough *daily* chi and you begin to restore your prenatal jing."

Chinese herbs used to increase our day-to-day vitality are *tonic* herbs. Examples of chi tonics are ginseng, American ginseng, cordyceps, codonopsis, and astragalus. Eleutherococcus root is known to increase oxygenation of the blood. When you increase oxygen, it reaches the mitochondria, those microscopic energy factories in each cell, and this increases chi.

Three Brothers is a liquid herbal supplement from Jing Herbs that combines three tonic herbs, each a superstar in its own right. The first of the three herbs is cordyceps (a favorite of martial artists and athletes). The second is astragalus (a premier herb that increases lung function and builds immunity by increasing white blood cells and natural killer cells). A study at the University of Texas showed that it prevents shortening of the telomeres on the end of DNA strands, greatly lengthening life span. The last is codonopsis, which supports digestion and helps keep lungs moist and protected. You could slip several droppers full of Three Brothers into any breakfast drink to wake you up instead of that morning cup of caffeine.

Finding that Yin/Yang Balance

*I*n Western medicine it is well understood that the adrenals produce our energy and sexual hormones. Chinese medicine views these organs slightly differently. The kidneys/adrenals are understood to house two separate yet interwoven energies. One is a cooling energy, and the other is warming.

The cooling energy (called *yin/water essence*) controls the fluids in the body, including the saliva; blood; sweat; tears; sexual, lymph, and spinal fluids; and overall moisture. When this adrenal/kidney cooling or yin essence is compromised, you tend to exhibit more sensation for "heat," with depleted body fluids, and dry skin, hair, and eyes. You are most likely often thirsty and become agitated easily and are more inflexible. **Three Sisters** is an example of a liquid herbal blend from Jing Herbs that was created to nurture balance by providing herbs that are cooling and nourish the fluids.

The warming energy (called the *yang/fire essence*) is responsible for sex drive, physical vitality, skeletal structure, willpower, courage, and overall energy. This warming energy enables all organs in your body to function; and when it is depleted, you are lethargic, tired, and introverted. Your immune system will be weak, and you will feel cold all the time. You will be very pale, have a frail voice, will not have a lot of spark in your personality, and will be more withdrawn in character. Urinary incontinence is a sign of weak adrenals or an adrenal/kidney yang deficiency. For this problem, Jing Herbs created what they call the **Deer Antler Essence.** As you might suspect from the name, it contains deer antler, which is considered very "yang" or strong. To create a balanced formula, two anti-aging herbs, *he shou wu* and *lycium* (goji), were added.

Take a look again at the symptoms you experience when your adrenal/kidney yin and adrenal/kidney yang essences are depleted. They are described in the two paragraphs above. Add the symptoms together and you have the perfect definition of an aging man or woman. It becomes clear, then, that restoring your adrenals is vital to rejuvenation! (To tonify or strengthen both essences in your adrenals, you would take both formulas.)

Adaptogens

Most of the tonic herbs are considered adaptogenic. To be called an "adaptogen," an herb must strengthen and provide energy. Examples of some of the most popular adaptogens are panax, Siberian and American ginseng, ashwagandha, shatavari, tribulus, maca, suma, mucuna pruriens, muira puama, rhodiola, schisandra, and matcha green tea.

While adaptogens energize, they also work by calming down negative energy. They help restore your sexual vitality and are excellent for your adrenals. Adaptogens and Chinese herbs work best when combined with the food and lifestyle changes recommended in the Baby Boomer Diet.

As we begin to have an even greater appreciation for how valuable adaptogens are for restoring youthful vitality, we'll probably seek out and discover more of them growing all over the Earth—especially in the Amazon rain forest—a potential "Garden of Eden."

Two special herbs worth singling out are holy basil and ashwagandha. Holy basil, also known as tulsi, is not related to the herb basil often used in cooking. It is revered in Tibetan and Indian medicine. It brings down elevated cortisol and sugar levels. It is highly recommended to take one or two capsules from Gaia Herbs if you feel your cortisol levels are too high, especially if you are having trouble falling asleep or staying asleep. Ashwagandha is an Ayurvedic herb that has also been shown to restore prenatal jing energy. To be effective, take 1,500 milligrams in the morning and again at bedtime.

As effective as tonic herbs and adaptogens can be, it is a waste of your money to take them while continuing to eat a high-sugar diet, over-indulging in caffeine or alcohol, and failing to manage the stress in your life.

As effective as tonic herbs and adaptogens can be, it is a waste of your money to take them while continuing to eat a high-sugar diet, overindulging in caffeine or alcohol, and failing to manage the stress in your life. Also, please understand that herbs are not substitutes for minerals and vitamins. They do different things in your body.

Stress

Boomers know all about stress, and we tend to take on a lot more of it than we can handle. Because we want to pack as much living as possible into a 24-hour day, we often ignore the toll stress and an overextended lifestyle are taking on our bodies. We forget to take time to decompress and honor our need for quiet and rest.

Stress weakens the immune system, making us more susceptible to a wide range of illnesses, from heart disease to depression. Unmanageable stress often leads to other unhealthy behaviors, such as overeating, drug and alcohol abuse, and destructive relationships.

A little stress is okay. Small amounts can increase the intensity of a good experience and heighten creativity and mental focus. But unmitigated stress—when it persists without the body having a chance to return to its resting state—may be what ages us most quickly. When the famous fight-or-flight response is on overdrive, we start to feel high-strung, irritable, and run-down.

What is happening to us in medical terms? Well, when we find ourselves in a highly demanding situation or an emergency, our bodies are flooded with cortisol, which boosts our immune response. However, cortisol must then inform the immune system that the emergency is over so that it can return to normal. Stress that doesn't die down keeps cortisol circulating in the body for too long, causing our immune cells to become sluggish and opening the door to infection.[1] Interestingly, cortisol also determines where the body will store fat, locating more of it on the belly, rather than on the hips and thighs, where it would be less harmful.

Stress-Management Tips

There are many stress-management techniques, but the most important thing to remember about stress is that we create a lot of it ourselves by trying to be superwoman or superman. Much of our anxiety can be alleviated if we choose to do less and delegate more. When we say, "I don't have time to exercise," or "I don't have time to relax," what we are really saying is "I am not a valuable person unless I am always busy."

Make quiet time for yourself a priority. Actively pursue those activities that support you emotionally and spiritually.

This might mean keeping a journal; working on a photo album of your grandchildren; listening to a little Mozart before you go to bed; taking a short, meditative walk in the early morning; or painting a watercolor. Set aside some time each day to do something nice for *you*.

When life becomes too overwhelming, turn to family and friends for support. Even if they can't solve your problems for you, sharing how you feel with an empathetic listener always helps you feel better and arrive at new perspectives and options you might not have been able to come up with on your own.

Massage Therapies

There are many kinds of massage, from Swedish and deep tissue to hot stone and craniosacral. All have a wide range of benefits. Below is a discussion of a special kind of massage called Ohashiatsu®, which is a unique combination of touch and acupuncture.

Ohashiatsu

Developed by a Japanese man named Ohashi who came to the United States in the early 1970s, Ohashiatsu is a special method of touch derived from traditional shiatsu, exercise, and Zen philosophy. Ohashiatsu manipulates the energy within the body, but places an emphasis on the special synergy between giver and receiver. When you receive Ohashiatsu, your posture, mobility, and overall well-being are improved, and it is an excellent way to relieve stress and enhance range of motion. When you give Ohashiatsu, you are energized and rejuvenated by your body's own dance-like movements and the meditative quality of your work. This massage involves deep but painless pressure applied to the acupuncture meridians, along with gentle stretches and limb rotations.

To learn more, go to: **www.ohashi.com/ohashiatsu.html**.

Meditation

People practice meditation for any number of reasons—to improve concentration and focus, to reduce stress, and to even overcome an addiction. Research reveals that meditation can literally "reshape" the brain and transform the body.

Meditation has been shown to reverse the buildup of plaque in the coronary arteries and to increase antibody levels in the bloodstream, boosting the immune system. It is often used to mitigate and manage pain associated with chronic health problems such as cancer, high blood pressure, and AIDS. Even more astonishingly, new research is showing that meditation and other relaxation techniques *actually turn off the genes that are associated with inflammation and cell aging.*[2]

Gone are the days when you had to be a mystic to meditate. More and more people are doing it! In 2008, data was released by the National Center for Complementary and Alternative Medicine that showed that 9.4 percent of adults surveyed in 2007 had tried meditation at least once during the previous 12 months! Simply sitting in silence for 10 to 30 minutes and concentrating on your breath, a word, or an image can clear away the cobwebs and shift the activity in the prefrontal cortex from the right hemisphere to the left, reorienting you from the typical fight-or-flight mode to greater acceptance and equanimity.[3]

Meditation can be divided into two types: *concentrative* and *mindful*. In concentrative meditation, you fix your attention on a particular object (a repetitive prayer or mantra), and empty your mind of all other thoughts. As you do this, you try to minimize distractions, continually returning to the chosen object. In mindfulness meditation, you can also focus on your breath or a word or an object, but in this case you keep your focus open. Distractions are not considered intrusions, but rather something to simply observe without judgment or analysis. The emphasis is on staying in the present.

Meditation Practices

There's a meditation practice to suit every need or disposition. Here are just a few of the options out there today:

1. **Mindfulness:** Beginning and ending with the breath, mindfulness practice teaches an evenhanded awareness toward whatever thought arises, by simply acknowledging it and returning to the breath.

2. **Compassion meditation:** The aim of compassion meditation is outward, designed to foster a feeling of loving-kindness toward a cause or person.

3. **Movement meditation:** An example of movement or motion meditation is "walking meditation," which involves walking very slowly, with deliberate and conscious awareness of every step. T'ai chi and qigong might also fall in this category.

4. **Transcendental Meditation (TM):** Many Boomers experimented with TM in the 1960s. This type of focused meditation often involves repeating a mantra over and over. Dr. Herbert Benson, author of *The Relaxation Response,* was doing something truly radical in 1967 when he ran various tests on a group of 36 TM practitioners to measure heart rate, blood pressure, and skin and rectal temperatures. He found that when they meditated, they used 17 percent less oxygen, lowered their heart rates by three beats a minute, and increased their theta brain waves (the brain waves that dominate during periods of deep relaxation).[4]

5. **Visualization:** This technique involves generating a mental image (a cross, a mandala, a journey, a safe place, or what have you); and can revolve around the achievement of a specific goal, such as losing weight, running a marathon, or curing a disease. This self-aware type of meditation often includes the repetition of an affirmation or intention.

Acupuncture/Acupressure for Rejuvenation

Any discussion of energy would be incomplete without the mention acupuncture, an ancient Chinese practice (dating to the 2nd century B.C.) used for a variety of physical and psychological issues. Acupuncture and herbs work hand in hand. The herbs can also stimulate the acupuncture points, especially when combined into formulas, but both together is ideal.

Acupuncture utilizes touch and very thin disposable needles to stimulate the body's own healing mechanisms. In a similar way, acupressure uses pressure from the palms, fingers, and thumbs to heal, but without the needles.

The last chapter talked about detoxification pathways in the body that must be unblocked in order for cleansing to occur. We also have energy pathways, called *meridians,* which are routes through which chi energy moves and flows throughout our bodies. Acupuncture points are specific areas along these

Boomers on the Cutting Edge

Qigong

Lower Your Blood Pressure with This Time-Honored Energy Practice

We know that stress ages us. It tires us out and weakens the immune system. Eventually, chronic stress will start to show up in our joints and aging skin. This makes qigong, an ancient energy practice from China, an especially effective anti-aging remedy, as it directly impacts our energy and replenishes our blood.

In China, qigong is the name given to the study, practice, and cultivation of chi, which we already know to mean "created energy." The word *gong* comes from *gongfu*, which refers to energy and time. Although there are different ways to perform qigong, most practices involve breathing exercises and a series of carefully choreographed movements or gestures designed to facilitate the flow of chi. A consistent qigong practice has the ability to strengthen physical power, increase mental alertness and endurance, and promote long life.

As it relates to longevity, qigong is especially important because, in addition to restoring and moving lost chi, it also replenishes the blood. As we age, our blood supplies dwindle; and our bodies become dry, brittle, and less elastic. In both Western and Chinese medicine, it is our bone marrow that maintains healthy levels of red and white blood cells—the fluid that protects and nourishes the body. Certain qigong exercises restore the suppleness of this marrow, which in turn strengthens the brain and enhances our mental capacity.

In addition, medical studies have found that qigong practice reduces sympathetic activity (the fight-or-flight response that is activated under stress) in the central nervous system. At the same time, qigong increases parasympathetic activity, which is restorative and most active during periods of rest. Qigong is considered a viable therapy for protecting the heart, lowering blood pressure, and reducing anxiety . . . all without the need for drugs![i]

---

[i] John Seim, "Qigong Reduces Stress in Computer Workers," *Natural News* website, February 25, 2008, **http://www.naturalnews .com/022718.html** (accessed 6/20/11).

routes where chi energy collects, which makes them especially significant for healing. These critical points on the body can be accessed through gentle pressure, heat, and more commonly, acupuncture needles.

Some people have likened chi meridians to a system of pipes through which water flows. The energy in these pipes can get stagnant, impeding or even stopping the easy movement of water. Just as our cleansing pathways must be open and unobstructed, so must our chi pathways be unblocked to allow the free flow of energy. When we are ill, one might say that a pathway has become dammed up somewhere. Acupuncture breaks up the dam.

Shown to increase energy and alleviate pain, acupuncture can also be used to address a variety of other conditions in which the body is in disharmony, such as hormone imbalances; sleep disorders, including insomnia; weight gain; chronic fatigue; anxiety; depression; jet lag; or susceptibility to illness.

The Five Tibetan Rites

The Five Tibetan Rites (also called the Five Rites of Rejuvenation) are another "must-have" in your growing toolbox of anti-aging remedies. Developed by Tibetan monks who condensed 21 yoga poses into 5 yoga movements, these rites were designed to stimulate our energy centers (also called chakras) that correspond to the endocrine glands in our bodies.

The "Rites" were first brought to American readers in a 1939 book entitled *The Eye of Revelation: The Original Five Tibetan Rites of Rejuvenation,* by Peter Kelder, who said he learned them from a wide-traveling retired British army colonel who had lived and studied with Tibetan monks. Subsequent editions of the book have brought these ancient "youthing" rites into the popular mainstream. They are believed to be Tibetan in origin because Tibetan yoga focuses on continuous movement *(Vinyasa)* rather than static poses. Each of the five movements is done 21 times because 21 is a mystical number in Tibet.

The rites lay a good foundation for any yoga practice and should be practiced with a focus on synchronizing the breath. Typically completed in about 15 minutes, the Five Tibetan Rites do not take as much time as a traditional yoga flow series. In a sense, they are the "best of the best."

> ## *Boomers on the Cutting Edge*
>
> ### Yoga Nidra
>
> For some of us, it can be nearly impossible to unwind after a stressful day. Our minds race, and our limbs feel restless and jumpy. Yoga Nidra is an ancient practice that means "yogic sleep," and it can be very calming for even the most frustrated insomniacs. When you practice Yoga Nidra, you are brought to a state of conscious deep sleep that is between wakefulness and dreaming. Although you are deeply calm, you are still awake and aware. During Yoga Nidra, the brain is at the delta brain-wave level, which is much slower and is the frequency of deep sleep. An excellent biofeedback practice, Yoga Nidra can involve breathing exercises, body surveys or "scans," and mental points of relaxation. It is ideal for stress reduction, insomnia, asthma, imaginative reveries, and even spiritual explorations.
>
> You can find out more about this unique practice at: **www.holisticonline.com/Yoga/yoga_nidra_home.htm**.

The benefits of the Tibetan Rites are many:

- They help detoxify and move the lymph system. (In fact, you may feel a little dizzy when you first start doing them as they move toxins around.)
- They enhance bone mass and help tone your muscles.
- They improve your posture and help create a more flexible spine.
- They flatten your abdomen and help you become more flexible.
- Many report that daily practice soon even eliminates an unattractive symbol of an aging body, the double chin.

A Word of Caution

If you do an Internet search on these exercises, you will discover that there is a lot of variation in how the poses are done and the speed at which they are done. If you are out of shape or unaccustomed to yoga, you might want to do the movements quite slowly at first. Many practitioners report struggling with the poses when they first try them, but then becoming stronger and more adept at them with practice. The important thing is to do them every day. It would be wise for any new practitioner to learn the proper way to do the movements so as to avoid injury. You might try Dr. Dariah Morgan's DVD, which shows the proper way to do the poses and offers modified poses depending on your level of fitness. It offers a warm-up and breathing exercises as well.

The Five Tibetan Rites are described below, with explanations taken from *The Eye of Revelation.*[5] Remember, each one must be done 21 times.

— The **First Rite** (spinning) strengthens the inner ear for balance. "Stand erect with arms outstretched, horizontal with the shoulders. Now spin around until you become slightly dizzy. There is only one caution: you must turn from left to right."

— The **Second Rite** (leg lifts) is for core (abdominal) strength. "Lie on your back full length on rug or bed. Place your hands flat down alongside your hips. Fingers should be kept close together with the finger-tips of each hand turned slightly toward one another. Raise your feet until the legs are straight up. If possible, let your feet extend back a bit over the body toward the head, but do not let the knees bend. Hold this position for a moment or two and then slowly lower the feet to the floor, and for the next several moments allow all of the muscles in the entire body to relax completely. Then perform the Rite all over again."

— The **Third Rite** (camel) activates the spine, opening the heart and solar plexus. "Kneel on a rug or mat with hands at sides, palms flat against the side of legs. Then lean forward as far as possible, bending at the waist, with head well forward—chin on chest. The second position of this Rite is to lean backward as far as possible. Cause your head to move still further backward. Your toes will prevent you from falling over backward. Your hands are always kept against the side of the legs. Next come to an erect (kneeling) position, relax as much as possible for a moment, and perform Rite all over again."

— The **Fourth Rite** (table) stimulates the sacral area and is excellent for building arm, leg, and gluteal strength. "Sit erect on rug or carpet with feet stretched out in front. Your legs must be perfectly straight—back of knees must be well down or close to the rug. Place your hands flat on the rug, fingers together, and the hands pointing outward slightly. Chin should be on chest—head forward.

"Now gently raise your body, at the same time bend your knees so that your legs from the knees down are practically straight up and down. Your arms, too, will also be vertical while your body from shoulders to knees will be horizontal. As your body is raised upward allow the head gently to fall backward so that your head hangs backward as far as possible when your body is fully horizontal. Hold this position for a few moments, return to first position, and RELAX for a few moments before performing the Rite again."

— The **Fifth Rite** (up dog and down dog) focuses on your upper-back muscles and is excellent not only for an immediate elevation in energy but for alleviating stress and depression. "Place your hands on the floor about two feet apart. Then, with your legs stretched out to the rear with your feet also about two feet apart, push your body, and especially your hips, up as far as possible, rising on your toes and hands. At the same time your head should be brought so far down that your chin comes up against your chest. Next, allow your body to come slowly down to a 'sagging' position. Bring your head up, causing it to be drawn as far back as possible."

Energizing Supplements for Endocrine Health

Well over 2,000 years ago, Hippocrates, the father of modern medicine, said, "Let food be thy medicine and medicine be thy food." And yet today, we have come to rely too much on synthetic drugs to cure what ails us. Even advocates of the "natural-foods movement" rely too heavily on vitamin and mineral supplements and components of plants. There are about 60 nutrients known at this time to be essential to human nutrition. Yet even if we swallowed a megavitamin/mineral pill consisting of generous quantities of all these nutrients, we could not maintain our health. This is because whole foods give us something we can't get anywhere else—they contain a live, spiritual essence that modern science has not yet identified.

Supplements can be healthy in the short term, until your inner ecosystem is reestablished. A wise way to supplement is to consider your personal lifestyle and habits and to follow the step-by-step process covered in Chapter 9. Answer these questions about the supplement:

- Does it create energy?

- Does it help correct digestion?

- Does it help conquer an infection?

- Does it help cleanse toxins from your body?

Remember—toxins are very damaging to the endocrine system. That's why the principles of cleansing set out in the previous chapter are an important first step in nurturing and healing the endocrine system.

The Adrenal-Thyroid-Pituitary Axis

When I first began studying Chinese medicine, every teacher and book referred to the kidneys as the root of "chi" or life force, supplying energy to all other organs in the body. After many years of relentless personal study, I now believe that this is a modern-day misinterpretation of this ancient system of healing. I believe that what ancient practitioners meant to convey is that *creating energy in a person's body is essential in order to establish, regain, or maintain health.* Certainly your kidneys are important organs, but if it is energy you seek, look to your adrenals.

The Adrenals

While not mentioned in the many textbooks I researched, the adrenals—and the thyroid—are the most important organs of focus if you want to regain youthfulness, health, and vitality. What happens when the adrenals and thyroid have lost their life force or "spirit"? Your digestive system, brain, sexual organs, heart, and central nervous system suffer.

Because of the stressful world we live in, and the confusion and negativity all around us these days, we are often in a fight-or-flight mode whether we realize it or not. This puts incredible stress on our adrenals. We have to find ways to calm them, and then nourish them back to health. In addition to stress-reducing techniques, like meditation and gentle exercise, the following supplements are indispensable to resetting the adrenals. Certain amino acids (GABA, tryptophan, DLPA, and tyrosine), holy-basil extract, B vitamins, and vitamin C help to calm down this fight-or-flight response so that you can then nourish the adrenals back to health. The *shen* herbs like reishi help calm the adrenals so that the tonic herbs can start to rebuild them.

Minerals are the most important part of the equation when nourishing your adrenals. Every second of your life, your adrenals must obtain the minerals they need from your bloodstream. How do we ensure that we have mineral-rich blood? An 80 percent plant-based, sugar-free, probiotic diet is a must. A healthy digestive tract that digests food and eliminates efficiently is also essential. While athletes try to replace minerals with sugary drinks like Gatorade, there are far better alternatives. (For more information on mineral supplements, visit: **www.bodyecology.com**.)

The Thyroid

Then there's the thyroid. Located slightly below the Adam's apple, the thyroid gland is intimately related to our metabolism and how quickly our bodies utilize energy. It helps us make protein, and it controls our sensitivity to the other hormones our bodies manufacture.

To function properly, your thyroid needs zinc, selenium, iodine, tyrosine, and good fats that contain vitamins A and D . . . all of which are found in egg yolks, butter, ghee, red-palm oil, and cod-liver oil. Coconut oil is excellent because it "warms" and "fuels" the thyroid. It also helps speed up metabolism, and can help you lose weight.

The Pituitary and Human Growth Hormone

There's been a lot of talk lately about human growth hormone (HGH), the most abundant hormone produced by the pituitary gland and the one responsible for the growth of nearly every cell and tissue of the body. HGH affects protein formation, cell differentiation, and cell growth. What most people don't realize is that the pituitary never stops producing growth hormone—even as we age. It simply stops *releasing* it.

> ## Do It Yourself
>
> *I*f you have more time in your schedule, you can make a wonderful, mineral-rich soup by slow-cooking organic vegetables and sea vegetables in water for several hours. Discard the vegetables, and you have a mineral-rich water that you can sip throughout the day. Use this over the course of a few days, or make more and freeze it for later use.

Although the impact of this hormone is most profound in the first 15 to 18 years of life, it will continue to influence the deposition of new bone on old bone throughout our lives. For adults, restoring HGH to its optimal youthful level is one of the most powerful of anti-aging therapies, as it causes our cells to regenerate, repair, and replicate.[6]

HGH increases the rate of protein synthesis and the mobilization of fat from fat cells in the body. It also decreases the rate of glucose use. As we age, we release less and less HGH, and by the time we are 60, we only have about 20 percent in our bodies. Diminishing HGH is called *somatopause,* and it contributes to many of those telltale signs of aging—lower energy and stamina, increased body fat, risk of osteoporosis, decreased sexual function, weight gain, and a greater tendency toward depression and anxiety.

HGH is also essential for hydration. In fact, you cannot correct dehydration in your body if you have low levels of HGH. As it slowly begins to decline, you become more dehydrated and wrinkled. HGH levels also affect your hair color. As the hormone wanes, there is also a gradual dying off of stem cells called *melanocytes* that provide a reservoir for the renewal of pigment-manufacturing cells. Without these pigment-manufacturing cells, your hair becomes gray and loses it shine.

Many people have started taking hormone-replacement therapy injections, which have some unpleasant side effects, including swelling of the arms and legs, water retention, high blood pressure, joint pain, and raised insulin levels.[7] These injections are also quite expensive. Ideally, we would begin to generate our own HGH through diet, lifestyle, and important supplements. The high-intensity, short-duration exercise program mentioned later in this chapter increases HGH.

A safer way to increase HGH is to take a secretagogue formula. As its name implies, a *secretagogue* is a substance that causes another substance to be secreted. Amino acids (like arginine, ornithine, lysine, glutamine, glycine, and GABA) and glandulars (usually the hypothalamus and anterior pituitary) are "stacked" or combined because together they work more efficiently to stimulate the release of your own naturally occurring HGH.

Bottom line . . . it is essential to evaluate, nourish and rejuvenate your entire endocrine team— your hypothalamus, pituitary, thyroid, adrenals and ovaries or testes.

Secretagogues have been on the market for at least a decade. Unfortunately, some of the more effective formulas come in a sachet packet and contain sugar or an artificial sweetener. If you use one of these, be sure to put the ingredients into three to four ounces of young coconut kefir or a probiotic liquid before drinking it. Adding a teaspoon of apple-cider vinegar to this mixture is also wise because HGH naturally depletes potassium and apple-cider vinegar is an excellent source of this mineral. These tips will help offset some of the negative issues associated with this type of secretagogue.

You can also purchase secretagogue formulas in capsule form and as a homeopathic liquid. These last two do not contain artificial sweeteners or sugar. Because of the recent popularity of secretagogues, more than 75 companies sell them, and there are inferior formulations offered at a low price, so buyers beware.

The anti-aging benefits of taking a secretagogue are all over the Internet. They appear to be true for many and include: increased energy and exercise endurance; weight loss; an improvement in skin texture and a reduction of wrinkles; darker, thicker hair; and stronger immunity. Most also report increase in sexual energy, better sleep, and a decrease in frequent nighttime urination.

Secretagogues are not recommended for children, teenagers, or pregnant or lactating women. It is not advisable for diabetics or borderline diabetics to use a secretagogue without the supervision of a physician, preferably one who specializes in anti-aging medicine, because HGH opposes the action of insulin. L-arginine and L-ornithine may improve or worsen diabetic conditions. There are no known side effects from taking a *homeopathic* version of HGH.

Hormone Therapy

Many people today reach for the quick fix of hormone-replacement therapy, but when they do, they are not addressing the *real* problem. Typical of our tendency toward narrow thinking, many endocrinologists are prescribing estrogen, progesterone, and perhaps testosterone and DHEA; however, your pituitary and hypothalamus glands are also part of your hormone-producing team. They need your focus and support as well. And of course, don't forget your liver. It *processes* your hormones, so the healthier it is, the healthier your entire endocrine system will be.

If your hormones have started to decline and you are seeing signs of a hormone imbalance, you must be asking yourself these questions: "Why have I become deficient in these youthening sexual hormones? How can I rejuvenate the organs that produce these hormones so that they'll begin to manufacture them once again?"

Bottom line . . . it is essential to evaluate, nourish, and rejuvenate your entire endocrine team—your hypothalamus, pituitary, thyroid, adrenals, and ovaries or testes in order to restimulate the production of HGH.

Women

Perimenopause can be a very difficult time for a woman today. When her hormones are out of balance, she'll feel quite unhinged until she finds her way to a savvy endocrinologist experienced in *bioidentical* hormone-replacement therapy. Most women believe that a decline in estrogen and progesterone is an inevitable part of menopause. But with proper diet and supplementation, it is possible to have healthy ovaries and adrenals (the two organs that produce most of your estrogen and progesterone) even if you have entered perimenopause or menopause.

Although a woman may benefit from testing and individualized hormone supplementation, the fact is that our hormones are always fluctuating throughout the day. Even bioidentical hormones, while a dramatic improvement over synthetic hormones, can never exactly mimic the fluctuations and rhythms of our own naturally produced hormones.

Testing your hormones at least twice a year is wise. However, you might consider postponing your next set of tests until *after* you've been on the Baby Boomer program for several months. Many women find that their hormones balance out significantly and that they no longer require hormone treatments, or they only need minimal amounts.

As a woman, you should know that when your estrogen levels drop, you will most likely suffer from low levels of two important, feel-good brain chemicals—serotonin and dopamine. These brain chemicals are very much related to mood and happiness.

Because low serotonin causes both depression and low self-esteem, you can see how this might negatively affect your relationships. Bad relationships seriously drain a woman's energy. Both stress and a diet of excessive animal protein are especially harmful for a woman, because they lower serotonin. A woman needs to feel calm and needs to eat much less animal protein than a man. Seasonal affective disorder (SAD), or a lack of exposure to sunlight, especially in the winter, also depresses serotonin levels.

With low serotonin levels you will find yourself craving carbohydrate-rich foods. You may have all the willpower in the world, but there is a true biological reason for your cravings for chocolate. Your brain is always trying to achieve balance and when stressed, wants to feel calm again. It's no surprise that chocolate is a woman's favorite food, as it increases endorphins and temporarily elevates both dopamine and serotonin.

Drugs that increase serotonin levels are not the answer. Low serotonin levels cause constipation, and while these "serotonin reuptake inhibitors" may temporarily relieve you of constipation, they soon *cause* it again as serotonin levels increase and then become too high. Healthier choices are the supplements 5HTP and tryptophan, an amino acid. Either can be taken in the morning or at bedtime to increase serotonin levels naturally.

While women have less dopamine in their brains than men do, you won't feel contented or at peace with life when your levels of this neurotransmitter are low. Declining levels of dopamine can lead to restless legs syndrome, fibromyalgia, or Parkinson-like symptoms. In midlife, this combination of declining estrogen and dopamine may create mood swings, severe hot flashes, night sweats, or sleep disturbances.

Fortunately, the amino-acid supplement tyrosine can help normalize dopamine levels in your brain. If you have cancer, do not take tyrosine, because certain types of cancer use amino acids to fuel their growth. If you are on an antidepressant medication, you should only take tyrosine under your doctor's supervision. Tyrosine affects mood, and you may need to adjust your dosage. Take tyrosine in the mornings as it can keep you up at night if you take it close to bedtime.

Mucuna pruriens, an ancient herb from India, also increases dopamine levels in the brain and can be taken at any time of the day. PEA (phenylalanine), the chemical found in chocolate and cocoa, increases dopamine as well. Klamath Lake blue-green algae is rich in PEA.

Clearly, because of the close connection between your hormones and your brain chemicals, it would be wise to have your doctor test your amino-acid levels to see what brain chemicals you may be deficient in.

Relationship expert John Gray, Ph.D., has written a fascinating book about our brain chemicals. It is a must-read for both men and women who want to better understand their emotions and behaviors and those of others. Dr. Gray's new book is called *Venus on Fire, Mars on Ice: Hormonal Balance—the Key to Life, Love, and Energy.*

Men

We sometimes forget that men also have their hormone challenges. Men should have their HGH, DHEA, and testosterone levels checked twice a year. In men, the hormone decline can be subtle and incremental. They may find that they aren't as self-confident or as motivated as they used to be, or may even struggle with depression or sadness. One day they wake up and find they're in the throes of the "grumpy old man" syndrome.

Acupuncture is an excellent therapy for balancing hormones in men, and Chinese tonic herbs mentioned earlier in this chapter help restore energy to the adrenal/kidney meridian in the body. Walking or other daily exercising is a must to keep levels of hormone like DHEA and HGH high, but even with exercise, it may be necessary to use a small amount of all three of these natural, *bioidentical* hormones.

Don't underestimate the importance of testosterone. It isn't just for sex drive and sperm count. It also helps maintain bone density, muscle mass, and red-blood-cell production. For most Baby Boomer men, a more noticeable decline in testosterone starts in the mid-40s, and so does this common yet unnecessary symptom of aging: a decrease in muscle mass with an increase in body fat. Unfortunately, reduced physical energy and endurance, gradually decreasing libido, loss of bone density, and an increase in cholesterol accompany this decline in testosterone. A deficiency of testosterone has even been cited as a precursor to cancer.

Dopamine is a brain chemical that is vital for a man's happiness, and it, too, decreases with age. Lower levels intensify the negative effects of low testosterone that are mentioned above. Anxiety, depression, cravings, or addictions all can be traced to low levels of dopamine. This neurotransmitter helps keep us alert, active, and motivated. Sexual desire and feelings of excitement and pleasure decline as dopamine declines. General symptoms of aging such as poor sleep; fatigue; depression; decreased muscle tone; and loss of cognitive functions, like memory, alertness, concentration, and decision making can become issues. A man with low dopamine levels loses his ability to make executive decisions.

Dopamine has a positive effect on heart and circulation. It keeps a man's metabolic rate high. As his metabolic rate declines he puts on weight. Dopamine is essential for control of movement. Numerous research studies have identified low levels of dopamine as a cause of Parkinson's disease. As mentioned previously, tyrosine, mucuna pruriens, and PEA from Klamath Lake blue-green algae help increase dopamine.

While today's Baby Boomer has the luxury of bioidentical hormones and natural supplements that increase neurotransmitters such as dopamine and serotonin, bioidentical hormones will soon be seen as merely a temporary bridge to something even better. With new inroads in stem-cell therapy, we will soon be able to produce these hormones again on our own.

Stem-Cell Therapy

There are few areas of medical science that are more fascinating and have as much potential for transforming how we think about healing, longevity, and quality of life than stem-cell research.

Whether used preventively or as an active intervention, stem cells are the latest anti-aging miracle. Found in almost all multicellular organisms, they are unique in that they not only have the capacity to renew themselves, but they are also able to *differentiate*—to develop into specialized cells that make up a variety of our organs and other tissues. They can literally transform themselves into any other type of cell in the body, which is why they have been called the "building blocks of nature," with potential to treat numerous diseases and traumatic injuries, as well as to regenerate entire organs.

You may not be aware of this, but you've been using stem cells your entire life. Think of them as the body's MASH unit—they see trauma and quickly mobilize to fix it. When you cut your finger or get a sunburn, it is stem cells that receive the alarm signal and rush in to repair the damage.

There are two basic kinds of stem cells—those found in most adult tissues and those found in the cells of three- to five-day-old embryos. Adult stem cells, found in brain, bone marrow, muscle, skin, blood, liver tissues, and especially adipose (fat) tissue, can change into most cell types.

The stem cells found in three- to five-day-old embryos (embryonic stem cells), on the other hand, are pluripotent—that is, they have the unique ability to develop into any of the 220 cell types in the human body.[8] But it's not just embryonic stem cells that have this ability—umbilical-cord and placental stem cells are also pluripotent. In fact, researchers have found strikingly similar characteristics between cells taken from the outer membranes of the amniotic sac and embryonic stem cells.

Bone-marrow transplants, a stem-cell therapy that has been used for many years as a treatment for leukemia and other types of cancer, is well known today. But as mentioned above, stem cells can also be derived from peripheral blood, umbilical-cord blood, the placenta, the Wharton's jelly in the lining of the umbilical cord, and even from menstrual blood.

But what does all this have to do with aging?

Boomers on the Cutting Edge

TA-65 Therapy
Startling Advances in the Science of Human Rejuvenation

*D*o you remember Leonard Hayflick from the chapter on the causes of aging? Well, he is intimately linked with a cutting-edge new anti-aging therapy that has had some amazing preliminary results. Hayflick was the pioneering scientist who believed that cells had a built-in obsolescence. He noted that even a healthy lifestyle could not ultimately stave off the slowing down and eventual cessation of cell division, which leads to death.

Some 35 years later, Elizabeth Blackburn and Jack Szostak discovered *telomeres* and the indispensable role they play in cellular protection. A few years later, in 1985, Carol Greider and Dr. Blackburn discovered the enzyme *telomerase* in the protozoa *tetrahymena*. They knew that telomerase synthesized in this organism, but they didn't know it was so intimately involved in human aging. Greider, Blackburn, and Szostak would go on to win the Nobel Prize in Medicine in 2009 for their explosive research.[i]

So what, in simple terms, do telomeres do? Some people have likened telomeres to the piece of plastic at the end of our shoelace that protects it from fraying. Over time that plastic wears down. Our cellular chromosomes are the same. They have a protective casing around them, like the skin around a grape. These protective end pieces are called telomeres, and they hold our chromosomes together and help them to replicate. In short, they are essential for maintaining the integrity or structure of our DNA.[ii]

As you know, our cells divide over and over again throughout our lifetime; and each time they do, these telomeres get a little shorter, and our chromosomes weaken. These shortened telomeres cause cell senescence (aging), which in turn leads to what used to be considered the "inevitable" signs of growing old, such as diminished sex drive, loss of energy, wrinkles . . . and eventually death. By the time we hit our 80s, our telomeres are quite short, and shorter still if we've neglected ourselves through bad food, lack of exercise, drug abuse, and so forth.

The only cells that have telomerase turned on permanently are reproductive cells. This makes sense, because without it, babies would not be born as babies. They would have telomeres as short as their aging parents. These shortened telomeres are also directly linked to some of the major illnesses we associate with aging, such as degenerative and rheumatoid arthritis, Alzheimer's and dementia, various cancers, myocardial infarction, and congestive heart failure.

So, what if there was a substance that could actually lengthen our telomeres? Well, there is! It's a Chinese herb called *astragalus*. Used in traditional Chinese medicine for thousands of years, astragalus actually *lengthens* these chromosomal end pieces.

A biopharmaceutical company named Geron Corporation set out to create an anti-aging therapy derived from astragalus. They called it TA-65®, and it is the first and only safe telomerase activator on the market today.

TA-65 is only available through a health-care professional who has been approved by T.A. Sciences, the company licensed to sell it. In other words, TA-65 is not an FDA-approved drug, but a nutritional supplement. However, a significant amount of clinical research backs up the early claims made for TA-65. It has been shown to lengthen the shortest telomeres (those most likely to put a cell into crisis), and improve immune function and bone mass. In double-blind, placebo-controlled studies, it was discovered that those who took the therapy saw improvements in eyesight, their immune systems, and their sexual performance. Their skin was restored to its former elasticity and youthfulness.[iii]

So far, TA-65 is considered safe. There have been no reports of toxicity, and no one has discontinued the drug because of adverse reactions.

For some years, TA-65 was prohibitively expensive and out of the reach of most people. Recently, this price has dropped considerably, and its anti-aging benefits are well worth the cost (approximately $600 per month).

Not only do I love the science behind TA-65, but it also helps me enjoy a deeper night's sleep and gives me that extra energy I need each day. I was so sold on its value—not only for Baby Boomers, but also for those who are nearing midlife and may have prematurely shortened their telomeres through poor lifestyle choices—that I became a licensed practitioner. Expect more products to come on the market that are targeted at lengthening our telomeres. Again, we live in an amazing time!

[i]T.A. Sciences Team, "T.A. Sciences Cell Rejuvenation through Telomerase Activation," *T.A. Sciences Educational Manual*, December 9, 2010: 4.

[ii]Natural Health Dossier Research Team, "Cracking the Genetic Code to Youth: The Chinese Herb That Can Turn Back Your Biological Clock 10–20 Years," **www.naturalhealthdossier.com** (accessed 6/9/11).

[iii]T.A. Sciences Team, "T.A. Sciences Cell Rejuvenation through Telomerase Activation," *T.A. Sciences Educational Manual*, December 9, 2010: 13–15.

Stem-Cell Therapeutics and Aging

The first implication for aging should be obvious. When organs fail or wear out over time, stem cells may have the capacity to bring them back to life again. In this sense, stem cells might be used to restore our prenatal energy, to grow new teeth, replace exhausted livers and kidneys, and repair damaged limbs. Imagine if our adrenals and glands such as the hypothalamus, pituitary, and pineal thyroid could be reenergized with stem cells? Phase III trials in the U.S. are revealing how stem-cell products might address a range of indications, including osteoarthritis, Alzheimer's, heart disease, Crohn's, and Parkinson's, particularly when treated in the early stages. Furthermore, in Panama there have been several cases in which spinal-cord injuries were reversed; and numerous cases of multiple sclerosis, rheumatoid arthritis, and autism markedly improving using both allogenic (donor) umbilical-cord cells and autologous (native) bone marrow, and adipose-derived stem cells.

And there are cosmetic impacts as well—for example, *mesenchymal* stem cells, which are particularly effective at rebuilding tissue, bolstering immunity, and combatting inflammation, have been used as anti-aging treatments, offering patients noted improvements in restoring hair to its original color, creating a smoother complexion, and reducing age-related pigmentation marks.[9]

Scientists have recently found a type of stem cell in hair follicles that is capable of making epidermis, sebaceous tissue, and more hair follicles—in short, new skin and hair. Paul Sanberg, professor of neurosurgery and director of the

University of South Florida Center of Excellence for Aging and Brain Repair, points out the profound implications this could have for cosmetic skin repair and grafting, and perhaps even for hair replacement.[10]

But there's a second, possibly more important thing to understand about stem cells. Research and early clinical studies have proven that stem cells can release nutritional or "trophic" factors that can be of great benefit. At the University of Buffalo in New York, mesenchymal stem cells (MSCs) were injected into hamster-leg skeletal muscles. Not only did the MSCs not migrate away from the target area, but they also released trophic factors that traveled to and repaired the severely damaged heart.

What's more, just injecting the trophic factors without the cells into leg skeletal muscle had about the same benefit as the cells did! This has huge clinical implications . . . think how wonderful it would be to treat heart disease and many other conditions with either intramuscular shots of MSCs or even just the trophic factors. For those interested in learning more, please see the free online article entitled "Heart failure therapy mediated by the trophic activities of bone-marrow mesenchymal stem cells: a noninvasive therapeutic regimen" (available at: **www.ncbi.nlm.nih.gov/pmc/articles/PMC2716100**).

As we get older, our stem-cell reserves decline, we aren't able to produce new ones, and the ones that we have become less robust. But scientists are discovering that the environment in which these cells exist also matters. If that environment is inflamed, it can impede the functionality of stem cells—they can no longer do what they are intended to do.

A study conducted at the University of South Florida has found that the injection of human umbilical-cord cells can assist an aging brain. When umbilical-cord blood cells (UCBCs) were injected into aged laboratory animals, improvements were found in the microenvironment of the hippocampus (an area of the brain that plays an important role in long-term memory and spatial navigation), and there was also a measurable rejuvenation of the neural stem/progenitor cells. "Brain cell neurogenesis (new cell development) decreases dramatically with increasing age, mostly because of a growing impoverishment in the brain's microenvironment," says study co-author Alison Willing, Ph.D., of the Center of Excellence for Aging and Brain Repair.

According to researchers, the decrease in neurogenesis that accompanies aging is a result of a decrease in proliferation of new stem cells, not the loss of existing cells. However, the improvements they saw did not come from direct replacement of cells but by changing the microenvironment of the brain in which the cells reside. Willing added: "The increase in neurogenesis we saw after injecting UCBCs seemed to be due to a decrease in inflammation."[11]

Once again we see the enormous role that inflammation plays in aging. Do you remember the factors that cause inflammation? (See Chapter 3.) Food with pesticides, environmental pollutants, mercury in the air we breathe, overuse of cell phones and computers, excess body fat, poor diet, lack of exercise, and even genetic predisposition can contribute to inflammation in the body. As we age and become more inflamed, our brains shrink, and the stem cells that might be on the ready to repair them just aren't functioning as well anymore.

In fact, any of the above can contribute to neurotoxicity, and can lead to disabling genetic defects in the neural stem cells. Research in rats has shown a 2-month-old rat will have about twice as many neural stem cells as a 24-month-old rat. This loss in brain stem cells is likely tied to most all neurodegeneration that occurs with advanced aging, or even earlier if there is enough neurotoxicity present.[12]

The implications of this should be obvious. People who live a healthy lifestyle have lower inflammatory markers, which prevent healthy stem cells from being released. Lifestyle can turn down the "hot-water faucets" of inflammation inside us and create the kind of healthy environment we need to get those stem cells activated.

If you eat well, sleep deeply, exercise regularly, are well hydrated, and have high/normal vitamin D levels, many more stem cells will be released from your bone marrow and you will age slowly. With this new understanding of stem cells, medical textbooks will now have to be rewritten to say that in many ways, death and aging are a sign of insufficient stem-cell production in your bone marrow. Viruses and toxins from heavy metals, pesticides, and chemicals cause mitochondrial failure in your bone-marrow cells so that they cannot produce healthy stem cells.

Exercise Mobilizes Stem Cells

It's especially important to note that exercise is one of the primary ways we can create new stem cells. When we exercise, there are six to eight times more stem cells present in our peripheral blood. Here's an example of what exercise can do for one area of the body in which we often see signs of aging—our brains.

As we age, our cortisol levels increase, and the hippocampus decreases in size. The hippocampus, as noted before, is related to memory and plays a big role in dementia. Exercise can help the hippocampus to regenerate. A stem cell will re-create the cell that is needed, in this case a neural cell, and at the same time it will replicate itself. Working with aged mice, researchers in Florida have demonstrated that a single injection of human umbilical cord blood mononuclear cells (HUCBMCs) can rejuvenate a mouse's hippocampus and supply of neural stem-cell progenitors. The aged mouse brains also began producing new nerves. And this type of therapy doesn't have to be invasive. It can be introduced into the peripheral veins (injected in the arm) rather than directly into the brain.[13]

So, basically we've added a new theory of aging—the *stem-cell theory*. We age because we stop releasing adequate numbers of stem cells. What we eat, how we think, the people we surround ourselves with, and how many toxins we are storing in our bodies all impede the activation of these cells. Rejuvenation begins with the reactivation of weaker, dying cells first, followed by the restoration of new stem cells that have been lost.

Other studies have shown that the optimal conditions for stem-cell release are related to being properly rested—this means that sleeping regularly and restoratively, managing our stress, and finding balance in our lives can affect the maximal release of stem cells. Paul S. Frenette, M.D., professor in the Department of Medicine at Mount Sinai School of Medicine, writes: "We don't know why stem cells circulate in the blood but the maximal release of stem cells in the circulation occurs when the animal is resting. This argues for a role in regeneration."[14]

One of the most exciting uses of stem cells has been the regeneration of tissues. Anthony Atala, M.D., the head of the regeneration program at Wake Forest University, stated that his researchers have grown nearly two dozen different types of body parts, including muscle, bone, and a working heart valve. He went on to say: "I think if we start combining things like better prevention, better care, doing things better for our body, and just with regenerative medicine, we may push [our life spans] up to 120, 130 years."[15]

New Discoveries on the Stem-Cell Frontier

Dr. Leonard Smith, medical advisor for this book, is a volunteer on the surgical staff at the University of Miami, and medical advisor for the University of Miami Department of Integrative Medicine. He is also a consultant for the Institute for Cellular Medicine, which specializes in research and clinical stem-cell therapy, and publishes articles on stem cells in peer-reviewed journals. Located in Panama City, Panama, the Institute has treated more than a thousand patients.

When researchers at the Institute began their work five years ago, they worked solely with umbilical-cord stem cells. Today, they also use bone-marrow cells and fat-derived stem cells from liposuction, with good results, especially in the area of autoimmune diseases. Promising outcomes have also been seen for autistic children and people suffering from multiple sclerosis, renal and heart failure, rheumatoid arthritis, and osteoarthritis. In addition, they have treated several paraplegics with spinal-cord injuries who are now recovering nicely, including walking again.

Now affiliated with several universities, the work done at the Institute may be on the cutting edge of stem-cell advances. (For more information on the Institute for Cellular Medicine, go to: **www.cellmedicine.com**.) There are increasing numbers of stem-cell clinical trials now taking place in the U.S., mostly at universities. There are, however, some publicly traded companies doing stem-cell trials. One such company, Osiris, is conducting ongoing clinical trials on type 1 autoimmune diabetes and graft-versus-host disease. As these trials continue, it will become obvious how stem-cell therapy has the potential to benefit humankind in many ways.

Classic Cell Therapy

Stem-cell therapy has marvelous potential for the treatment of our most feared illnesses, but it is primarily aimed at a single disease process or traumatic injury. There is another kind of cell therapy that offers anti-aging benefits. It complements stem-cell therapy because it doesn't just treat a single organ or gland, but reaches into *all* organs, endocrine glands, and connective tissues. We call this more comprehensive kind of cell rejuvenation "classic cell therapy" to differentiate it from stem-cell therapy.

Classic cell therapy was introduced by Dr. Paul Niehans of Montreux, Switzerland, in 1931, when he injected calf parathyroid into a patient whose parathyroid glands had been damaged during thyroid surgery. The patient survived and went on to live a healthy life into her 90s. Variations of this method have been practiced in the 80 years since then, and during his lifetime, Dr. Niehans went on to treat many heads of state and movie stars of the World War II era and beyond.

The goal of classic cell therapy is to slow, and even reverse, biological aging. The focus is on the immune and endocrine systems, as well as connective tissue. Breakdown in these areas is the cause of aging and is responsible for most chronic disease.

The cells used in classic cell therapy are slightly more mature than stem cells, resulting in an organ-specific cellular serum. The tremendous advantage to this is that the cellular serum can be administered intramuscularly and will migrate to the target organ—that is, heart to heart, lung to lung, and so forth. This has been demonstrated by radioisotope tracing studies.

Further studies at the Pathological Institute of Munich University have shown that protein biosynthesis in the targeted organ will increase by up to 100 percent compared to untreated organs, resulting in renewed vitality and function, commensurate with a younger biological age.

My good friend Judi Smith, with the International Clinic of Biological Regeneration, has developed a protocol reflecting more than 30 years of experience in the field and major pharmaceutical advancements. This protocol is designed to treat the body as a whole, and then to target specific organs/glands relating to immune and endocrine function, the connective tissue, and skin, as well as the pituitary, hypothalamus, and adrenal glands, to support immune function and reduce inflammation. Other serum preparations can be customized to address the specific concerns of the individual patient. This combination, particularly when administered periodically, can have significant positive impact on both appearance and vitality.

The idea is to look and feel as great as you can, as long as you can, and to have the vital energy to pursue your interests and passions. While classic cell therapy can't prevent aging entirely, it can slow it down considerably. And now, of course, you hold a "bible" in your hands that provides you with all you must do to actually reverse the "hands of time."

Our knowledge of stem-cell, trophic, and gene therapy is evolving at a tremendous speed. With new insights being reported every day, this is an exciting time to be alive—for Boomers and every generation.

Healthy Sexuality—Doing It Without Drugs

For many people "life after 40" includes more satisfying and meaningful sexual relationships. The urgent hormonal drives we experienced when we were younger will have abated a bit, and most of us are no longer focused on conception and starting a family. But these changes in lifestyle and drive don't mean we no longer want, or can't have, fulfilling intimate relationships. In fact, with more of us single today than at any other time, we Boomers are more willing to enjoy our sexuality and meet each other in nontraditional ways, such as online social-media sites. And because women of this generation tend to be more educated, career-oriented, and affluent, they aren't necessarily dating in order to "settle down" and get married. They view their sexual relationships as just one more aspect of a fulfilling life.

It should be noted, however, that many Boomers, who came of age before the HIV epidemic, don't have a sense of the dangers of sex that younger generations do. Women over 50 are at risk of developing HIV from heterosexual sex because their thinner vaginal walls are more susceptible to cuts and tears. The number of new HIV infections among older women is rising, and AIDS cases among women 50 and older nearly doubled between 1988 and 2000.[16]

And what about sexual-performance issues, particularly in men, whose problems with erectile dysfunction dramatically increase with age? Too often, Boomers have a "quick fix" approach to sexual problems or waning sexual energy. If something isn't working, or isn't working as it did when we were 18, we reach for a pill. But magic pills like Viagra and Levitra don't address the underlying conditions that may be producing sexual dysfunction, and for many, they simply don't work at all.

Al Sears, a Fort Lauderdale physician, has developed a 12-minute exercise program called PACE, which advocates shorter bursts of intense exertion as a healthier means of losing weight and staying fit. It has the added benefit of improving one's sexual performance. Short bursts of vigorous exercise cause an increase in blood flow and boost the supply of nitric oxide in the body. Being able to release nitric oxide is critical to erection of the male penis and female clitoris for sexual responsiveness. Our supply of nitric oxide declines as we age, and this is one reason why older men and women often report declining performance in the bedroom.

High-intensity workouts are a great way of improving nitric-oxide production, but as we grow older this can be more challenging, as we have less stamina during rigorous exercise. Sears recommends a more incrementally intensive program that allows exercisers to control and manage their own progression.

Sears's PACE program increases endorphins—those feel-good chemicals in the body—as well as brain chemicals, like serotonin and dopamine, which make us feel content yet excited about life. Peri- and postmenopausal women, in particular, can be quite low in endorphins and brain chemicals because these decline as estrogen declines. HGH and testosterone levels also increase dramatically when we exercise.

The PACE program is a form of interval training that uses running as the mode of exercise. This is fine, but for many people over age 40, running may be too stressful on the joints, ligaments, and tendons. Rapid walking may be more appropriate and is just as effective. Interval training with swimming, with elliptical cross-training machines, and even with weights can be done. *The key is to exercise at maximum or near maximum intensity for 10 to 60 seconds and then rest or go slower for 30 seconds to two minutes, and then go fast again.* Interval training increases the release of HGH, insulin-like growth factor one (IGF-1), and testosterone; and helps lower blood sugar and sensitize insulin receptors. All of these are critical for optimal sexual performance for both men and women.

In addition, this program increases the intake of oxygen by increasing the capacity of our lungs and preventing them from shrinking with age. This in turn ensures that our energy levels rise; excess fat is burned; and the anti-aging process is

Boomers on the Cutting Edge

Tantric Sex

*M*any people have misguided notions about tantric sex, assuming it must involve never-before-discovered erogenous zones, techniques, and positions. Basically, tantric sex is "What's the hurry?" sex. For most people, the typical sexual experience lasts approximately 15 minutes, yet most women take at least 20 minutes to climax. What's wrong with this picture? Tantric sex is *sensual sex,* intimacy that focuses on extending the sexual experience and satisfying your partner on a spiritual and emotional level, as well as on a physical one.

activated by the dynamic regeneration of cells and tissues inside the body, including increasing the number and function of mitochondria, our energy producers.

Like most exercise, interval training will also decrease total body inflammation as long as you don't overdo it. Remember to start slowly, then gradually increase the intensity and decrease the amount of time in between each exercise.

Here is a PACE outdoor-running workout proposed by Dr. Sears.[17]

1. **Warm up.** Warm up for about one or two minutes.

2. **Start.** Once you're warmed up, start at low to moderate intensity, and increase the level of intensity after each set. Start first by running (or walking rapidly) for two minutes.

3. **Recover.** Now relax. Notice your heartbeat, and keep track of how long it takes to get back to normal.

4. **Repeat.** Then run for 90 seconds, followed by rest. Repeat this; and decrease the exertion period each time from 90 seconds to 45 to 30 and then to 20 seconds for a total of six sets. This shouldn't take more than eight to ten minutes.

Whole-Body Vibration
A Way to Enjoy the Benefits of Exercise

When you hear the words *vibration machine,* you might get a mental image of an overweight woman wearing a wildly vibrating belt that shakes and bounces the cellulite from her hips. Fortunately, we've come a long way from those funny contraptions of the 1950s! In fact, vibration technology is said to be the medicine of the future and the ideal anti-aging tool. I own a machine and love it.

The first generation of whole-body vibration machines appeared on the market in the '70s, and today there are more than 30 different companies making them, ranging in price from $700 to $15,000. They can be found in the homes of professional athletes, dancers, entertainers, physical therapists, doctors, and authors. However, it pays to do your homework before purchasing one.

How Whole-Body Vibration Works

With most whole-body vibration machines, you stand on a platform that vibrates rapidly with a motor that creates either a vertical, a vertical and horizontal, or a seesaw movement. On the motor-driven machines, you stand on a platform and do workout sessions and resistance-training exercises. This produces very effective results in a shorter time than without the machine. While motor-driven machines are mostly for exercise, they do cleanse your lymph system and stimulate circulation. A professional trainer will give you the best results and customize workouts for your unique body type, changing them as needed. All machines come with educational materials that demonstrate how to use the equipment in your home.

Motor vs. Sound-Wave Vibration

The safest and most medicinal whole-body vibration machines use sound waves under the platform to create a vertical vibration that can be adjusted, offering a wider range of vibrational frequencies and medicinal benefits. You can stand or sit on these machines and can practice qigong or meditate. If you have a weaker constitution or an injury, or are struggling with osteoporosis, this is the vibration machine for you. The motor-driven ones can be injurious to hips and knees, while the sound-vibration ones are softer and gentler—perfect if you have physical limitations. And if you just won't exercise because you lack the time or desire, sound-vibration machines provide the benefits of exercising without the exercising.

My own sound-wave-vibration machine—the TurboSonic X5—stands proudly in my home (**www.turbosonicusa.com**).

The Benefits of Whole-Body Sound Vibration

In addition to feeling and looking vibrant when you step off of a sound-vibration machine, you will immediately notice improvements in balance, a common problem as we age. The gentle vibration stimulates the middle ear so your sense of equilibrium improves; while you also build muscle, tendon, and ligament strength. But there are many other benefits:

- Cleanses the lymph system and stimulates circulation

- Improves blood pressure, digestion, sleep, stress, and overall mood

- Stimulates healthier, more resilient cells

- Creates stronger, better-defined muscles

- Lowers cortisol and naturally increases bone density, testosterone, and growth hormone

- Promotes cellular waste removal, increasing your ability to detoxify

Exercise is just one way to bolster healthy sexuality. Dr. Ridwan Shabsigh, a certified urologist specializing in sexual health, encourages people to see their sex lives in the context of better overall health. He points to the conditions that can contribute to sexual dysfunction—from diabetes and obesity; to cardiovascular disease, depression, and drug and alcohol abuse. Dr. Shabsigh's holistic approach looks at overall lifestyle choices—diet, exercise, supplements, stress reduction, avoidance of self-destructive behaviors, and commitment to a partner—and how these issues can positively or negatively affect sexual function.[18]

There's no reason why sex can't be "sensational" as we age, argues Shabsigh, and for many, sexual intimacy is better than ever before because we've learned and grown wiser from past relationships. We are much more in tune with our bodies now, and we are, in turn, more attuned and attentive to the needs of our partners.

As the years come and go, you may no longer have the sexual motivation you used to have. You may be resigned to this and feel that your desire for sex has become a lesser priority than other things, like self-discovery, grandchildren, friendship, and travel. Perhaps you've been told that as you age your sexual energy will become directed outward to more spiritual and service-oriented activities.

True, this has been the norm for previous generations, because they did not have the resources to stop the decline in hormones, endorphins, and brain chemicals that keep us looking and feeling sexy. But healthy levels of sexual hormones, equal to those present when we were in our 20s, give us a love for life that can still be directed into both service-oriented activities *and* an active sex life.

Indeed, sexual energy *is* spiritual energy. Sexual energy is the sacred energy of creation. As members of an extraordinary generation that has brought about so much change, we certainly can and should enjoy healthy sexuality throughout our lives.

Chapter 27

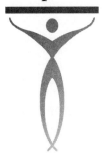

What Survives of Us: Our Mission for the Next 50 Years

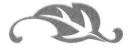

For Baby Boomers, always transforming and defying expectations, our greatest test will be how we handle and redefine aging.
How will we live . . . and what will survive of us?

I began writing the first chapter of this book sitting on the white, pristine beaches in Jupiter, Florida. Four years later, as I write the last one, I sit on the opposite coast of this great country, near Venice Beach, California.

It's interesting how reflective you become when you sit near the ocean. It is so vast and permanent—an ever-changing witness to millions of years of life. It humbles me, because unlike these ancient waters, my life is transient.

Scientists say that approximately 6,000 years ago a great flood occurred and the earth was completely covered with water. This flooding is depicted in the biblical tale of Noah's ark and in the legends of many other cultures. With the real threat of famine, disease, polluted water and air, infertility, childhood diseases, and on and on, it seems we may once again need a modern "ark" as our means of survival.

We have certainly been made aware of these dangers for some time.

In 1962, while the oldest Baby Boomers were still in high school and the youngest were learning to talk, a scientist named Rachel Carson wrote a forward-looking and penetrating book called *Silent Spring.* Carson warned us then that human-made chemicals were interfering with the development of our own offspring. She was right. Her book had huge pre-publication sales, was serialized in the *New York Times Magazine* prior to publication, and was on the *New York Times* bestseller list for more than 30 weeks. Reaction to its content was loudly and publicly debated. It also inspired a small group of field biologists to begin observing widespread evidence of damage in the birds, fish, and other wildlife throughout the Great Lakes. For their efforts they were reprimanded and given lateral transfers, and their findings were stuffed away in the bottom drawer of a supervisor's desk . . . never published.

> *Our universal purpose as a generation and as individuals is to become a doorway for change and to help nourish righteous action so that a superior way of life is born.*

Thirty-five years later, Theo Colborn wrote a book that picked up where *Silent Spring* left off—*Our Stolen Future.* She, too, warned us that human-made chemicals interfere with the natural ones that tell our cells, tissues, and organs how to develop and function. In her acceptance speech for the Rachel Carson Leadership Award in 1997 she said:

> Scientists now realize that although effects have been reported in adults who were directly exposed to some of these chemicals, the most sensitive period to exposure occurs prenatally and shortly after birth. The damage is insidious and irreversible and expressed in offspring as inconspicuous loss of function. These are population-wide effects, unlike cancer, acute toxicity, and obvious birth defects. Your children, their children, and all future children are at risk.[1]

It Falls to Us to Change Our Direction

Once the enormous wave of Baby Boomers began entering this world, we changed it forever. In some ways, it is a better place—in many other ways, it is not.

Clearly, our influence as a generation cannot be denied. If we choose, our ability to continue to effect enormous change on this planet is far from over.

Many of us born between 1946 and 1964 are finally waking up to the fact that we are heading in the wrong direction and cannot continue on this flawed path any longer. I am quite concerned about the younger generations and *their* future. I am sure you are as well.

Over the course of more than 20 years of training and working in the area of natural foods and healing, I have wondered why we are not doing more to stop the suffering we see around us. For many decades to come, there will be a great deal of pain and heartbreak for all of us because those who suffer the most will be the younger generations.

So far, we haven't really taken heed of the red flags all around us, yet we still have great potential to reverse our course. Like Noah, let's create an "ark" together and try to save our own families, friends, and the animals we share the planet with. The Body Ecology Way of Life can be a kind of "ark," with answers that will lend us strength through these troubled times.

But how does each one of us give purpose to our time spent here on Earth? First, we need to experience a calling, a true and passionate conviction about what we want our lives to *mean*.

Finding Your Passion

As teens, we asked the questions *Who am I?* and *Why am I here?* As adults, we are still asking ourselves questions, but they have changed, and we have more of them.

We are now asking: *Who have I become? Has my existence really mattered? I'm here now, but how much time do I have left? Will I leave behind a meaningful legacy? Is there more I need to do?*

Science won't give us the answers to those questions . . . but if we look with our "spiritual eye," the answers become crystal clear.

Our *universal purpose* as a generation and as individuals is to become a doorway for change and to help nourish righteous action so that a superior way of life is born.

We are willing to make personal sacrifices to get things back on track. After all, the lives of our children and grandchildren depend upon it.

We *will* change . . . because survival is the strongest force in nature, and if we don't change, we humans won't survive. This ocean in front of me will once again be witness to the ending of another civilization.

So, how do you want to use your current interests, skills, and passions to influence the world around you?

About 20 years ago, it began to dawn on me that we were created to serve, and that we are happiest when we are making a difference in the world around us. While you may have purchased this book to learn the secrets to recapturing your constitutional "prenatal jing," there is an even more deep-seated reason for us to recapture the vibrancy of our youth—we must regain the power we had in our youth to transform this planet before we leave.

Indeed, it is why we came. We cannot become a burden to the younger generations who will have to care for us if we are no longer able to care for ourselves. Clearly, we must focus our intention on a common purpose, and we cannot leave here until our mission is complete.

Finding Your Tribe

In the past, a tribe was a clan of people who descended from a common ancestor. A tribe today can be defined as a group of people or a "subfamily" that holds common interests or a collective passion. Together they share knowledge and find and implement solutions.

In Seth Godin's book *Tribes,* he talks about how the *individual* has more power than ever before to create change. When people have a shared interest and a shared way of communicating that interest, "miracles" happen. The legacy of the Boomers—to challenge the status quo and act from a place of vision—is now bringing an entirely new business and social-change culture to the world. As Godin says, *heretics* have become the new leaders. These new leaders don't "manage." They connect and inspire. They are not concerned with earnings reports. They are concerned with leveraging skills and resources in ways that make palpable change in suffering lives.[2]

Baby Boomers are a powerful tribe.

With our enormous resources . . . our wisdom, our talents, and our wealth . . . we are more ready than ever to have an intentional and positive impact in the world.

And we are generous.

According to the Corporation for National and Community Service, volunteering in America is at a 30-year high. In fact, the number of Americans volunteering in their communities jumped by 1.6 million in 2009, the largest increase in six years.[3] And Baby Boomers have made more charitable contributions than any other age-group. Their interest in and commitment to volunteerism are the primary reasons for a 37 percent increase in volunteering among midlife Americans since 1989 (from 23.2 percent in 1974 and 22 percent in 1989 to 30 percent in 2005).[4]

What makes the way we give unique? Well, first, we are noticeably more engrossed in making use of our existing expertise and interests, and we want our volunteer activities to reflect our beliefs and what we care about. We have high expectations, want diversity of choice, and tend to bypass opportunities that we don't find interesting or challenging. "Making a difference" is the top reason why we volunteer, and because we see retirement as a new chapter to our lives rather than an ending, we are more upbeat about the future and always on the lookout for ways to stay involved and learn new skills.[5]

Sweeping and transformative change is not something that only Boomers do. In fact, our children may be even more successful at it than we are.

More and more universities are changing the focus and curriculum of their business programs. Why? Because their students are demanding it! Schools like the University of Maryland have made social entrepreneurship a priority, giving students the opportunity to align entrepreneurial vision and problem solving with philanthropy and social change. See: **www.rhsmith.umd.edu/svc**.

Baby Boomers won't follow the sedentary ways of our aging parents, nor will we allow ourselves to become as isolated. In the 1960s, some of us became hippies and tried to live in communes or ashrams, but we weren't mature enough to make these succeed. Still, we have retained that deep need to connect with others and build community. And today we are creating new communes and tribes where we can be bonded with passionate members like ourselves—even if they live across a vast ocean—by using technology such as online social networks.

Mother Teresa often said that isolated people are the poorest people on the planet. Don't let loneliness and separation enclose your life as the years fly by. Get involved. Become a member of a tribe that shares *your* passions.

Envisioning the "Coffee Shop" the Body Ecology Way—a New Kind of Fast Food

*M*ore and more people are working virtually. Today, as many as one in five employees avail themselves of some type of telework, and this number will only grow as we become more technologically self-sufficient. For the self-employed or the telecommuter, the coffee shop has become an all-important meeting place to network and conduct business. But with the typical coffee shop serving caffeinated beverages and fatty/sweet pastries, what is the health-conscious person supposed to do? Many diets fail because they are by nature "antisocial"—they force people to avoid social situations where unhealthy and fattening food is served. This isolation causes many dieters to feel despondent, which in turn makes them want to eat and return to their old habits! For the healthy Baby Boomer today, the coffee shop has become a Catch-22.

But what if someone were to start a chain of "probiotic cafés"—places where people could meet in a more communal setting, socialize, do their work, and eat healthfully at the same time? Instead of a caffeine buzz, customers would enjoy the rush of a CocoBiotic cocktail or a green smoothie, or an anti-aging soup. Wouldn't it be great if you could order your favorite fermented foods as takeout, or enjoy a dessert that satisfies the munchies but doesn't pack on the pounds?

What Is Your Passion? Where Is Your Tribe?

Is your passion food? Consider taking a workshop on how to use whole foods to make quick, inexpensive meals. You can pass on what you've learned to your busy adult children.

Is your passion sustainable agriculture? Join your local Slow Food movement (**www.slowfoodusa.org**), or get involved in your community's farmers' market. If none exists, start one!

Is your passion exercise? Perhaps you will be the person who develops a radical new and fun program to motivate sedentary people to become active and strong so that they are not as prone to injury and illness in their later years.

Is your passion educating children? Why not start a garden at a nearby school or in your community? These local gardens are a great way to get kids outdoors and to teach them about vegetables and other healthy foods. They can actually see the food growing; it helps them make a connection between what's on their plates and where it came from.

Is it your passion to go back to school and learn? I love to learn, and I love to teach. And I am passionate about changing the way the world eats because I know how important this is. I think my greatest love is to teach young women how to create beautiful, healthy babies. I also love giving online classes and teleseminars to explain the Body Ecology Way to anyone and everyone who wants to learn.

Find something that ignites your passion and do it. Your chances of being successful are very high because you have earned wisdom from your successes and failures.

Our Final Chapter—a New Beginning

In another 30 years, the oldest of us Boomers will be hitting our 90s; the youngest of us will only be in our 70s. Imagine what *you* can accomplish with another 30 years of energy to pursue your dreams. Imagine what we will have accomplished as a generation in that much time as we harmonize our amazing resources!

Never underestimate the power of one person! *You* can make a huge difference in the world—and with social-media outlets such as blogs, Facebook, and Twitter, it has never been easier to do. A new idea or theory, new research, and especially new solutions can find their way around the world in a matter of minutes.

An eternal optimist, I know we can overcome the many challenges facing us, and I am certain that you know this, too. That is why I wrote this book.

I want us *all* to have the energy we need to create a healthier, happier world by serving in the way each of us is trained or is called to do. I wrote this book for *you*.

Yes, Baby Boomers are witnessing an era coming to an end. Yet, as we all know so well, every ending is also a new beginning. We are the generation given the task to open the door to a new and much better way of life. You are alive now in these ending/beginning times; and when you focus on restoring *your* vital energy to serve, you can help herald a shiny, bright new beginning. . . .

Nourish your body and your soul well . . . and when you draw your last breath, you can proudly say, "*My life really mattered. I'm glad I came.*"

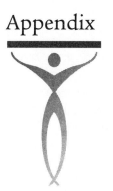

Appendix

The Body Ecology
Diet Shopping List

Buy organic foods whenever possible.

A sensitivity to any one of the foods in this list, while uncommon, is *not* uncommon when you have digestive problems and immune deficiency. As you create a healthy inner ecosystem, and strengthen your digestion and immune system, you should soon be able to enjoy most of these foods. But remember the Principle of Uniqueness. Find foods that work best for your unique body. We have carefully examined the ingredients in the brand names mentioned below and have given them the Body Ecology stamp of approval (Υ). As we learn about new safe and delicious foods and products that help you become even healthier, we will expand and update this list.

ANIMAL PROTEIN
(Free from antibiotics or hormones)
Eggs, from free-range poultry (the best come directly from the farmer)
Fish and fish eggs (roe), cold-water, fresh, and frozen
Premium grass-fed ground beef (one supplier we like is White Oak Pastures [Bluffton, GA], available at Whole Foods and Publix Markets)
Free-range poultry
Natural beef and turkey hot dogs and sausage (Applegate Farms: **www.applegatefarms.com**)

—◦◦◦—

BAKING PRODUCTS
Alcohol-free flavoring extracts
(Frontier: **www.frontiercoop.com**; St. John's Botanicals: **www.stjohnsbotanicals.com**; and The Spicery Shoppe)
Baking powder
(Hain Pure Foods: **www.hainpurefoods.com**)
Pure vanilla powder (Nielsen-Massey Vanillas, Inc.: **www.nielsenmassey.com**)

—◦◦◦—

BUTTER/GHEE
(Preferably from grass-fed cows; many grass-feeding farmers advertise butter in *Wise Traditions in Food, Farming, and the Healing Arts*, the journal of the Weston A. Price Foundation)
Body Ecology's **Culture Starter**
(for homemade cultured butter—even raw)
X-Factor Gold High-Vitamin Butter Oil
(Green Pasture Products: **www.greenpasture.org**)
Butter (raw best)
Ghee, also called clarified butter
(Purity Farms is organic: **www.purityfarms.com**)

—◦◦◦—

DAIRY*
(Visit **www.realmilk.com** for sources near you)
Hawthorne Valley Farm raw cow's milk
(NY: **www.hawthornevalleyfarm.org**)

Claravale Farm raw cow's milk
(CA: **http://claravaledairy.com**)
Organic Pastures raw cow's milk
(CA: **www.organicpastures.com**)
Sweetwoods Dairy raw goat's milk (NM: 505-465-2608)
Peaceful Pastures raw cow's and goat's milk (TN: **www
.peacefulpastures.com**)

—∿∿—

ENZYMES

Body Ecology's **Assist™ Full Spectrum Plant Digestive
Enzyme Formula** (for vegetarian meals)
Body Ecology's **Assist™ Dairy & Protein**
(effectively digests animal-protein meals)
Body Ecology's **Assist SI™**
(digests protein, carbs, and fats in small intestines; use
at every meal)

—∿∿—

FERMENTED FOODS

Body Ecology has starter cultures for making raw cultured
vegetables, cultured butter, and sour cream, as well
as kefir starter for making traditional milk kefir,
young coconut kefir, and kefir cheese. Body Ecology
also has fermented probiotic liquids (**InnergyBiotic,
CocoBiotic, Whole Grains Biotic,** and **Dong Quai**).
Dilute these liquids with sparkling mineral water
and they make an ideal replacement for soft drinks
when sweetened with Body Ecology's **Stevia Liquid
Concentrate**.
Potent Proteins (100% fermented protein powder
with 50% fermented spirulina) is a very sour, very
potent way to nourish your liver, increase iron and
magnesium levels, and significantly boost energy. It
provides powerful probiotic benefits.
Raw cultured vegetables are now available in many stores
around the U.S. There are also private "artisans" who
make them and will ship to you.
(See **www.bodyecology.com** for listings.)
Raw miso*
Raw natto (no MSG)*

—∿—

FRUIT

Black currant juice from Austria (Austria's Finest,
　　Naturally: **www.austriasfinestnaturally.com**)
Cranberries, fresh or frozen
Cranberry juice concentrate, pure and unsweetened
Lemons, fresh
Limes, fresh
Pomegranate juice or from concentrate
Noni, mangosteen, and açaí juices, unsweetened (Genesis
　　Today: **www.genesistoday.com**)

—∿—

GRAINS

(Remember to soak 8–24 hours)
Amaranth buckwheat (also called kasha)
Cream of Buckwheat cereal
　　(Pocono: **www.poconofoods.com**)
Millet
Puffed Millet Cereal, dry
　　(Arrowhead Mills: **www.arrowheadmills.com**)
Quinoa and Quinoa Flakes
　　(Ancient Harvest: **www.quinoa.net**)

—∿—

STEVIA, SALT, HERBS, AND SPICES

Stevia: Body Ecology's own great-tasting liquid herbal
　　concentrate with no aftertaste.
Seasoning salts: Herbamare and Trocomare (A.Vogel: **www
　　.avogel.com**).
Garden herbs (fresh or dried). All traditional land herbs and
　　spices are on The Diet, including antifungal herbs like
　　cinnamon, coriander, curry, garlic, ginger, and turmeric.
Seasonings from the ocean: Maine Coast Sea Seasonings
　　Dulse, Dulse with Garlic, Kelp with Cayenne (good
　　substitute for salt and pepper) (**www.seaveg.com**).
Sea salt: The special sea salts we use in our Body Ecology
　　test kitchens are the most medicinal of salts and have
　　a superior "vibrational energy." We recommend you
　　use fine-grind and gray Celtic sea salt for cooking and

Hawaiian Deep Sea Salt at the table (Selina Naturally: **www.SelinaNaturally.com**).

———

LAND VEGETABLES

All land vegetables except for cooked beets, mung bean sprouts, mushrooms (dried shiitake is okay), parsnips, green peppers, yams, and potatoes (red-skin is okay)

———

NUTS AND SEEDS

Always soaked and dehydrated

———

OCEAN VEGETABLES

Agar, arame, dulse, hijiki, kelp, kombu, nori, sea palm, and wakame (Maine Coast Sea Vegetables: **www.seaveg .com**; Eden: **www.edenfoods.com**; and other brands)

———

ORGANIC, UNREFINED OILS

Extra-virgin olive oil (Rallis [**www.rallisoliveoil.com**] has a premium, early-harvest *extra*-extra-virgin oil with a nearly flawless <0.14% acidity—needless to say, it is delicious and our absolute favorite)

Wild Alaskan Sockeye Salmon Oil
(Vital Choice: **www.vitalchoice.com**)

Coconut oil

Pumpkin-seed oil (Austria's Finest, Naturally: **www .austriasfinestnaturally.com**)

X-Factor Gold High-Vitamin Butter Oil and Blue Ice Fermented Cod Liver Oil (both from Green Pasture: **www.greenpasture.org**)

Fish oil

Flaxseed oil (Barlean's Organic Oils: **www.barleans.com**)

Flax with borage

The Essential Woman or Omega Man (both from Barlean's Organic Oils: **www.barleans.com**)

Macadamia-nut oil

Red-palm oil

———

SALAD DRESSINGS AND CONDIMENTS
Mustards made with apple-cider vinegar (Tree of Life's
Whole Grain, Eden's mustard, Anne's Original
Mountain Herb, Zake's Fire Country, True Natural
Taste organic mustards: 800-559-2998)
Cindy's Kitchen Organic Creamy Miso salad dressing
(**www.cindyskitchen.com**)
Spectrum salad dressings (**www.spectrumorganics.com**)

TEAS
(Read labels carefully. There are many great herbal teas
available, but green tea is an excellent choice. Avoid
teas with citric acid and from fruits like raspberry;
raspberry leaf, stem, or root is fine.)
Body Ecology's **Tea Concentrates**
Traditional Medicinals Weightless, Organic Ginger
Aid, Organic Mother's Milk, Organic Echinacea
Plus, Organic Echinacea Elder, Pau d'Arco, Organic
Chamomile, Organic Raspberry Leaf
(**www.traditionalmedicinals.com**)

PERSONAL-CARE PRODUCTS
(Antimicrobial)
Thursday Plantation Tea Tree Suppositories
(**www.thursdayplantation.com**)
Tea tree oil castile soap, dental floss, shampoo,
mouthwash, and lip balm
NutriBiotic Dental Gel (**www.nutribiotic.com**)
Desert Essence Natural Tea Tree Oil & Neem Toothpaste
(**www.desertessence.com**)
ProSeed Feminine Rinse (douche concentrate);
ProSeed Nail Rescue (antifungal nail formula);
ProSeed Healthy Gums
(all from Imhotep, Inc.: **www.imhotepinc.com**)
Vita-Myr Zinc-Plus Toothpaste (herbal toothpaste with
myrrh, clove, and grapefruit seed extract) (**www
.vitamyr.com**)

ANTIFUNGAL, ANTIVIRAL, ANTIBACTERIAL IMMUNE BOOSTERS

Oil of oregano
ProSeed Soothing Ear Drops
    (Imhotep, Inc.: **www.imhotepinc.com**)
Olive-leaf extract

—⁓—

OTHER VALUABLE PRODUCTS

Body Ecology's **Vitality SuperGreen™** (preferred to a multiple vitamin, it is designed to help restore your inner ecosystem and supply a wide spectrum of easily digested nutrients)

Body Ecology's **Ocean Plant Extract™** (nourishes the thyroid to increase energy for healing, helps eliminate mercury, and protects against radiation—a must for pregnant women and those with an underactive thyroid)

Body Ecology's **LivAmend™** (helps support a healthy liver, increases bile flow, and improves bowel elimination)

Body Ecology's **Ancient Earth Minerals™** (chelated from ancient plant matter; and an excellent source of energy minerals, trace elements, and amino acids)

Body Ecology's **EcoBloom™** (100% natural chicory extract, a prebiotic to feed friendly flora; can be added to salad dressings, drinks, baked goods, and cultured foods before fermenting)

Genesis Today's 4 Fiber (has flaxseeds, hemp seeds, noni fiber, and excellent herbs to promote better elimination; **www.genesistoday.com**)

Lecithin granules (tossed into a salad or salad dressing, this adds creaminess, aids fat metabolism, and is good for the brain and nervous system)

Morningstar Minerals Energy Boost 70 (a liquid fulvic acid, chelated from ancient plant matter, it's a great tasteless liquid source of minerals, trace elements, and amino acids that nourish your adrenals and thyroid . . . add to any food or drink you prepare; **www .msminerals.com**)

Morningstar Minerals Vitality Boost HA (great to implant after your colon-cleansing sessions; **www.msminerals.com**)

Xanthan gum (add to salad for thickening)

—⚬⚬⚬—

KEFIR PRODUCTS

(Commercially produced are of poor quality and cannot compare to fresh, delicious homemade kefir)

Body Ecology's **Kefir Starter** (for homemade milk kefir or for fermenting the liquid and spoon-meat of the young coconut)

—⚬⚬⚬—

PROBIOTICS

Your local health-food store carries many excellent probiotic supplements. They all are far more effective when taken with the fermented foods on the Body Ecology Diet. Our favorite brand is Probulin. It not only includes an inulin prebiotic and well-researched strains of probiotics, but also an acid-protection technology to ensure the safe passage of bacteria through the stomach (**www.bodyecology.com/ probulin**).

—⚬⚬⚬—

OTHER BOOKS YOU'LL WANT TO READ

The Body Ecology Diet: Recovering Your Health and Rebuilding Your Immunity, by Donna Gates, with Linda Schatz

The Stevia Cookbook: Cooking with Nature's Calorie-Free Sweetener, by Ray Sahelian, M.D., and Donna Gates

*These foods are not tolerated by everyone. Avoid them the first six weeks, then introduce them by rotating them into your diet once every four days and eat them with alkaline, nonstarchy vegetables; avoid eating them alone.

Many of the products listed here are available in your local health-food store. Body Ecology's products (appearing in bold) are available online at **www.bodyecology.com** or by calling 866-4BE-DIET (423-3438). Your local health-food store can also order them for you.

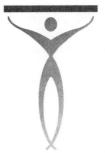

Endnotes

Chapter 1

1. David Masci, "Baby Boomers at Midlife," *CQ Researcher,* Congressional Quarterly, July 31, 1998: 659.

2. Randall Fitzgerald, *The Hundred-Year Lie: How Food and Medicine Are Destroying Your Health* (New York: Penguin Group, 2006): 3.

3. AARP, *Boomers at Midlife: The AARP Life Stage Study* (Washington, D.C.: AARP, 2005): 3.85.

4. Rob Stein, "Baby Boomers Appear to be Less Healthy Than Parents," *The Washington Post,* April 20, 2007: 1–3, **washingtonpost.com**.

Chapter 2

1. Randall Parker, "Cancer-Proof Mouse with Anti-Cancer Immune System Discovered," *FuturePundit,* April 30, 2003, **http://www.futurepundit.com/archives/003846.html** (accessed 10/20/09).

2. Heather S. Oliff, "Astonishing Advances in Tissue Regeneration," *Life Extension,* March 2006: 63–68.

3. Randall Parker, "Mini-Livers Grown from Umbilical Cord Stem Cells," *FuturePundit,* October 30, 2006, **http://www.futurepundit.com/archives/003846.html** (accessed 10/20/09).

4 Paul T. Sharpe and Conan S. Young, "Test-Tube Teeth," *Scientific American,* August 2005: 36–41.

5 Bruce H. Lipton, *The Biology of Belief* (Carlsbad, CA: Hay House, Inc., 2008): 125.

6 Meryl Ann Butler, with Gregg Braden and Dr. Bruce Lipton, "A Romp through the Quantum Field," *Awareness Magazine*, 2006–2007, **http://www .awarenessmag.com/sepoct06/so06_a_romp_through_the_quantum. htm** (accessed 10/20/09).

7 Rhonda Byrne, *The Secret* (New York: Atria Books, 2006).

Chapter 3

1. **http://en.wikipedia.org/wiki/Necrosis** (accessed 12/1/09).

2. "Anti-Aging Theories," *New Beauty*, 2004: 70–74.

3. Graham Simpson, M.D., Stephen T. Sinatra, M.D., and Jorge Suarez-Menendez, M.D., *Spa Medicine: Your Gateway to the Ageless Zone* (North Bergen, NJ: Basic Health Publications, 2004): 116.

4. **http://www.antiaging-systems.com/extract/mitochondrial.htm** (accessed 12/1/09).

5. Simpson, Sinatra, and Suarez-Menendez, *Spa Medicine: Your Gateway to the Ageless Zone:* 119.

6. Prof. Serge Jurasunas, "Mitochondria and Cancer," *Townsend Letter*, August/September 2006: 85.

7. "Mitochondria and the Evolution of Human Longevity," as published in *Life Extension*, February 2006, **http://www.lef.org/magazine/ mag2006/feb2006_report_mitochondria_01.htm** (accessed 12/1/09).

8. S. Dukic-Stefanovic, R. Schinzel, P. Riederer, and G. Munch, "AGES in brain ageing: AGE-inhibitors as neuroprotective and anti-dementia drugs?" *Biogerontology* 2(1) (2001): 19–34, as published in *Life Extension*, February 2006, **http://www.lef.org/magazine/mag2006/feb2006_report_ mitochondria_01.htm** (accessed 12/1/09).

9. R. F. Loeser, Jr., "Aging cartilage and osteoarthritis—what's the link?" *Science of Aging Knowledge Environment* 29 (2004): e31, as published in *Life Extension*, February 2006, **http://www.lef.org/magazine/mag2006/ feb2006_report_mitochondria_01.htm** (accessed 12/1/09).

10. J. L. Wautier and A. M. Schmidt, "Protein glycation: a firm link to endothelial cell dysfunction," *Circulation Research* 3 (2004): 233–238, as published in *Life Extension*, February 2006, **http://www.lef.org/magazine/ mag2006/feb2006_report_mitochondria_01.htm** (accessed 12/1/09).

11. J. E. Rofina, K. Singh, A. Skoumalova-Vesela, et al., "Histochemical accumulation of oxidative damage products is associated with Alzheimer-like pathology in the canine," *Amyloid* 2 (2004): 90–100, as published in *Life Extension*, February 2006, **http://www.lef.org/magazine/mag2006/ feb2006_report_mitochondria_01.htm** (accessed 12/1/09).

12. Simpson, Sinatra, and Suarez-Menendez, *Spa Medicine: Your Gateway to the Ageless Zone*: 118.

Chapter 4

1. Ram Chaudhari, Ph.D., "Fortifying Foods for the Baby Boomer Market," technical paper for *Fortitech*, June 1, 2006: 5.

Chapter 5

1. Andrew Martin, "Will Diners Swallow This? On Your Plate: A Battle between Profit and Portions," *The New York Times*, March 25, 2007: 9.

2. Cheryl Simon, "Eat Less, Live Longer? The Quest to Learn Why Slashing Calories Extends Life," *Genome News Network*, July 9, 2004, **http://www.genomenewsnetwork.org/articles/2004/07/09/calorierestriction.php** (accessed October 19, 2009).

3. Xi Zhao-Wilson, Ph.D., and Paul C. Watkins, SM, "Longevity Genes and Caloric Restriction: Scientists Say Rapidly Advancing Technologies Hold the Key to Extending the Human Life Span," *Life Extension*, July 2006: 70.

4. David A. Sinclair and Lenny Guarente, "Unlocking the Secrets of Longevity Genes," *Scientific American*, March 2006: 48–57.

5. "Psychoeducational principles in the treatment of eating disorders," in *Handbook for Treatment of Eating Disorders*, eds. D. M. Garner and P. E. Garfinkel (New York: The Guilford Press, 1997): 145–177.

6. S. Margolis and P. V. Rabins, "Depression and Anxiety," *The John Hopkins White Papers* (1995): 16.

7. Lia Huber, "Eat to Live Longer: Nutrition Secrets of Okinawa," *Fitness*, April 2006: 1, **www.okinawaprogram.com/news/20060401_fitness.html**.

8. Ibid.

9. Julia Ross, M.A., *The Mood Cure* (New York: Viking Penguin, 2002): 133–134.

Chapter 6

1. Fritjof Capra, *The Turning Point: Science, Society, and the Rising Culture* (New York: Bantam New Age Books, 1982): 253–257.

2. **http://www.soil-net.com**.

3. Nancy Appleton, Ph.D., *The Curse of Louis Pasteur* (Santa Monica, CA: Choice Publications, 1999): 30–32.

4. Ibid., 34.

5. "In-Hospital Deaths from Medical Errors at 195,000 per Year, HealthGrades' Study Finds," HealthGrades Press Release, *American Iatrogenic Association*, July 27, 2004, **http://health.groups.yahoo.com/group/iatrogenic/message/1451** (accessed October 19, 2009).

6. Appleton, *The Curse of Louis Pasteur*: 109.

Chapter 7

1. National Geographic Channel, *In the Womb,* Pioneer Film and TV Productions, Ltd., 2005.

2. Michael D. Gershon, *The Second Brain: A Groundbreaking New Understanding of Nervous Disorders of the Stomach and Intestine* (New York: HarperCollins Publishers, 1998): 177.

3. Ker Than, "Talking Bacteria, and How to Shut them Up," *Whitehead Institute for Biomedical Research,* March 10, 2005, **http://www.livescience. com/animals/050310_talking_bacteria.html** (accessed 10/28/09).

4. **http://en.wikipedia.org/wiki/Ilya_Ilyich_Mechnikov**.

Chapter 8

1. Sue Woodman, "Sex, Drugs & Rock 'n' Roll: The Damage Done: A Health Report," *AARP* magazine (originally published in *My Generation*), 2003: 1–3, **http://www.aarpmagazine.org/lifestyle/Articles/a2003-01-21-sdr.html** (accessed 10/19/09).

2. James D. D'Adamo, *The D'Adamo Diet* (Toronto: McGraw-Hill Ryerson, 1989).

3. Peter J. D'Adamo, *Eat Right 4 Your Type: The Individualized Diet Solution to Staying Healthy, Living Longer & Achieving Your Ideal Weight* (New York: G.P. Putnam's Sons, 1996).

Chapter 10

1. "Environmental Toxins Found in Newborns' Blood," an Environmental Working Group study published in *Daily News Central,* July 15, 2005, **http://health.dailynewscentral.com/content/view/1294/62** (accessed 10/23/09.).

Chapter 14

1. Omraam Mikkael Aivanhov, *The Yoga of Nutrition* (Los Angeles: Prosveta U.S.A., 1991): 40.

2. Ibid., 41.

Chapter 15

1. Sonia Pavan, Pierre Desreumaux, and Annick Mercenier, "Use of Mouse Models to Evaluate the Persistence, Safety, and Immune Modulation Capacities of Lactic Acid Bacteria," *Clinical and Vaccine Immunology,* Vol. 10, No. 4 (July 2003): 696–701, **http://cdli.asm.org/cgi/content/full/10/4/696** (accessed 12/15/09).

2. Stephen Daniells, "Probiotic may prevent respiratory illnesses: study," **NutraIngredients.com**, November 7, 2008, **http://www .nutraingredients.com/Research/Probiotic-may-prevent-respiratory- illnesses-study** (accessed 12/15/09).

3. Mitchell Lawrence Jones, Hongmei Chen, Wei Ouyang, Terrence Metz, and Satya Prakash, "Microencapsulated Genetically Engineered *Lactobacillus plantarum* 80 (pCBH1) for Bile Acid Deconjugation and Its Implication in Lowering Cholesterol," *Journal of Biomedicine and Biotechnology,* Vol. 1 (April 27, 2004): 61–69, **http://www.ncbi.nlm.nih.gov:80/pmc/ articles/PMC545656/** (accessed 12/15/09).

Chapter 16

1. Benjamin P. Sandler, *Diet Prevents Polio* (Milwaukee, WI: Lee Foundation for Nutritional Research, 1951), as found in "Low Blood Sugar and Susceptibility to Polio," **http://www.whale.to/v/sandler4.html** (accessed 12/15/09).

2. "Diet is Major Factor in Polio Prevention, Dr. Sandler Believes," *The Asheville Citizen,* August 5, 1948, **http://www.whale.to/v/sandler13.html** (accessed 12/15/09).

3. Joe Mercola, "Killer Sugar: Suicide with a Spoon," posted January 9, 2009, **http://articles.mercola.com/sites/articles/archive/2000/01/09/ killer-sugar-suicide-with-a-spoon-sugar-dangers.aspx** (accessed 12/15/09).

4. Charlotte Eyre, "Glucose-free increases lifespan, says study," *Decision News Media,* October 3, 2007, **http://www.ap-foodtechnology.com/ Publications/Food-BeverageNutrition/ConfectioneryNews.com/ Formulation/Glucose-free-increases-lifespan-says-study** (accessed 12/14/09).

5. Lorraine Heller, "Sugary drinks linked to Alzheimer's, says study," *Decision News Media,* December 10, 2007, **http://www.foodnavigator.com/ Science-Nutrition/Sugary-drinks-linked-to-Alzheimer-s-says-study** (accessed 12/15/09).

6. Fiona Macrae, "Babies hooked on junk food in the womb," *The Daily Mail,* September 28, 2007, **www.dailymail.co.uk/pages/live/articles/ health/healthmain.html?in_article_id=475375&in_page_id=1774** (accessed 12/14/09).

7. H. J. Roberts, *Aspartame (NutraSweet®): Is it Safe?* (Philadelphia: Charles Press Publishers, Inc., 1992): 11.

Chapter 17

1. **http://en.wikipedia.org/wiki/Crisco**.

2. "Link Between Obesity And Memory? Researchers Examine Hormone That Turns Off Hunger," Saint Louis University study, *Science Daily,* June 14, 2006, **http://www.sciencedaily.com/ releases/2006/06/060614090511.htm** (accessed 12/22/09).

3. Ibid.

4. Lorraine Heller, "Trans fats linked to infertility, reveals new study," *Decision News Media,* January 23, 2007, **http://www.foodnavigator.com/ Publications/Food-Beverage-Nutrition/FoodNavigator-USA.com/ Science-Nutrition/Trans-fats-linked-to-infertility-reveals-new-study** (accessed 12/22/09).

5. Richard Gibson, "Why Trans Fats Are Still Dining Out," *The Wall Street Journal,* June 7, 2006, **http://online.wsj.com/article/ SB114964917892673457.html?mod=health_hs_research_science** (accessed 12/22/09).

6. Kalyana Sundram, Tilakavati Karupaiah, and K. C. Haynes, "Stearic acid-rich interestified fat and trans-rich fat raise the LDL/HDL ratio and plasma glucose relative to palm olein in humans," *Nutrition and Metabolism,* January 18, 2007, **http://www.nutritionandmetabolism.com/ content/4/1/3** (accessed 12/22/09).

7. Stephen Daniells, "Toxic weed could boost omega-3 from fish," **NutraIngredients.com**, August 24, 2006, **http://www.nutraingredients .com/Research/Toxic-weed-could-boost-omega-3-from-fish** (accessed 12/22/09).

Chapter 18

1. Mark Brittman, "Rethinking the Meat Guzzler," *The New York Times,* January 27, 2008, **http://www.nytimes.com/2008/01/27/ weekinreview/27bittman.html** (accessed 12/20/09).

2. Eric Schlosser, *Fast Food Nation* (New York: Houghton Mifflin Company, 2001): 195.

3. Rob Stein, "Daily Red Meat Raises Chances of Dying Early: Study is First Large Analysis of Link with Overall Health," *The Washington Post,* March 24, 2009: A01.

4. "Is Soy Healthy?" from **Healingdaily.com** website, **http://www .healingdaily.com/detoxification-diet/soy.htm** (accessed 1/19/10).

5. Thomas Jefferson to Dr. Vine Utley, 21 March 1819. Source: **www.monticello.org/reports/life/vegetarian.html**.

6. Bess Dawson-Hughes, Susan S. Harris, and Lisa Ceglia, "Alkaline diets favor lean tissue mass in older adults," *The American Journal of Clinical Nutrition,* Vol. 87, No. 3 (2008): 662–665.

Chapter 19

1. **http://en.wikipedia.org/wiki/Popeye** (accessed 1/30/10).

2. **http://encyclopedia.vestigatio.com/Spinach** (accessed 1/30/10).

3. Lindsey Tanner, "Study: Vegetables May Keep Brains Young," *The Associated Press,* October 24, 2006, **http://www.washingtonpost.com/ wp-dyn/content/article/2006/10/24/AR2006102401033.html** (accessed 1/30/10).

4. Sidney MacDonald Baker, M.D., "The Metaphor of an Oceanic Disease," *Integrative Medicine,* Vol. 7, No. 1, February/March 2008.

5. Susan Owens, in e-mail correspondence with Donna Gates, March 2010.

6. C. Campieri, M. Campieri, V. Bertuzzi, E. Swennen, D. Matteuzzi, S. Stefoni, F. Pirovano, C. Centi, S. Ulisse, G. Famularo, and C. De Simone, "Reduction of oxaluria after an oral course of lactic acid bacteria at high concentration," Department of Nephrology, S. Orsola University Hospital, Bologna, Italy, PubMed—indexed for MEDLINE, PMID: 11532105.

7. "Genetically Modified Foods are Inherently Unsafe," Institute for Responsible Technology, **http://www.responsibletechnology.org/utility/ showArticle/?objectID=212** (accessed 1/30/10).

Chapter 20

1. Karen Hursh Graber, "Mexico's Cooking with Amaranth," **http:// www.manataka.org/page1688.html** (accessed 12/20/09).

2. "The Health Benefits of Buckwheat," from *Healthy Reader* website, July 19, 2006, **http://www.healthyreader.com/2006/07/19/the-health-benefits-of-buckwheat/** (accessed 12/20/09).

3. Karen Railey, "Whole Grains: Millet (Gramineae/Poaceoe)," from *Chet Day's Health & Beyond* website, **http://chetday.com/millet.html** (accessed 12/20/09).

4. "Millet," from *The World's Healthiest Foods* website, **http://www .whfoods.com/genpage.php?tname=foodspice&dbid=53** (accessed 12/20/09).

5. Trevor Ellestad, "Quinoa Grain History and Nutrients: Exploring the Origins and Health Benefits of the Mother Grain," July 4, 2007, **http:// food-facts.suite101.com/article.cfm/quinoa** (accessed 12/20/09).

6. E. A. Oelke, D. H. Putnam, T. M. Teynor, and E. S. Oplinger, "Quinoa," *Alternative Field Crops Manual,* **http://www.hort.purdue.edu/ newcrop/afcm/quinoa.html** (accessed 12/20/09).

Chapter 21

1. Homer, *The Iliad,* translated by Samuel Butler, Book XIV.

2. "Miraculous Messages from Water," from *Water Secrets Revealed* website, **http://www.life-enthusiast.com/twilight/research_emoto.htm** (accessed 2/27/10).

3. F. Batmanghelidj, M.D., *Water for Health, for Healing, for Life* (New York: Warner Books/Time Warner Group, 2003): 25.

4. Stefan Kuprowsky, M.D., "The Body Matrix: Your Key to Health," *Vista Magazine Online,* **http://www.vistamagonline.com/vista_articles/ page.php?tp=3&p=1&id=56&s=the_body_matrix_your_key_to_health** (accessed 2/27/10).

5. "Effects of Dehydration," from *Symptoms of Dehydration* website, **www
.symptomsofdehydration.com/effects-of-dehydration.htm** (accessed
2/27/10).

6. Batmanghelidj, *Water for Health, for Healing, for Life:* 32–35.

7. Mike Adams, "The Water Cure: An Interview with Dr. Batmanghelidj.
Part I—Discovery of the Water Cure," *Natural News,* **http://mrgreenbiz
.wordpress.com/2009/05/23/the-water-cure-an-interview-with-dr-
batmanghelidj** (accessed 2/27/10).

8. Stefanie Schoppen, Ana M. Pérez-Granados, Ángeles Carbajal,
Pilar Oubiña, Francisco J. Sánchez-Muniz, Juan A. Gómez-Gerique, and
M. Pilar Vaquero, "A Sodium-Rich Carbonated Mineral Water Reduces
Cardiovascular Risk in Postmenopausal Women," *Journal of Nutrition* 134
(May 2004):1058–1063, as found on John Briffa, M.D., website, "The health
benefits of drinking sparkling (yes, SPARKLING) water," posted January
23, 2005, **http://www.drbriffa.com/blog/2005/01/23/sparkling-water**
(accessed 2/22/10).

9. "Fine Waters Minerality," posted October 2, 2005, on *Fine Waters*
website, **http://www.finewaters.com/Bottled_Water_Etiquette/Flavor_
of_Water/FineWaters_Minerality.asp** (accessed 2/22/10).

10. R. Siener, A. Jahnen, and A. Hesse, "Influence of a mineral water
rich in calcium, magnesium, and bicarbonate on urine composition and the
risk of calcium oxalate crystallization," *European Journal of Clinical Nutrition,*
58 (February 2004): 270–276.

11. Batmanghelidj, *Water for Health, for Healing, for Life:* 227.

12. "Green Tea," from *Silk Road Teas* website, **http://www.silkroadteas
.com/servlet/the-template/greentea_gateway/Page** (accessed 2/22/10).

13. "Pomegranate inhibits hormone-dependent breast cancer
cell growth," posted January 8, 2010, on *Life Extension* website,
**http://www.lef.org/newsletter/2010/0108_Pomegranate-
Inhibits-Hormone-Dependent-Breast-Cancer-Cell-Growth.
htm?source=eNewsLetter2009Wk51-2&key=Archive&l=0** (accessed
2/22/10).

Chapter 22

1. "Vinegar supplementation lowers glucose and insulin responses and
increases satiety after a bread meal in healthy subjects," *European Journal
of Clinical Nutrition,* 59 (2005): 983–988, published online June 29, 2005,
http://www.nature.com/ejcn/journal/v59/n9/abs/1602197a.html#aff1
(accessed 3/4/10).

2. B. B. Aggarwal and S. Shishodia, "Suppression of the Nuclear Factor-
kappaB Activation Pathway by Spice-Derived Phytochemicals: Reasoning
for Seasoning," *Annals, New York Academy of Sciences,* 1030 (2004): 434–441,
found at **http://www.ncbi.nlm.nih.gov/pubmed/15659827** (accessed
3/4/10).

Chapter 24

1. Cedric F. Garland, et al., "Could sunscreens increase melanoma risk?" *American Journal of Public Health,* 82, No. 4 (April 1992): 614–15.

2. *People Against Cancer: Finding the Best Cancer Treatment,* from the *People Against Cancer* website, **http://www.peopleagainstcancer.com/pdfs/ news/20080916n3.pdf** (accessed 10/11/10).

3. Guy B. Mulligan and Angelo Licata, "Taking vitamin D with the largest meal improves absorption and results in higher serum levels of 25-hydroxyvitamin D," *The Journal of Bone and Mineral Research,* Department of Endocrinology, Diabetes, and Metabolism, Cleveland Clinic Foundation, Cleveland, OH, **http://www.jbmr.org/view/0/index.html** (accessed 7/19/10).

4. Swami Ambikananda Saraswati, *Breathwork* (Hong Kong: HarperCollins Publishers, LTD, 2001): 14.

5. Ibid., 20.

6. Paul G. Harch and Virginia McCullough, *The Oxygen Revolution,* (New York: Hatherleigh Press, 2007) 156–174.

7. Robert Preidt, "Errands Tomorrow? Sleep May Help You Remember," *HealthDay News,* originally published in *Psychological Science,* July 2, 2010, **http://www.medicinenet.com/script/main/art.asp?articlekey=117753** (accessed 7/19/10).

8. *North Carolina Driver's Handbook,* Division of Motor Vehicles, Department of Transportation: 37.

9. F. P. Cappuccio, L. D'Elia, P. Strazzullo, and M. A. Miller, "Sleep Duration and All-Cause Mortality: A Systematic Review and Meta-Analysis of Prospective Studies," *Sleep,* 33 (2010): 585–592, **http://www .journalsleep.org/ViewAbstract.aspx?pid=27780** (accessed 10/6/10).

10. The National Sleep Foundation, "How Much Sleep Do We Need," from the *National Sleep Foundation* website: **http://www .sleepfoundation.org/article/how-sleep-works/how-much-sleep-do-we- really-need** (accessed 10/14/10).

11. Roni Caryn Rabin, "Behavior: Napping Can Prime the Brain for Learning," *The New York Times,* February 22, 2010, **http://www.nytimes .com/2010/02/23/health/research/23beha.html?em** (accessed 10/6/10).

12. Mark Stibich, Ph.D., "Tips for Great Naps," from **About.com** website, December 6, 2008, **http://longevity.about.com/od/sleep/a/ napping_tips.htm** (accessed 10/6/10).

Chapter 25

1. Mary Carmichael, "Strong, Faster, Smarter," *Newsweek,* March 26, 2007: 40–46.

2. Michael Craig Miller, M.D., "Exercise is a State of Mind," *Newsweek,* March 26, 2007: 48–55.

3. Mikkel Aaland, "Finnish Sauna: History of the Nordic Bath," ©1997, http://www.cyberbohemia.com/Pages/historyofnordic.htm (accessed 6/1/10).

4. "Health Benefits of Saunas," *Doctorline: The Ultimate Directory,* www.doctorline.com/sauna.htm (accessed 6/1/10).

5. Cheryl Richardson, *Take Time for Your Life* (New York: Broadway Books, 1999) 188–189.

Chapter 26

1. Nancy Smith, "Manage Your Stress," from *Real Simple* website, http://www.realsimple.com/health/mind-mood/stress/manage-stress-10000001550513/index.html (accessed 10/6/10).

2. Michelle Andrews, "How to Beat Stress and Angst Through Meditation," *US News & World Report,* December 29, 2008: 2.

3. Joel Stein, "Just Say Om," *Time,* August 4, 2003: 53.

4. Ibid., 52.

5. Peter Kelder, *The Eye of Revelation* (1946), ed. J. W. Watt, Booklocker.com, Inc.: 1st Reprint Edition, January 10, 2008.

6. Dr. Dicken Weatherby, *Naturally Raising Your HGH Levels* (Jacksonville, OR: Bear Mountain Publishing, 2005): 1–22.

7. Ibid.

8. Christine Vestal, "The Science Behind Stem Cell Research," *The Pew Forum on Religion and Public Life,* July 17, 2008, http://pewforum.org/Science-and-Bioethics/The-Science-Behind-Stem-Cell-Research.aspx (accessed 10/6/10).

9. "StemCellTherapy21 Launches $15,000 Anti-Aging Therapy with Umbilical Cord Blood Mesenchymal Cells," *PR Log,* July 20, 2009, http://www.prlog.org/10287130-stemcelltherapy21-launches-15000-antiaging-therapy-with-umbilical-cord-blood-mesenchymal-cells.html (accessed 10/6/10).

10. Amanda Gardner, "Scientists Find Stem Cells in Hair That Can Become Skin," *HealthDay News/Bloomberg Business Week,* March 11, 2010, http://www.businessweek.com/lifestyle/content/healthday/636896.html (accessed 10/6/10).

11. Mohit Joshi, "Human Umbilical Cord Blood Injection Helps Rejuvenate an Aging Brain," **TopNews.in**, March 11, 2008, http://www.topnews.in/health/human-umbilical-cord-blood-injection-helps-rejuvenate-aging-brain-21412 (accessed 10/6/10).

12. Alexander Y. Maslov, Tara A. Barone, Robert J. Plunkett, and Steven C. Pruitt, "Neural Stem Cell Detection, Characterization, and Age-Related Changes in the Subventricular Zone of Mice," *The Journal of Neuroscience,* 24 (2004): 1726–1733.

13. Al Fin, "Brain Rejuvenation Using Stem Cells From Cord Blood," *Future Blogger,* April 3, 2008, **http://www.memebox.com/futureblogger/show/317-brain-rejuvenation-using-stem-cells-from-cord-blood** (accessed 10/6/10).

14. "Bone Marrow Stem Cell Release Regulated By Brain's Biological Clock," *Science Daily,* February 7, 2008 (reprinted with editorial adaptations by *Science Daily* staff from materials provided by Mount Sinai Medical Center, via *Newswise*), **http://www.sciencedaily.com/releases/2008/02/080206212051.htm** (accessed 10/6/10).

15. "High-Tech Ways to Extend Your Life," **Oprah.com** website, March 24, 2009, **http://www.oprah.com/health/Life-Extension-Technology-and-Tissue-Regeneration/print/1** (accessed 10/6/10).

16. Barbara Kantrowitz, "Sex and the Single Baby Boomer," *Newsweek,* February 20, 2006, **http://www.newsweek.com/2006/02/20/sex-love-the-new-world.html** (accessed 10/6/10).

17. Al Sears, M.D., "Better Blood Flow Where You Need It," *Power for Healthy Living* website, **http://www.alsearsmd.com/better-blood-flow-where-you-need-it** (accessed 10/6/10).

18. Bruce Scali, "Optimal Sexual Health for a Lifetime," *Life Extension,* September 2007: 3.

Chapter 27

1. Theo Colborn, "Acceptance Speech by Theo Colborn Upon Receiving the Rachel Carson Leadership Award," Chatham College, Pittsburgh, PA, June 19, 1997, **http://www.pmac.net/rctc.htm** (accessed 9/14/10).

2. Seth Godin, *Tribes* (New York: The Penguin Group, 2008): 11.

3. Corporation for National & Community Service, Office of Research and Policy Development, *Volunteering in America: 2007 Trends and Rankings in Civic Life* (Washington, D.C., 2007): 1.

4. Corporation for National & Community Service, Office of Research and Policy Development, *Volunteer Growth in America: A Review of Trends Since 1974* (Washington, D.C., 2010): 2.

5. "Great Expectations: Boomers and the Future of Volunteering," *A VolunteerMatch User Study,* MetLife Foundation, 2007.

Index

Note to readers of E-books:
The page numbers listed in this index refer
to the printed version of the book.

Acknowledgments

It's just perfect that Hay House is publishing my second book. Louise, your words of encouragement have been in my head for the four years it has taken Lyndi and me to write this book, especially your advice to "keep it positive." Following the Principle of Balance, I've tried to do so, but also wanted Baby Boomers to realize the negative impact our sheer numbers have had on the world, in the hopes that we will take the right steps to correct the problems. When you said you felt that you were "holding a treasure" in your hand, that meant everything to me.

I'm deeply grateful, too, to Lyndi for your insistence on giving this book an almost poetic energy. I know working with a perfectionist is difficult, but I hope you will be eternally proud of what we have accomplished together. Kenneth Storey, you must be the most patient man on the planet. Thank you for making our book beautiful. Carole Addlestone meticulously edited the first part of our manuscript, and when she became too busy, Stephanie Marr did a brilliant job with the second half and with the index. Alex Freemon gave a final polish to everything. Thank you all for your hard, committed work.

I am very fortunate to have an incredible Body Ecology team working with me, helping me bring Body Ecology's message to the world. Without even being asked, they go above and beyond the call of duty, because they believe so much in this work. I can feel confident that you as the reader will find your life enhanced with the information in this book. Please help all of us spread Body Ecology's message; and let's work together to create a happier, healthier world.

I am always deeply grateful to the Force that guides me, opens the right doors, and helps me reach the most amazing people—all who are ready to hear this message.

About the Authors

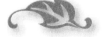

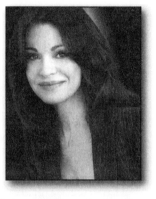

DONNA GATES has helped hundreds of thousands of people overcome immune-system disorders and other health issues and achieve peak health. She is known as the teacher to the teachers, and her insights continue to guide many of today's most renowned natural-health physicians and other professionals. An expert on candidiasis (CRC) and related immune disorders, she has done extensive research on how these debilitating conditions affect the body, mind, and spirit. She developed and tested the Body Ecology Diet on many different people, who have all improved their health by following the basic principles of The Diet.

Donna is a nutritional consultant, home economist, and founder of Body Ecology, Inc., a leading nutrition company. She has studied with the top macrobiotic teachers and graduated from Lima Osawa's cooking academy in Japan. She holds an M.Ed. in Counseling from Loyola University and a B.S. in Early Childhood Development from the University of Georgia.

Donna is credited with leading some of the most important innovations in natural health, including inventing young coconut kefir, being at the forefront of probiotics and fermented foods, and bringing stevia/reb A (powder and liquid), along with other products, into the U.S.

Donna's free newsletter, available at **www.bodyecology.com**, is one of the most widely read and respected natural-health publications in the world.

LYNDI SCHRECENGOST is a professional writer and marketing consultant specializing in health, fitness, education, and environmental advocacy. Co-founder of FLUENT Communications, LLC, a Washington, D.C.–based writing firm, she has worked for more than two decades as a communications professional for a wide range of commercial and nonprofit clients. Lyndi has a strong interest in all aspects of alternative health and has co-written a number of books on the topic. In addition to *The Baby Boomer Diet*, she is co-writer of *The Genius of Flexibility: The Smart Way to Stretch and Strengthen Your Body, with Bob Cooley*. She will be assisting Donna Gates on her forthcoming book, *The Body Ecology Approach to Detoxification*. Lyndi holds a B.A in Communication Arts, an M.A. in Literature, and is a graduate of the University of Denver's Publishing Institute. She currently resides in Chapel Hill, North Carolina.

The Body Ecology Mission

As the leader in fermented foods and nutrition, our mission at BODY ECOLOGY is to change the way the world eats, thus ending disease. We want every home in America to be using the healthy foods we recommend in this book. We want all children to be born with perfect health. With advances in modern genomics coupled with Body Ecology's Seven Universal Principles and our BED foods . . . especially fermented foods . . . this can be our future.

Please help us spread the word:

✔ Eating a variety of cultured foods found all around the world helps create a healthy inner ecosystem and contributes to a long, healthy lifespan.

✔ Organic, unrefined seed oils, coconut oil, extra-virgin olive oil, raw butter, and raw cream are the best fats to eat. Avoid bleached, refined, and deodorized vegetable oils commonly found in most foods. Also avoid margarine.

✔ Stevia is an excellent choice to satisfy your sweet tooth.

✔ Taking an alkaline, mineral-rich superfoods formula is even better than man-made supplements for reversing protein, mineral, and essential fatty acid deficiencies.

✔ Raw apple cider vinegar is the only really healthy vinegar.

✔ Ocean vegetables and organic land vegetables should make up a significant portion of each meal.

✔ Cold-water fish, free-range poultry, and eggs from free-running, fertile chickens are your best sources of animal protein.

BEDROK and Autism

Body Ecology Diet Recovering Our Kids

The Body Ecology Diet (BED), developed by Donna Gates, has been in use for over 15 years to address immune-system issues, including viral and fungal infections, various autoimmune diseases, nutritional deficiencies, and digestive disorders (IBS, ulcerative colitis, and Crohn's disease). For the past several years it has been used experimentally within the autism community with very positive results. BEDROK children improve dramatically when their parents introduce our principles and our foods into their way of life.

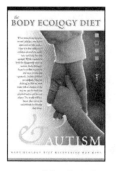

The BED views autism as a combination of disorders—all correctable. A gut-brain infection in the early stages of the disorder distances the child from his surroundings. The goal of dietary intervention is to bring him back into our world and back to his true self.

Donna Gates has a passion for helping children. BEDROK (Body Ecology Diet Recovering Our Kids) is a program she is developing together with parents of children with autism. BEDROK has a strong spiritual component to it. Donna truly believes that the children coming into our world today are highly evolved beings and need to be treated as such. She explains, "Our planet is in such turmoil at the moment, and many children in this new generation carry priceless information and solutions to our most serious problems. But these highly evolved souls will come of age unable to fulfill their missions on earth unless we correct the conditions that threaten to hold them back."

Autism has multiple causes, including:

• Undetected infections (fungal and viral)
• Environmental toxins inherited from several previous generations
• Weak endocrine organs (adrenal and thyroid)
• Blocked detoxification pathways that prevent toxins from leaving the body
• Congested livers
• Nutritional deficiencies coupled with vulnerable immune systems due to the lack of an "inner ecosystem"

All these form a complex disorder that takes our children away from us and ultimately will prevent them from accomplishing their spiritual purpose. It is our responsibility to bring them back. The world needs this generation; we can't afford to lose them.

Please visit us at www.bodyecology.com to learn more about Body Ecology Diet research on autism, chat about autism and ADD, and browse a wide range of information and products to recover your inner ecology. Or call 866-4BE-DIET.

Stay Connected with Body Ecology!

You can make a difference in the world by simply joining Body Ecology in its mission to change the way the world eats. The Body Ecology tribe can be found on Facebook and Twitter.

www.facebook.com/bodyecology   BodyEcology

The Body Ecology Facebook fan page is teeming with activity. Great health topics are addressed, and support with helpful suggestions are offered from thousands of health-minded "friends and fans." How can you impact your family, friends, and community? Start living the Body Ecology lifestyle! Learn our system of health and healing, and put it into practice step by step – just watch the difference it will make in your life and in the lives of those around your. Learn more on Facebook and Twitter!

Subscribe to Body Ecology's FREE e-Newsletter

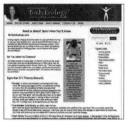

The Body Ecology Health & Wellness e-Newsletter is cherished by readers around the world and widely considered one of THE most important newsletters available. It's an essential read for anyone committed to improving their health. Once you subscribe, you will find health insights and solutions with a strong focus on natural and alternative health angles – long before you read them elsewhere. In fact, many of the world's most renowned and respected natural health physicians and dietary experts have referred to Body Ecology to learn essential insights that are then incorporated into their own health programs and publications.

Even more important, the health and wellness insights you'll discover in every free issue REALLY WORK. The natural/dietary-health-focused articles you'll read are a combination of scientific research, common sense, and factual data. Tens of thousands of people have genuinely seen their health *dramatically improve* through the well-researched and easy-to-understand insights provided by Body Ecology.

Sign up today for FREE at www.BodyEcology.com

We hope you enjoyed this Hay House book. If you'd like to receive our online catalog featuring additional information on Hay House books and products, or if you'd like to find out more about the Hay Foundation, please contact:

Hay House, Inc., P.O. Box 5100, Carlsbad, CA 92018-5100
(760) 431-7695 or (800) 654-5126
(760) 431-6948 (fax) or (800) 650-5115 (fax)
www.hayhouse.com® • **www.hayfoundation.org**

—◊◊◊—

Published and distributed in Australia by: Hay House Australia Pty. Ltd., 18/36 Ralph St., Alexandria NSW 2015 • *Phone:* 612-9669-4299 • *Fax:* 612-9669-4144 • www.hayhouse.com.au

Published and distributed in the United Kingdom by: Hay House UK, Ltd., 292B Kensal Rd., London W10 5BE • *Phone:* 44-20-8962-1230 • *Fax:* 44-20-8962-1239 • www.hayhouse.co.uk

Published and distributed in the Republic of South Africa by: Hay House SA (Pty), Ltd., P.O. Box 990, Witkoppen 2068 • *Phone/Fax:* 27-11-467-8904 • www.hayhouse.co.za

Published in India by: Hay House Publishers India, Muskaan Complex, Plot No. 3, B-2, Vasant Kunj, New Delhi 110 070 • *Phone:* 91-11-4176-1620 • *Fax:* 91-11-4176-1630 • www.hayhouse.co.in

Distributed in Canada by: Raincoast, 9050 Shaughnessy St., Vancouver, B.C. V6P 6E5 • *Phone:* (604) 323-7100 • *Fax:* (604) 323-2600 • www.raincoast.com

—◊◊◊—

Take Your Soul on a Vacation

Visit **www.HealYourLife.com®** to regroup, recharge, and reconnect with your own magnificence.
Featuring blogs, mind-body-spirit news, and life-changing wisdom from Louise Hay and friends.

Visit **www.HealYourLife.com** today!

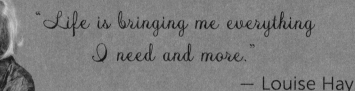